Biological and Medical Significance of Chemical Elements

Authored by

Irena Kostova

Department of Chemistry
Faculty of Pharmacy
Medical University-Sofia
2 Dunav St.,
Sofia 1000,
Bulgaria

Biological and Medical Significance of Chemical Elements

Author: Irena Kostova

ISBN (Online): 978-981-5179-00-2

ISBN (Print): 978-981-5179-01-9

ISBN (Paperback): 978-981-5179-02-6

First published in 2023.

need for a court order if at any point you breach any terms of this License Agreement. In no event will any delay or failure by Bentham Science Publishers in enforcing your compliance with this License Agreement constitute a waiver of any of its rights.

3. You acknowledge that you have read this License Agreement, and agree to be bound by its terms and conditions. To the extent that any other terms and conditions presented on any website of Bentham Science Publishers conflict with, or are inconsistent with, the terms and conditions set out in this License Agreement, you acknowledge that the terms and conditions set out in this License Agreement shall prevail.

Bentham Science Publishers Pte. Ltd.
80 Robinson Road #02-00
Singapore 068898
Singapore
Email: subscriptions@benthamscience.net

BENTHAM SCIENCE

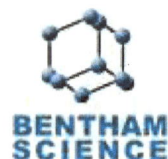

CONTENTS

PREFACE

This book attempts to highlight the current knowledge of the biological role of chemical elements of the periodic table in organisms' life. The first part covers the occurrence in the body and the environment, the chemical properties, and biological functions of all the chemical elements of the periodic table in detail. The second part focuses on the effects of chemical elements on human health. It describes the beneficial effects of the incorporation of chemical elements in drugs including the latest trends in the development of new pharmaceuticals. Essential elements useful in diagnosis and therapyand notable features in their chemistry related to their biological activity are emphasized.

The book deliberates the importance of chemical elements in the lifecycle from both chemical and biological perspective and their role in biological pathways. The biochemistry of the essential non-metals oxygen, nitrogen, carbon, hydrogen, sulfur, and phosphorus is well studied, but all other elements in the periodic table have multiple functions and a serious influence on life processes despite their lower amounts in the body. Their biological role is of great importance and should be considered, especially the functions of the biogenic metals Na, K, Mg, Ca, Cu, Zn, Fe, Co, Mn, and Mo. Many other chemical elements, though non-essential, are present in biological systems and some of them are in higher amounts than some essential ones. However, non-essential elements are bioactive, having either beneficial (healthy) or harmful (toxic) effects depending on concentration. Each element is buffered in a certain range of quantities in order to minimize interference with the other elements or biomolecules and to obtain its required specificity of action. Many transition and trace metal ions and some biometalloids are constituents of naturally occurring metal-based biomolecules with fundamental biological roles in enzyme catalysis, in the structures and interactions of macromolecules of the body, in the regulation of metabolic pathways, in biomineralization processes, etc.

A periodic table of the elements, required for life, commonly includes all the elements observed in life functions for human, animal, and plant health. Although the journey through the periodic table illustrates the specific functions of biogenic elements, there are some elements whose functions in living systems are poorly understood. Research demonstrates that we need to know more about all elements and address their functions, even those that are considered non-essential. Inorganic compounds have been used in medicine for many centuries, but often only in an empirical way with little or no understanding of the molecular basis of their mechanisms of action and in many cases with little experience in designing targeted biologically active compounds. Diagnostic and therapeutic nuclear medicine uses many elements representing a large part of the periodic table. For many of them, it is necessary to find out in more detail the negative side effects. The information about the complex pathways of biological processes where various elements of the periodic table play important roles will help in understanding various diseases and treatment options.

Moreover, the duality that exists in the biology of the elements in the groups of the periodic table is also of great importance for the protection against the biochemical mimicry and competition of chemically similar elements. Conditions of overload and deficiency pose a risk of accumulating, toxicity or various disease obstructions. Many drug molecules and metal-based complexes have been discovered in recent years for diagnostic and therapeutic purposes, which also highpoint the importance of metal ions and the synergistic functions of elements in humans and other organisms. Many exciting challenges remain in this field. The aim of the current book is to give a comprehensive, authoritative, critical, and appealing account of general interest to the chemistry community.

The Author

Irena Kostova
Department of Chemistry
Faculty of Pharmacy
Medical University-Sofia
2 Dunav St.
Sofia 1000
Bulgaria

CHAPTER 1

Occurrence and Classification of Chemical Elements

OCCURRENCE OF CHEMICAL ELEMENTS IN NATURE

The study of the influence of various chemical elements on the body of animals and humans, as well as the study of chemical elements as permanent components of tissues and biological fluids of living organisms began in the second half of the XIX century. Since then, a lot of scientific literature has appeared concerning the distribution of chemical elements and their biological role.

The chemical elements found in nature are elements with atomic numbers from 1 through 98, however around ten of them occur in extremely small quantities, especially the elements with atomic numbers 93-98. Although many elements of the periodic table occur in nature, they might not exist in pure or native form [1, 2]. The only pure native elements in nature are the noble gases, noble metals (gold, silver), and carbon, nitrogen, and oxygen from nonmetals. Most of the elements that occur naturally are not in pure form and can be found in their chemical compounds.

Studying the geochemical transformations in the earth's crust, it has been established that the changes occurring in the upper layers of the earth's crust have a certain effect on the chemical composition of living organisms and the development of bioreactions in them [3 - 5]. Living organisms, in turn, cause regular migrations of chemical elements in nature. The science that studies the role of living organisms in the geochemical processes of migration, distribution, scattering, and concentration of chemical elements in the shells of the biosphere is called biogeochemistry.

The biosphere is a shell of the Earth, containing the entire set of living organisms and that part of the planet's matter that is in continuous exchange with these organisms. The biosphere covers the lower part of the atmosphere, the hydrosphere, and the upper part of the lithosphere (up to a depth of 5 km).

The atmosphere is the lightest shell of the Earth, which borders outer space, through the atmosphere, there is an exchange of matter and energy with the cosmos. The atmosphere has high mobility, variability of its constituent components, and uniqueness of physical and chemical processes. The thermal regime of the Earth's surface is determined by the state of the atmosphere. The ozone layer in the atmosphere protects our planet from the effects of ultraviolet radiation from the Sun. As a result of the activity of living organisms, geochemical phenomena, and human economic activity, the composition of the atmosphere is in a state of dynamic equilibrium. The main components of the atmosphere are nitrogen (78%), oxygen (21%), argon (0.9%), and carbon dioxide (0.04%) - in the surface layer [1 - 5]. The atmosphere includes the troposphere, stratosphere, and ionosphere. The troposphere and stratosphere are usually combined into the lower layers of the atmosphere (height 9-17 km), which differ significantly in composition from the upper layers (ionosphere). In the lower layers of the atmosphere, about 80% of the gases and all water vapor are concentrated.

The troposphere is a non-equilibrium chemically active system. As a result of geological and biological processes and human activities, most of the gaseous impurities released from the Earth's surface into the troposphere are in reduced form or in the form of some oxides: NO, NO_2, H_2S, NH_3, CO, CH_4, SO_2, *etc.* Impurities returned to the Earth's surface turn into compounds with a high degree of oxidation - H_2SO_4, HNO_3, sulfates, nitrates, CO_2, *etc.* Thus, the troposphere plays the role of a global oxidative reservoir on the planet.

The hydrosphere is the water shell of the Earth. Water penetrates everywhere into various natural formations, and even the purest atmospheric water contains 10-50 mg/l soluble substances. In the hydrosphere, 96.54% of the mass is oxygen and hydrogen, and 2.95% is chlorine and sodium [1 - 5].

The lithosphere is the outer solid shell of the Earth, consisting of sedimentary and igneous rocks. The surface layer of the lithosphere, in which the interaction of living matter with mineral (inorganic) matter occurs, is the soil. The remains of organisms after decomposition passes into the humus (fertile part of the soil). In the lithosphere, oxygen is the most common (47% of its mass), followed by silicon (29.5%), aluminum (8.05%), iron (4.65%), calcium (2.96%), sodium (2.50%), potassium (2.50%) and magnesium (1.65%). These eight elements account for more than 99% of the mass of the lithosphere [1 - 6]. In nature, there is always a cycle of chemical elements, where living organisms play a large role. Living organisms continuously cause the movement of chemical elements - this is their geochemical function. Any movement of chemical elements in the Earth's crust is called the migration of chemical elements. When this migration occurs with the participation of living organisms, it is called biogenic migration. Among the most important tasks of biogeochemistry are the exchange of substances between living matter and matter of the planet, biogenic migration of chemical elements in the biosphere, biogenic properties of elements, biogenic concentrations of chemical elements that determine the normal conditions for the development of organisms [6].

It is estimated that 98% of the body mass of men is made up of nine nonmetallic elements. In the average chemical composition of a living being, the part of oxygen, carbon, hydrogen, and nitrogen, makes up most of its mass [7]. The important feature of these chemical elements is their greater reactivity. These four elements have one property: they easily form covalent bonds typical for biosystems. In addition, carbon, nitrogen, and oxygen form single and double bonds, thanks to which they can give a wide variety of chemical compounds. Carbon atoms are also capable of forming triple bonds with both other carbon atoms and nitrogen atoms. This explains the great diversity of carbon compounds in nature. Phosphorus, sulfur, chlorine, bromine, iodine, calcium, sodium, potassium, magnesium, *etc.* are also strongly captured and accumulated by organisms. Approximate percentages by weight of some chemical elements in the hydrosphere, lithosphere and in the human body are given in Table **1**.

Table 1. Percentages of biogenic elements in the hydrosphere, lithosphere, and in the human body and their biological importance.

Chemical element	Hydrosphere	Lithosphere	Human body	Biological importance
Oxygen	85.82	47.20	62.40	O plays a crucial role in respiration, immune function, and photosynthesis in living organisms.
Hydrogen	10.72	0.15	9.80	H forms H-bonds, crucial for the life-supporting
Nitrogen	$1 \cdot 10^{-5}$	0.01	3.10	properties of water and the operation of enzymes;
Carbon	$2 \cdot 10^{-3}$	0.10	21.15	controls protein folding, and opening of active
Phosphorus	$5 \cdot 10^{-6}$	0.08	0.95	sites in hydrophilic and hydrophobic
Sulfur	0.09	0.09	0.25	environments.
Chlorine	1.89	0.045	0.15	N - the essential constituent of proteins, enzymes,
Calcium	0.04	3.60	1.50	DNA, RNA; N-fixation by plants is the key
Sodium	1.06	2.64	0.15	reaction in the nitrogen cycle; N-based
Potassium	0.04	2.60	0.35	biocompounds.
Magnesium	0.14	2.10	0.05	C plays a key role in the formation of organic molecules; CO_2 in photosynthesis; respiration supplies O_2 for the conversion of carbohydrates and other organic compounds back to CO_2.
				P creates a bridge between sugar units in DNA and RNA for cell replication; ATP - the major source of energy in all biological processes.
				S - important constituents of plant and animal proteins holding amino acids - cysteine, cystine, methionine involved in metabolic reactions.

(Table 1) cont.....

Chemical element	Hydrosphere	Lithosphere	Human body	Biological importance
				Cl⁻ ions regulate or control the acid-base equilibrium, fluid balance, and osmotic pressure; major constituents of plasma and cerebrospinal fluid; in the formation of HCl in gastric juice. Ca - the major constituent of bone and teeth; important in neuromuscular function, interneuronal transmission, maintenance of cell membrane integrity, and blood coagulation. Na⁺ ions participate in transmitting nerve signals, regulating water flow across the cell membrane, and the transport of sugars and amino acids into cells. K⁺ ions activate enzymes, which participate in the oxidation of glucose to ATP. Transmission of nerve signals. Mg in photosynthesis, in storing energy; enzymes catalyzing replication and transcription of DNA; in nerve impulse transmission, muscle contraction, and metabolism of carbohydrates. Ca - the major constituent of bone and teeth; important in neuromuscular function, interneuronal transmission, maintenance of cell membrane integrity, and blood coagulation. Na⁺ ions participate in transmitting nerve signals, regulating water flow across the cell membrane, and the transport of sugars and amino acids into cells. K⁺ ions activate enzymes, which participate in the oxidation of glucose to ATP. Transmission of nerve signals. Mg in photosynthesis, in storing energy; enzymes catalyzing replication and transcription of DNA; in nerve impulse transmission, muscle contraction, and metabolism of carbohydrates.

The largest share in the composition of living organisms' matter falls on oxygen (62.4%), carbon (21.15%), and hydrogen (9.8%) and much less nitrogen, silicon, aluminum, iron, calcium, manganese, sulfur, phosphorus, chromium, magnesium, potassium, sodium, chlorine and other elements. Most of them are those chemical elements that easily form gases and water-soluble compounds that are very mobile in the biosphere [8]. Those elements that do not produce easily soluble compounds in the biosphere are found in organisms in negligible quantities, *e.g.,* aluminum, silicon, titanium, which are among the most common elements of the earth's crust. In contrast, hydrogen, carbon, nitrogen, and phosphorus, found in very small amounts in the Earth's crust, form soluble compounds and are largely concentrated in organisms. Most trace elements are found in living matter in much smaller quantities than in the earth's crust. For example, silicon and titanium, due to the low solubility and availability of their compounds, are contained in organisms in thousands and tens of thousands of times smaller quantities than in the earth's crust. This is also the case for Fe and Al, which form insoluble hydroxides. There are organisms that selectively accumulate certain elements so that they can serve as "indicators" of chemical environmental conditions.

Biological Role of Elements, Depending on their Position in the Periodic Table

The ability to link the need of organisms for certain chemical elements with the structure of their atoms is of exceptional interest [9]. In general, the quantitative content of chemical elements in living matter is inversely proportional to their serial numbers (Table **1**). The availability of elements for organisms is determined by the ability to slight solubility and volatility, chelation and oxidation-reduction reactions. In the vast majority of cases, the transition from light to heavy elements within the same subgroup increases the toxicity of the elements and, in parallel, their content in the biomass decreases. So, in the human body there are mainly ions of light metals Na^+, K^+, Mg^{2+}, Ca^{2+}, related to s-elements, and ions Mn^{2+}, Fe^{2+}, Co^{3+}, Zn^{2+}, related to d-elements and belong to the so-called biogenic metals with biological functions sustaining the life of living organisms.

The biological activity of the elements is largely determined by their position in the periodic table, *i.e.,* depending on the atomic structures of the chemical elements [10]. However, not all aspects of this relationship are well-studied. Among the s-elements of the IA group of the periodic system, a special place is occupied by hydrogen, which is part of the absolute majority of important molecules and macromolecules (proteins, nucleic acids, polysaccharides). Attention is drawn to the quantitative distribution of sodium and potassium ions between cells and extracellular fluid: sodium ions are concentrated mainly in the extracellular fluid, and potassium ions are concentrated inside cells. For part of the s-elements of the IIA group, there are phenomena of replacement of normal structural components of bone (Ca, Mg) with some elements of this group that are not part of bone tissue (Sr, Ba, Ra). Of the biological functions, the effects of calcium ions on blood clotting, neuromuscular excitability, and heart muscle have been studied in sufficient depth. It should be pointed out that with the increase in atomic mass, the toxicity of the s-elements of the IIA group increases, and their percentage in the body decreases (for example, the strontium content in the human body is $10^{-3}\%$, barium - $10^{-5}\%$, radium - $10^{-12}\%$). Similar relationships can be observed in the examples of p-elements [10, 11]. Thus, boron does not have significant toxicity to animal organisms, while thallium is one of the strongest poisons. Similarly, the light p elements of the IVA, VA and VIA groups (C, N, O, P, S) are the most important biogenic elements, while the heavy p elements of the same groups (Sn, Pb, As, Sb, Bi, Se, Te) are highly toxic to living organisms. In the p-elements of the VIIA group (F, Cl, Br, I), there is an increase in the ability to form biologically active organic compounds due to the increase in atomic mass (iodine is part of the thyroid hormone - thyroxine). Many d elements are the most important biogenic trace elements (Cu, Zn, Cr, Mn, Fe, Co, Mo, *etc.*) which exert large effects on health, acting as macrominerals and participating in many catalytic and oxidation-reduction bioreactions. Like s- and p-elements, d-elements are characterized by a general pattern, which consists of the fact that with an increase in atomic mass, the toxicity of elements in this group of periodic table increases, and their percentage in the body decreases. Thus, in the human body, less toxic zinc is about 10^{-3}%, more toxic cadmium - 10^{-4}%, and the normal content of mercury (the most toxic element of this group) does not exceed 10^{-6}%. Moreover, the elements have dual functions and can be both good and bad for life. For example, copper, a vital trace element, plays numerous roles in human physiology, including the growth of connective tissue, bone, and nerves, but occasional chronic and acute copper toxicity can lead to liver damage and some gastrointestinal effects [11].

Chemical elements participate in all life processes. The main biological functions of the biogenic elements can be classified as follows [2 - 11]:

1. Structural function - as components of body tissue of the hard structures - this function is characterized mainly by Ca^{2+}, Mg^{2+} cations and anions of P, O, C, Si, S, F, *e.g.*, PO_4^{3-}, F^-, CO_3^{2-}, NO_3^-, SiO_3^{2-} *etc.*;

2. As charge carriers for electrical impulses in nerves and for activating muscle contractions - this function is typical for simple monoatomic ions like Na^+, K^+, and Ca^{2+};

3. Electron transfer, essential for energy transfer - this function is representative of transition metals with various oxidation states enabling the transfer of electrons (Cu^+/Cu^{2+}, $Fe^{2+}/Fe^{3+}/Fe^{4+}$, $Mo^{4+}/Mo^{5+}/Mo^{6+}$, $Mn^{2+}/Mn^{3+}/Mn^{4+}$);

4. In the maintenance of acid-base balance;

5. In the regulation of body fluids;

6. In metabolism, including the synthesis and degradation of organic-based compounds-catalyzation of these biochemical processes is performed by enzymes that involve microelements like Zn, Fe, Ni, and Mn;

7. Activators of small molecules - this function is typical for microelements (transition metals) to enable the transport of gases with different reactions at physiological conditions, e.g.:

- Fe, Cu in the transport and storage of O_2;
- Ni, Fe in the reduction of CO_2 to methane;
- Mo, Fe, V in the fixation of N_2 and conversion to ammonia;

8. Numerous specific functions − Co in vitamin B_{12}, Mg in chlorophyll, hormonal activity (triiodothyronine and thyroxine), and many other functions.

Destruction of the balance of biogenic macro- and microelements leads to various changes in the state of the body. Some of them are essential for enzyme reactions where they attract and facilitate the conversion of substrate molecules to specific end products. Others have structural roles and are responsible for the stability of important biological molecules. Some of them donate or accept electrons in oxidation-reduction reactions that are of primary importance in the generation and utilization of metabolic energy. Additionally, some of the trace elements have important specific activities throughout biological processes. For illustration, children lag behind in physical development if in their body there is a lack of any one of such elements as K, Mg, Ca, Fe, Zn, Cu, Co, or Cr. A decrease in immune force is observed when the balance of K, Ca, Cu, Mn, Co, and Se is disturbed in the body. The condition of the teeth depends on the content in the body of Ca, Mg, Fe, Zn, Cu, and P. Therefore, the composition of food should include mineral substances, due to which the body realizes its need for chemical elements. In fact, although biogenic elements are essential components of biological activities, excessive levels of these elements can be toxic to body health and may lead to many fatal diseases, even such as cancer. The lack or excess of certain chemical elements in the human body allows the specialist to conclude whether the patient eats properly, whether the environment in which he lives is safe, and whether his gastrointestinal tract, kidneys, and the liver function properly. [12]. Additionally, humans are exposed to metal-based drugs for therapeutic and diagnostic purposes (Pt, Ru, Au). The use of Si implants, Co prostheses, and Hg dental fillings also has implications for living systems.

There are elements that are vital to only some organisms, like vanadium, found in some nitrogenases and halo-peroxidases in algae and fungi; Ni - in bacteria and plant enzymes; W - in thermophilic bacteria enzymes. These elements are not recognized to be essential for animals and humans. Lanthanides are found as cofactors of methanol dehydrogenase of methanotrophic bacteria in place of calcium, although rare earth elements are of limited significance for animal and human nutrition [13].

Our knowledge about the role of chemical elements in life remains very limited and open-ended. Attempts to establish a connection between the biological significance of elements and the structure of their atoms, as well as the search for evidence that some elements necessary for life have certain common properties of the atomic structure, will undoubtedly continue. There is every reason to believe that as our knowledge expands, it will be possible to enter into the most interesting regularity of the relationship between the structure of the elements and their biological activity and to collect a periodic table of the biological properties of the elements.

CLASSIFICATION OF BIOGENIC ELEMENTS

Various classifications have been proposed by different authors on chemical elements, both essential as well as trace elements [1 - 4].

All elements that play an important physiological role and have a key function in helping plants and animals live and be healthy are biogenic elements [14]. Biogenic elements, by definition, are chemical elements that are constantly part of organisms and have a certain biological significance. These elements are necessary for the construction and vital activity of various cells and organisms. Biogenic elements are required for life and their absence results in death. Of all elements of the periodic table, the ten metals - Na, K, Mg, Ca, Zn, Mn, Fe, Co, Mo, Cu and six organogens - H, C, N, O, P, and S, play a particularly important role in the implementation of various physiological and pathological processes and form the basis of all biologically important molecules and macromolecules. Currently, it is assumed that almost every one of the chemical elements of the periodic table plays some role in Earth's living systems and are found in living organisms, however, only around 25 elements are required by most, if not all, biological systems [3, 4]. Therefore, with the improvement of methods of determination, the knowledge of the presence of chemical elements in a living substance will expand.

Chemical elements can be classified into two main groups: essential elements and non-essential elements. An element is considered essential when a lack of that element produces an impairment of function and the addition of the element restores the organism to a healthy state. Essentiality can be defined by the next criteria: physiological deficiencies arise when the element is removed from the diet; deficiencies are alleviated by the addition of this element to the diet; specific biological functions are related to that element [11 - 13]. According to the content of elements in the human body, the elements are divided into three main groups:

- Macroelements ($> 10^{-2}$%) - C, H, O, N, P, S, Na, Ca, K, Cl;

- Microelements ($< 10^{-2}$%) - Mg, Cu, Zn, Mn, Co, Fe, I, Al, Mo, *etc.*;
- Ultra-microelements ($< 10^{-12}$%) - Ra, Hg, Au, U, *etc.*

Essential biogenic elements, which are crucial to maintaining the normal living state of the body, are divided into macroelements and microelements according to their abundance in organisms.

Macroelements constitute 60-80% of all inorganic minerals in the body and they include 12 elements in total - carbon, hydrogen, oxygen, nitrogen, sodium, potassium, calcium, magnesium, iron, phosphorus, sulphur, and chlorine. Macroelements can be further subdivided into two groups: the group of stable primary elements (O, C, H, and N) and the group of stable secondary elements (Na, K, Ca, Mg, P, S and Cl) which provide essential ions in body fluids and form the major structural components of the body. The first four elements are present in considerable amounts in every body tissue and together with phosphorus and sulfur, provide the building blocks for major cellular components including proteins, nucleic acids, lipids, carbohydrates, and metabolites [11 - 14]. These six elements (C, H, O, N, S, and P) combine with each other to form molecules that are the building blocks of the body. The four main electrolytes namely sodium, magnesium, potassium, and calcium, constitute about 1.89%. These macroelements maintain osmotic pressure, pH of the medium, ionic equilibrium, acid-base balance, *etc.* Macroelements can be subdivided into:

a. A group of stable primary bulk elements (elements found in all of Earth's living systems, often in relatively large quantities, from 2 to 60% of the total organism weight). These elements are O, C, H and N. They constitute the bulk of the human diet and tens of grams per day are required for humans;

b. A group of stable secondary elements, referred to as macrominerals (elements found in living systems in relatively small quantities, from 0.05 to 2% of the total organism weight). These elements are Na, K, Ca, Mg, P, S and Cl. As they are present in the organism in rather smaller amounts than the bulk elements, consequently lower levels are required in the diet, correspondingly.

Unlike the chemical elements that make up the bulk of a living being, the so-called macronutrients (C, O, H, N, P, S, Ca, Na, Mg, *etc.*), minerals, the content of which in organisms is very small and is between 10^{-3} - 10^{-12}%, are called trace elements. Microelements (trace elements) are required in very small amounts by the body and are present in the organism in amounts ranging from a few grams to a few milligrams. Microelements include the group of metals (Fe, Cu, Zn, Mn, Co, Ni, Mo, V, W) and the group of semimetals (or metalloids) and nonmetals (B, Si, F, I, Se). Trace elements play an important role in enzymatic activity. These elements, together with enzymes, hormones, vitamins, and other biologically active substances, are involved in the processes of growth, reproduction, metabolism of nucleic acids, proteins, fats, carbohydrates, *etc*. It is well known that the metal ion concentration of trace elements (Fe, Cu, Zn, Mn, Co, Ni, Cr, Mo, V) in human plasma is much higher than that of seawater, for instance. This observation designates that the biosystems have well-organized mechanisms for the accumulation, storage, and transport of these trace elements, which explains their specific functions and their role in life evolution [11 - 14]. Although these elements account for only 0.02% of the total human body weight, they play significant biological roles. Most of the microelements mediate vital biochemical reactions by acting as cofactors or catalysts for many enzymes. They also act as centers for building stabilizing structures such as enzymes and proteins. Microelements (trace elements) can be subdivided into:

a. group of metals: Fe, Cu, Zn, Mn, Co, Ni, Mo, V, W;
b. group of semimetals (metalloids) and nonmetals: B, Si, F, I, Se.

The biological functions of trace elements in living organisms are mainly associated with oxidation-reduction reactions and the processes of complexation occurring between biological ligands and ions of the corresponding metals. The transition metal trace elements have unfilled or partially filled d-orbitals, hence their oxidation states in the compounds are variable, which elucidates their affinity to take part in a great range of oxidation-reduction reactions. All these trace elements have a high ability to form coordination complex compounds because of their free s- and p-orbitals and partially vacant d-orbitals, which allows them to form donor-acceptor bonds in the complexes thus acting as perfect complexing ions [11 - 14]. The formation of organometallic complexes is of great biological importance since they take an active part in the metabolic processes occurring in the body. It is known that the ability of trace elements to catalytic action increases millions of times if they form metal-organic complexes. The accumulation of metal microelements or deficiency of these elements may stimulate an alternate pathway which might produce different pathologies.

Measurable levels of some of the remaining elements of the periodic table are found in humans but are not required for growth or health, accordingly called non-essential elements [11 - 13]. Non-essential elements found in organisms at very low concentrations (less than 10^{-12}%) are sometimes called ultra-microelements. Their function in the body is yet unknown, at least as far as we know today. Nonnegligible quantities of apparently non-essential elements such as Br, Al, Sr, Ba, or Li and toxic elements such as As, Pb, Cd, or Hg are also present in the body due to the chemical similarity with the significant essential elements (Li^+ is similar to Na^+ and K^+; Sr^{2+} and Ba^{2+} are similar to Ca^{2+}; Br^- shows similarity to Cl^-; Al^{3+} is like Fe^{3+}; Cd^{2+} and Pb^{2+} are similar to Zn^{2+}). For example, rubidium and strontium with similar chemistry to that of the essential elements potassium and calcium, are absorbed by the body, although they have no known biological function.

There is another classification of the elements, which is consistent with the importance of chemical elements for the vital activity of humans [13]:

1. Irreplaceable elements, which are constantly in the human body. These are C, H, O, N, K, P, S, Na, Ca, Cl, Mg, Cu, Zn, Mn, Co, Fe, I, Mo, V, *etc.* The deficiency of these elements leads to disorders of the vital activity of the organism;

2. Impurity elements that also could be found in the human body, but their biological role has not always been identified or is still little studied. These are Ga, Sb, Sr, Br, F, B, Be, Li, Si, Sn, Cs, As, Ba, Ge, Rb, Pb, Ra, Bi, Cd, Cr, Ni, Ti, Ag, Th, Hg, Ce, Se;

3. Micro-impurity elements, which are found in the human body, but there is no evidence about their content in the body or their biological roles. These are Sc, Tl, In, La, Pr, W, Re, *etc.*

Criteria of counting the chemical element of essential biogenic elements are created on many years investigations of specific elements' pathways and mechanisms. The classification is not completed yet and it can be reformed on the basis of new information and knowledge [6 - 10]. Low content of trace elements in the composition of the body does not at all indicate that these substances are accidental impurities or contaminants. On the contrary, the toxicity of essential elements often depends on its chemical form - for instance, only certain chromium compounds are toxic (Cr^{+6} in chromate), whereas others are often added in mineral supplements (Cr^{+3}), having beneficial functions and little toxicity. Every single element has three possible levels of nutritional intake - deficient, optimum, and toxic levels. Very low intake levels cause deficiency symptoms. Higher intake levels produce symptoms of intoxication. Each organism tends to maintain its tissue concentration of the elements at levels that optimize the respective biological functions. Finally, the most important biological functions of many of the most studied trace elements are being revealed increasingly fully every year.

Chemical Classification of the Elements

The main characteristics of the chemical elements (the structure of the electron shells, the oxidation state, the ability to form coordination complexes, *etc.*) are determined by the position of these elements in the periodic table. The same characteristics underlie the physiological and pathological role of elements in the human body.

Based on the modern quantum mechanical interpretation of the periodic table of elements, the classification of elements is carried out in accordance with their electronic configuration. It is based on the degree of filling of various electron orbitals (s, p, d, f) with electrons. Accordingly, all elements are divided into s-, p-, d-, and f-elements [15].

s-Elements are filled with electrons in the s-subshell. Depending on the degree of filling of the s- subshell, s-elements are classified into two main groups of the periodic table: s^1-elements (alkali metals) and s^2-elements (alkaline earth metals) which are located in groups IA and IIA, respectively.

In the groups of p-elements, the p-subshell is filled with electrons. In the periodic table, p-elements are located in groups IIIA-VIIIA. In atoms of s- and p-elements, the valence electrons are localized at the external energy level.

In d-elements, the d-subshell is filled with electrons. They are located in the IB-VIIIB groups of the periodic table of the elements. In the atoms of d-elements, the valence electrons are situated on the s-subshell of the outer and d-subshell of the preexternal energy levels.

f-Elements are chemical elements in whose atoms electrons build up the f-subshell of the third of the outside energy level. In the periodic table, f-elements are located outside the table and make up the families of lanthanides and actinides.

CHAPTER 2

Biological Functions of Elements of Main Groups General Characteristics of s-Elements and Their Compounds

s-Elements are placed in IA and IIA groups of the periodic table (except for helium, which is in the VIIIA group). At the external electronic level, they have one or two electrons for s^1- and s^2-elements that their atoms give up easily, producing one- and two-charged cations. As the amount of valence electrons increases at the energy level, the ionization energy of atoms increases (ionization energy is the energy needed to separate the least bound electron from an atom), and consequently, the reducing properties of atoms decrease. Therefore, s^2-elements are weaker reducing agents than s^1-elements. In the group, the reducing activity of s-elements increases from the top to the bottom, as the number of electron layers in atoms increases and the ionization energy decreases in the same direction [3, 4].

The radii of ions in the subgroups from the top to the bottom increase, and in the period moving from s^1 to s^2-elements, the radii decrease. The regularities of the radius changes of s-element ions in the group and period and the structure of their electron shells affect the nature of the relationship between the anions and cations of s-elements and the solubility of their salts. Since the ions of s-elements have a stable electron configuration such as that of inert gases, they have a small ability to polarize and are themselves weak polarizers. Polarization is the displacement of the electron cloud of an anion (polarized anion) under the influence of a positive charge of the ion.

The polarizing capacity (ρ) of the ion (*i.e.*, its ability to deform the electron cloud of the anion) depends on the charge of the cation and its size is proportional to the charge density on the ion: ρ is equal to the charge of the cation divided by the radius of the cation. From this relationship, it can be seen that the greater the charge of the ion and the smaller its radius, the greater the polarizing effect of the ion and the less it is capable of polarization.

The polarizing power of cations of s-elements decreases moving from Li^+ to Cs^+ in the IA group. Due to the high polarizing power of the Li^+ cation, lithium compounds have the least pronounced ionic character compared to the same type of compounds of other alkali metals. With an increase in the polarizing properties of cations, the bond strength with the anion rises and the solubility of the compounds decreases. If the s^1-elements have the lowest charge (+1) and the greatest radius in their period, so cations do not polarize themselves and have a low polarizing ability. Most of their salts are water-soluble due to the high polarity of the bond, which is close to ionic, because possible precipitation can be formed only with large, easily polarized anions [3, 4].

Sodium and potassium are vital biogenic metals and their biochemical behavior is similar, though Na^+ and K^+ cations are different based on their hydration enthalpies and ionic radius. In cell membranes, the specific protein pumps for these cations (Na/K ATPases) maintain their concentration gradient in the plasma and in the intracellular matrix which helps in generating the electro-potential gradients important for the nerve impulses.

When moving to cations of s^2-elements, the polarizing properties are enhanced as the charge (+2) increases and the radius of the ion decreases. This leads to an increase in the bond strength (the bond approaches covalent), and the solubility of the salts decreases. Cations of s^2-elements form insoluble precipitates of chromates, carbonates, sulfates, oxalates, *etc.,* which are of analytical importance and are used to separate and detect individual cations of s^2-elements.

Like sodium and potassium, magnesium and calcium are also plentiful elements in the body [7 - 10]. Bones, teeth, skeletal muscles, and soft tissues hold around 95% of the total Ca^{2+} and Mg^{2+} ions existing in the body. Mg^{2+} ion, representing 1% in extracellular fluid, acts as a vital cofactor activating many enzymes involved in transcription, replication, and translation processes. Both Ca^{2+} and Mg^{2+} ions participate in the stabilization of nucleic acids, lipid membranes and in the regulation of the contractions of skeletal and cardiac muscles. Dysregulation of calcium and magnesium leads to many disease conditions including gastrointestinal, coronary heart disease, diabetes, osteoporosis, and neurological indications.

In water, the cations of s-elements are hydrated and form aqua-complexes ($[Ca(H_2O)_6]^{2+}$) due to the electrostatic attraction of water dipole molecules. Since the electron shell of the ions of s-elements has a stable configuration of inert gases and ligands (water molecules) have a little effect on the state of electrons, all of them in aqueous solutions are colorless [3, 4].

Looking at the dependence of hydration enthalpies of the cations of s-elements on their size, it can be seen that with an increase in the charge of ions, the energy of their hydration increases, and with an increase in the size of the ions, it decreases.

Ions of s-elements in aqueous solutions form coordination compounds with inorganic and organic ligands, for example, with 8-oxyquinoline (LiOx, $MgOx_2$, $BaOx_2$) and with ammonia $[Mg(NH_3)_4]Cl_2$. Nevertheless, the stability of these complexes is small, since s-elements form a bond with the ligands, which is approaching the ionic bond. The least stability of complex compounds is observed in cations with a large radius and a small charge (s^1-elements). In the cations of s^2-elements with a decrease in radius and an increase in charge, the stability of the complexes increases.

The variation in the radius of the ion has a great influence on its basic properties. Hydroxides of s-element cations have pronounced basic properties (except for $Be(OH)_2$), which are explained by the fragility of the ionic bond E-OH. That is why s-elements are called alkaline and alkaline earth metals. The basic properties of hydroxides increase with an increase in the ion radius, since this weakens the mutual attraction of metal and hydroxide ions, which facilitates the process of ionization of the compound [3, 4]. Therefore, in the group, the basic character of s-element hydroxides increases from the top to the bottom (for example, from LiOH to CsOH), and in the period, it increases with the transition from s^2- to s^1-element. Thus, in the second period, LiOH is a strong base, $Be(OH)_2$ is amphoteric; in the third period, NaOH is a strong base; $Mg(OH)_2$ is a medium-strength base; in the fourth period, KOH is a strong base, $Ca(OH)_2$ is a strong base with less pronounced basic properties than that of KOH.

The solubility of s-element hydroxides is also associated with the change in the radius of the ion. With an increase in the polarizing capacity of the cation, the bond strength of the ion with the hydroxide anion increases and the solubility of the base decreases. Therefore, the hydroxide of the s^2-element cation has a lower solubility than the hydroxide of the cation of s^1-elements of the same period.

Salts of s-elements undergo hydrolysis when the salt is obtained by a strong base (alkaline and alkaline earth metals) and a weak acid. When such a salt is dissolved in water, the cations undergo strong hydration and the salt completely dissociates. The resulting anions of a weak acid, being a strong base, are protonated by water molecules, forming a weak acid and hydroxide ions:

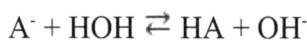

$$A^- + HOH \rightleftarrows HA + OH^-$$

Solutions of such salts have an alkaline reaction in the medium. Hydrolysis in this case goes by anions. Thus, the hydrolysis of sodium carbonate can be expressed by equations in molecular and ionic form. The first stage:

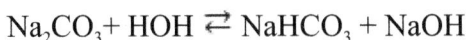

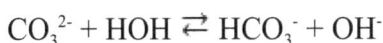

$$Na_2CO_3 + HOH \rightleftarrows NaHCO_3 + NaOH$$

$$CO_3^{2-} + HOH \rightleftarrows HCO_3^- + OH^-$$

The second stage:

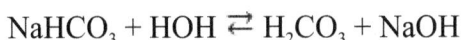

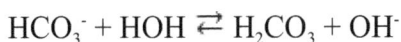

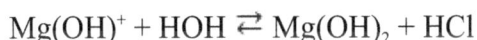

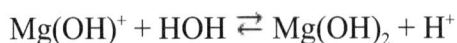

$$NaHCO_3 + HOH \rightleftarrows H_2CO_3 + NaOH$$

$$HCO_3^- + HOH \rightleftarrows H_2CO_3 + OH^-$$

However, under normal conditions, hydrolysis is practically limited to the first stage. This is because HCO_3^- ions dissociate much more difficult than H_2CO_3 molecules. Only with strong dilution and heating hydrolysis of the resulting acid salt is possible.

With a decrease in the strength of the base of the s-element, the ability of the cation to enter into protolithic interaction with water molecules increases [3 - 10]. Therefore, magnesium salts are able to hydrolyze along the cation to form the basic salt if the salt is formed by an anion of a strong acid. The first stage:

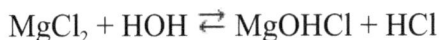

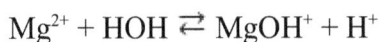

$$MgCl_2 + HOH \rightleftarrows MgOHCl + HCl$$

$$Mg^{2+} + HOH \rightleftarrows MgOH^+ + H^+$$

The second stage:

$$Mg(OH)^+ + HOH \rightleftarrows Mg(OH)_2 + HCl$$

$$Mg(OH)^+ + HOH \rightleftarrows Mg(OH)_2 + H^+$$

Hydrolysis is limited to the first stage. Solutions of such salts have an acidic reaction in the medium.

Ions of s-elements are resistant to the oxidants' and reducing agents' action and oxidation-reduction reactions are not characteristic of them.

In terms of radius and many chemical properties, ammonium ions NH_4^+ are close to the cations of s^1-elements, so their analytical properties are considered in common with the properties of the cations of s^1-elements [3 - 10]. Aqueous solutions of ammonia have an alkaline reaction in the medium, since ammonia partially reacts with water molecules, forming a conjugate acid-base pair:

$$NH_3 + HOH \rightleftarrows NH_3 \cdot H_2O \rightleftarrows NH_4^+ + OH^-$$

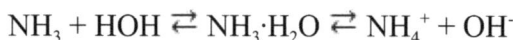

The attachment of a proton to an ammonia molecule occurs because of the electrons lone pair of N atoms by the type of donor-acceptor interaction. Ammonium salts undergo hydrolysis along the cation to form a hydrated proton (oxonium ion) and ammonia, as a result of which their solutions have an acidic reaction in the medium:

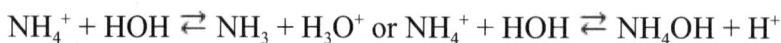

$$NH_4^+ + HOH \rightleftarrows NH_3 + H_3O^+ \text{ or } NH_4^+ + HOH \rightleftarrows NH_4OH + H^+$$

BIOLOGICAL ROLE OF S-ELEMENTS

s-Elements of the IA Group

Hydrogen

The main forms of hydrogen present in the biosphere are natural waters, gases, and organic substances [16]. Free H_2 is nearly absent in the biosphere, even though it is the most plentiful chemical element in the cosmos. In organisms, H_2 is a constituent of bioorganic substances and biopolymers and is the 3rd most abundant chemical element in the body (around 10%). This element is practically a physiologically inert gas. Its lethal dose for humans has not been determined.

The lightest element in the periodic table, which can be placed in either group IA or VIIA, has an important role in biological processes, nonetheless, it can form only a single bond. It can exist in the form of a H^+ cation, which stands alongside alkali ions, and in the form of a hydride H^- anion, similar to the anions of the VIIA group. H^+ cation is important for the pH control in the body. pH is strongly regulated by the proton pump and is held at pH 7.4 in the body fluids and tissues, and a substantial deviation from this value represents a kind of distress. The pH can reach 6-7 in tumor tissues [17], 5.5 in endosomes, and 4-5 in lysosomes [18]. pH plays a crucial role in the release of Fe^{3+} from its protein transferrin, which is also controlled by the concentration of H^+ cation [19]. In the stomach, the value of pH reaches 1-3. The regulation of pH is realized by amino acids and by buffering (carbonic acid/bicarbonate buffer) in the human blood. Hydride anion is also vital for the body functions not in the form of a free H^- anion, but as donated by the reduced coenzymes. Several redox enzymes use cofactors such as nicotinamide adenine dinucleotide phosphate (NADP), (Fig. **1**), nicotine adenine dinucleotide (NAD), flavin adenine dinucleotide (FAD), and flavin mononucleotide (FMN) which may transfer e^- and can provide H^- anion in the reduction stage of enzyme cycles. In bacteria, the enzyme hydrogenase may produce H_2 gas, a useful reductant for the survival of many bacteria.

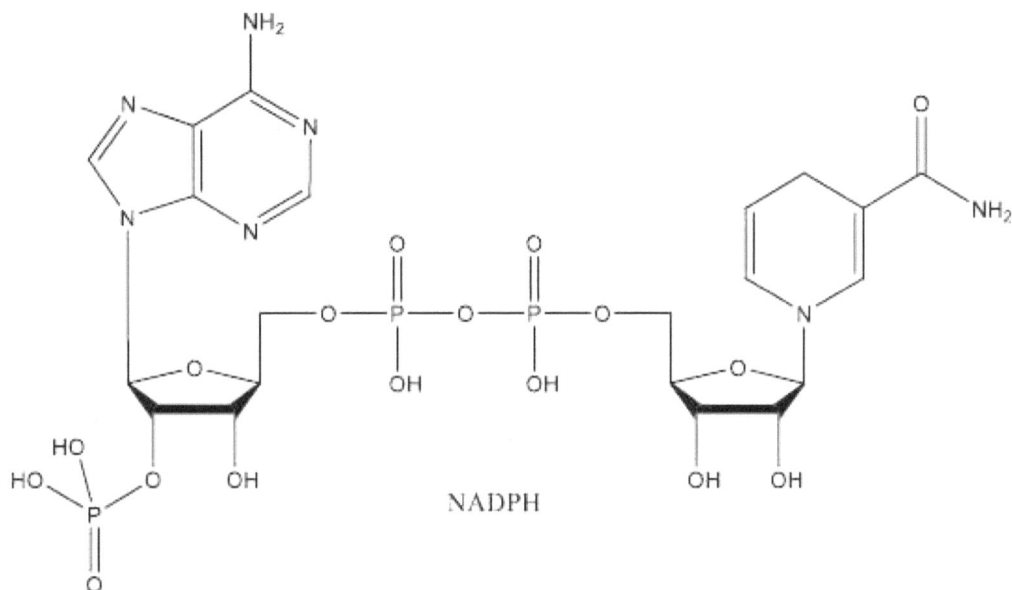

Fig. (1). The structure of NADPH.

Hydrogen has a significant role in biochemical oxo-reduction reactions. In the human body, the biological chains of oxo-reduction reactions occur at a specific redox potential. Biochemical oxidation-reduction processes are typically catalyzed by oxidoreductases. The degradation of saccharides, lipids, and proteins is based on the gradual oxidation of C to CO_2. The energy obtained by this oxidation is regularly released and thus it is maximally utilizable.

Some illustrations of oxo-reduction systems in the human body are listed below [3, 4]:

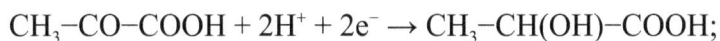

$$CH_3-CO-COOH + 2H^+ + 2e^- \rightarrow CH_3-CH(OH)-COOH;$$

Pyruvic acid (oxidized form), Lactic acid (reduced form)

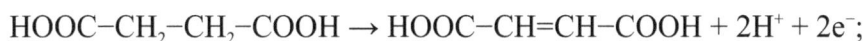

$$HOOC-CH_2-CH_2-COOH \rightarrow HOOC-CH=CH-COOH + 2H^+ + 2e^-;$$

Succinic acid (reduced form), Fumaric acid (oxidized form)

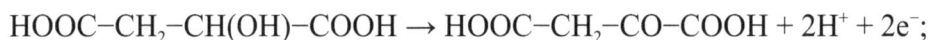

$$HOOC-CH_2-CH(OH)-COOH \rightarrow HOOC-CH_2-CO-COOH + 2H^+ + 2e^-;$$

Malic acid (reduced form), Oxaloacetic acid (oxidized form)

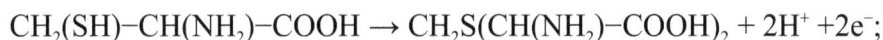

$$CH_2(SH)-CH(NH_2)-COOH \rightarrow CH_2S(CH(NH_2)-COOH)_2 + 2H^+ + 2e^-;$$

Cysteine (reduced form), Cystine (oxidized form)

Ubiquinone $+ 2H^+ + 2e^- \rightarrow$ Ubiquinol;

Ascorbic acid: oxidized form $+ 2H^+ + 2e^- \rightarrow$ Ascorbic acid: reduced form;

Cytochrome $(Fe^{3+}) + e^- \rightarrow$ cytochrome (Fe^{2+}) and others.

The most common oxidation process in biological systems is dehydrogenation. H atoms separated from the substrates bind to cofactors of the oxidoreductases [3,4,16]. The typical cofactors consist of nicotinamide adenine dinucleotide (NAD$^+$) and flavin adenine dinucleotide (FAD). H atoms bound to cofactors are transported to the respiratory chain localized in the mitochondrial membrane.

$NAD^+ + 2H^+ + 2e^- \rightarrow NADH + H^+$

$FAD + 2H^+ + 2e^- \rightarrow FADH_2$

The coenzyme NAD transports H to the human body by the reaction:

$NADH \leftrightarrow NAD^+ + H^+ + e^-$

Biochemically important NAD enzymatic redox reactions are:

- oxidation of ethanol in the liver: $C_2H_6O + NAD^+ \rightarrow CH_3CHO + NADH + H^+$;

- anaerobic glycolysis: pyruvate $+ NADH + H^+ \rightleftarrows$ lactate $+ NAD^+$;

- conversion of ketone: acetoacetate $+ NADH + H^+ \rightleftarrows$ β-hydroxybutyrate $+ NAD^+$.

The β-oxidation of fatty acids by FAD enzymatic redox reaction and the reaction of the citrate cycle can be expressed by equations:

$R\text{-}CH_2\text{-}CH_2\text{-}CO\text{-}CoA + FAD \rightarrow R\text{-}CH{=}CH\text{-}CO\text{-}CoA + FADH_2$

succinate $+ FAD \rightleftarrows$ fumarate $+ FADH_2$

Electrons obtained from H atoms are directed from the carriers with negative values of potential to positive potentials, and lastly to the dioxygen molecules. The released energy is used in the associated oxidative phosphorylation process to synthesize adenosine triphosphate (ATP), (Fig. **2**) [3,4,16].

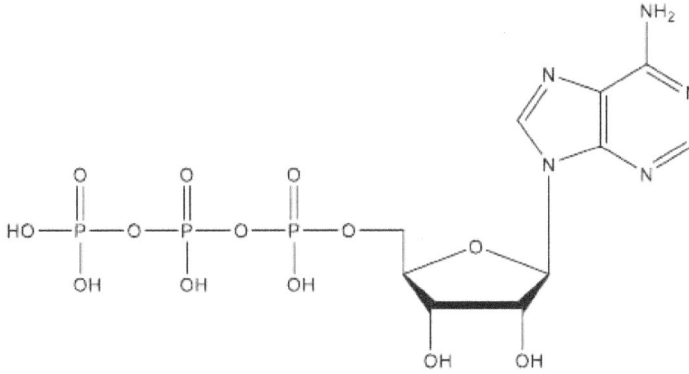

Fig. (2). Adenosine triphosphate (ATP).

Additional enzyme systems and the corresponding cofactors different in their redox potentials are listed below:

- Hydroxylation of phenylalanine: phenylalanine + O_2 + BH_4 → tyrosine + BH_2 + H_2O
- Reduction of H_2O_2 in erythrocytes: H_2O_2 + 2GSH → $2H_2O$ + G-S-S-G
- Reaction of glycolysis: glyceraldehyde 3-P + P_i + NAD^+ ⇌ 1,3-BPG + NADH + H^+

Where BH_4 -tetra -hydro biopterin, BH_2 -di -hydro biopterin, 1, 3-BPG-1, 3-bis - phos -phoglycerate, GSH- reduced glutathione, G-S-S-G - oxidized glutathione, (Fig. **3**).

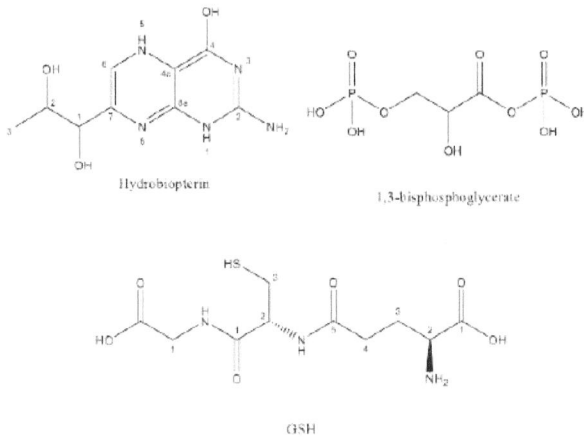

Fig. (3). Structures of dihydrobiopterin, 1,3-bisphosphoglycerate and GSH.

Gaseous dihydrogen H_2 is a product of bacterial fermentation in the colon [16]. Hydrogen gas is partially resorbed and breathed out.

Water

The transfer of hydrogen from organic biomolecules to O_2 with the formation of H_2O is the principal bio-oxidation, throughout which the organism gains energy in the form of ATP, an energy-carrying compound occurring in cells of all living beings.

The major amount of hydrogen is enclosed in water, which accounts for more than 90% of the mass of a living cell and more than 70% of the human body. Water is the main solvent in cellular systems. The human body, whose mass is 70 kg, contains approximately 45 liters of water.

Water dissolves the life-supportive organic and inorganic compounds and transfers them to liquids in and outside the cells. Water is a unique solvent for inorganic ions and compounds, for organic biomolecules including low-molecular compounds as carboxylic acids, for organic salts, amino acids, nucleic acids, proteins, mono- and polysaccharides and many others. H_2O is a medium for colloid and coarse particles of different dispersion systems.

Water has unique properties (high boiling temperature, specific heat capacity, and high heat of evaporation) which are connected with chemical bonds called "hydrogen bonds" - widespread bonds in living bodies that have a significant role in numerous life processes [20, 21]. Hydrogen bonds hold complementary strands of DNA together. They are basic for the three-dimensional structures of enzymes, proteins, and antibodies.

Water is a very polar compound that can cause electrolyte dissociation. Electrolytes possess a vital role in the organisms. Biological liquids for instance blood, urine, gastric juice, intracellular, and extracellular fluids are electrolytes. Blood contains Na^+, K^+, Ca^{2+}, Mg^{2+} *etc.* cations, as well as anions Cl^-, HCO_3^-, $H_2PO_4^-$, HPO_4^{2-}, SO_4^{2-}. In the body, there are two main types of fluid with different compositions of electrolytes, namely: intracellular, in which the predominant cation is potassium, and extracellular with a predominance of sodium cations. Electrolytes take part in maintaining the osmotic pressure, in influencing the proteins' solubility [3, 4, 16, 21]. Low molecular compounds catalyze the metabolism of blood clotting. Osmotic pressure variations are possible only within 1%. In the human body, 1-2% lowering of the osmotic pressure with a large amount of water, or a loss of salts leads to cramps, dizziness and vomiting. Growing the osmotic pressure by the introduction of a large quantity of salts causes a feeling of thirst and dehydration due to swelling of the mucous membrane. The constant value of osmotic pressure in the body is called isoosmosis or isoosmia. It is maintained by the liver, which keeps water and salt subcutaneous fat and retains water in the human body. It is supported also by the skin and the kidneys, which eliminate water from the body. The simple blood substitutes are 0.9% solution of NaCl (isotonic saline) or 4-5% glucose solution, as their osmotic pressures are equal to the blood osmotic pressure. The solution whose osmotic pressure is greater than the osmolality of the standard solution is called hypertensive or hypertonic solution. A solution that has osmotic pressure less than the osmotic pressure of the solution or other standard is called a hypotonic solution. Plasmolysis occurs when the blood cells are placed in a hypertonic solution, which results in the movement of water out of the cells through osmosis. The blood cells lose their normal shape and shrink. Hemolysis occurs when the blood cells are placed in a hypotonic solution, which leads to the movement of water into the cells through osmosis. The cells increase in size and some of them may hemolyze. Osmotic phenomena are also important for animals and plants.

Water is also a place in which many vital reactions occur in living organisms and is a substrate or product of many bioreactions (cellular respiration, photosynthesis). Hydrolysis, hydration, and oxidation-reduction reactions occur in an aqueous medium in the body, for example:

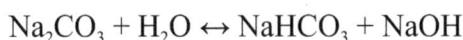

$$Na_2CO_3 + H_2O \leftrightarrow NaHCO_3 + NaOH$$

Water takes part in biosynthetic, catalytic, osmotic, and swelling processes. It transfers nutrients and displays metabolic products. It participates in the thermoregulation of the body. The loss of 1-2 liters of H_2O causes thirst. The loss of 6-8% of H_2O disturbs body metabolism, it slows oxidation-reduction processes, rises blood viscosity and the temperature of the body, and accelerates breathing. The loss of 10% H_2O is an irreversible process that can lead to the death of the organism. Water is spread unequally in organs and tissues of the body [3,4,16]. A significant indicator is water inflexibility, caused by the presence of calcium and magnesium sulphates, hydro-carbonates, and chlorides. Hard water influences the digestive processes by reducing gastric juice production. In this case, the calcium salts are deposited in the blood joints and vessels. Hard water is incompatible with some drugs, particularly sulphonamides.

In humans, the H^+ concentration in most fluids is usually kept within a very close range. Water plays a predominantly vital role in the preservation of acid-alkaline chemical balance [20, 21], because many vital reactions include proton H^+ exchange between soluble substances. Shifts in the acid-base balance to the acidic side are named acidosis and to the basic side-alkalosis. Acidosis is usually observed in the next cases: a) lung diseases when carbon dioxide removal is problematic; b) cardiac ischemia; c) diabetes or blood saturated with unoxidized glucose cleavage products (organic acids); d) in some inflammatory locations, where acidic decomposition products of proteins are accumulated. Alkalosis is observed in case of uncontrollable vomiting, intake of excessive amounts of antacids, *etc.* Acidosis and alkalosis are serious conditions that require serious attention since all equilibrium reactions which involve H^+ are sensitive to pH values.

Acid-base balance in the body maintains buffers; helps the kidney to remove hydrocarbons and acidic phosphates, and makes it easy to eliminate an excess of CO_2. Water is a fundamental factor to acid-base balance, providing the stability of the cell's internal environment which possesses a stabilizing and buffering capacity.

The pH is a significant characteristic of biofluids of the entire organism. The pH values of some biological fluids are listed in Table **2** [3, 4].

Table 2. pH of biofluids.

Biofluid	pH
Blood	7.36 -7.44
Gastric juice	0.90 - 1.50
Pancreatic juice	7.50 - 8.80
Urine	4.80- 7.50
Duodenal juice	6.50 - 7.60
Saliva	6.35 - 6.85
Intestinal juice	9.00 - 10.00
Bile	6.50 - 7.30
Spinal fluid	7.35 - 7.80

The pH values of the body cells are usually different from the neutral point (erythrocytes, pH= 7.00; prostatic cells, pH= 4.50; skeletal muscle cells, pH= 6.90; platelets, pH= 7.30; osteoblasts, pH= 8.50). Cells maintain a precise and constant cytosolic pH. The pH of the body fluid is kept constant, in the human blood in the narrow limits around 7.4 ± 0.04. Small alterations beyond this range are destructive for the cells [3, 4]. The displacement of blood pH to the acidic side in case of acidosis and the shift of blood pH to the basic side in alkalosis are harmful. The pH of urine is dependent on the food the person consumes. In case of animal food, urine becomes more acidic, as in the proteins' hydrolysis, amino acids are produced. When vegetable food is used, the pH of urine moves to the alkaline region because of the hydrolysis of the salts of weak organic acids in the vegetable juices, which produces an alkaline reaction.

The pH affects the activity of enzymes. Enzymatic activity is at its maximal value at the optimal pH. If the pH values are increased above or decreased below the optimal pH, the enzymatic activity decreases [3, 4]. Enzymes work within quite a narrow pH range. Pepsin, which breaks down proteins in stomach acid conditions, has an optimal pH with low values. Catalase has an optimum pH of 9. Most of the other enzymes work within a pH range of around 5-9 with neutral pH being the optimum. Extremely high or small pH values commonly result in a complete loss of enzyme activity. The pH also disturbs the microorganisms' functions. For instance, *Vibrio cholerae* grows at pH= 7.50-9.20. Consequently, people with gastric juice acidity are not infected with cholera. The optimal pH values for the action of some enzymes are presented in Table **3**.

Table 3. Optimal pH values for some enzymes.

Enzyme	Substrate	pH
β - fructofuranosidase	Saccharose	4.5 - 6.5
Pepsin	Protein	1.5 - 2.0
Urease	Urea	6.7
Arginase	Arginine	9.5 - 9.9

Practically, every biochemical process depends on pH. A slight alteration in pH results in a great change in the reaction rates. In order to keep the biological fluid pH constant, the bodies possess protection mechanisms for keeping the acid-base homeostasis, in particular, the presence of buffer systems. Some buffers are involved in preserving the constant pH of biofluids. In different compartments, they work with varied applications cooperating with each other. The buffer keeps the pH constant by acceptance or by releasing protons [3, 4, 16, 21]. The addition or elimination of H^+ is removed by different buffers equivalently to their capacities. This is correct not only for the interactions with H^+ cation, but also for bioreactions in which H^+ cation does not participate. The buffer solution typically contains almost equal concentrations of weak bases and salts of the conjugate acids or weak acids and salts of the conjugate bases. The buffer pH remains constant when minimal quantities of a strong base or a strong acid are added. The most significant buffers and their presence in biofluids are listed below.

Hydrogen carbonate buffer consists of H_2CO_3 and $NaHCO_3$ and has the greatest significance in the blood [3, 4, 16, 20]. It is the chief buffer of the extracellular environment, making up more than half of the buffer capacity of the blood, which depends on the equilibrium of H_2CO_3, $NaHCO_3$, and CO_2, presented below:

$$CO_2 + H_2O \rightleftarrows H_2CO_3 \rightleftarrows H^+ + HCO_3^-$$

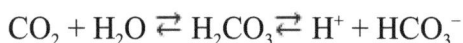

CO_2 formed as an end metabolism product is distributed into the blood erythrocytes. Then it is transformed into HCO_3^- anion. This process is catalyzed by carbonic anhydrase. The mechanism of action of hydrogen carbonate buffer can be expressed by the equations:

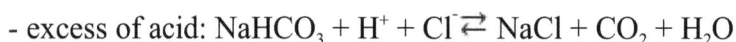

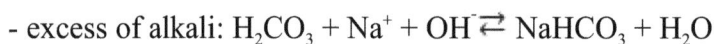

- excess of acid: $NaHCO_3 + H^+ + Cl^- \rightleftarrows NaCl + CO_2 + H_2O$

- excess of alkali: $H_2CO_3 + Na^+ + OH^- \rightleftarrows NaHCO_3 + H_2O$

If the pH of the blood decreases in excess of hydrogen ions, the concentration of HCO_3^- reduces because of CO_2 formation that enters the gas phase and is removed by the lungs. If the blood pH increases, the reverse process is observed. Excess of $NaHCO_3$ in this circumstance is excreted by the kidneys. Thus, under physiological conditions, the blood does not change with the increase or decrease of pH. Hydrogen carbonate buffer provides around half of the blood buffer capacity.

Hydrogen phosphate buffer, composed of the weak acid NaH_2PO_4 and the conjugate base Na_2HPO_4, has the highest impact in urine, digestive juices, and partially in blood [3, 4, 16, 21]. It acts in the cytoplasm of the cells. The mechanism of action of phosphate buffer can be represented by the next reaction equations:

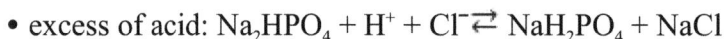

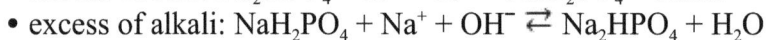

- excess of acid: $Na_2HPO_4 + H^+ + Cl^- \rightleftarrows NaH_2PO_4 + NaCl$
- excess of alkali: $NaH_2PO_4 + Na^+ + OH^- \rightleftarrows Na_2HPO_4 + H_2O$

The $H_2PO_4^-$ produced in the reaction of HPO_4^{2-} in low pH values is excreted by the urine.

The main protein buffer system in the blood is hemoglobin/oxyhemoglobin. *Hemoglobin buffer* (HHb + KHb) and *oxyhemoglobin buffer* ($HHbO_2$ + $KHbO_2$) are blood (erythrocytes) and make up roughly 35% of buffering [3,4,16,20]. Hemoglobin HHb and oxyhemoglobin $HHbO_2$ are weak acids. Oxyhemoglobin is a stronger acid than hemoglobin. Therefore, at oxygenation of HHb in the lungs, the produced $HHbO_2$ releases protons. On the other hand, in the tissues, $HHbO_2$ is converted into HHb, which behaves as a proton acceptor. Ionization and binding of protons can be performed by the imidazole group of histidine residues of globin.

$HHb \rightleftarrows Hb^- + H^+$

$HHbO_2 \rightleftarrows HbO_2^- + H^+$

The observed changes in the ionization process of hemoglobin correlate with the formation and ionization of H_2CO_3 in the case of hydrogen carbonate buffer.

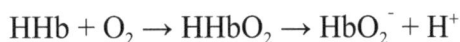

$HHb + O_2 \rightarrow HHbO_2 \rightarrow HbO_2^- + H^+$

The released protons during oxygenation in the lungs bind to bicarbonate ions and carbonic acid is formed. H_2CO_3 decomposes to carbon dioxide and water by carbonic anhydrase and CO_2 is removed by pulmonary ventilation, thus allowing constant transport of CO_2.

The mechanism of action of hemoglobin buffer can be expressed by the equations:

- excess of acid: $KHb + H^+ + Cl^- \rightarrow HHb + KCl$
- excess of alkali: $HHb + K^+ + OH^- \rightarrow KHb + H_2O$

An analogous effect is shown in the $HHbO_2$ buffer.

Protein buffer consists of Pt-H and Pt-K (protein and protein salt) and occurs in the blood and different tissues [3,4,16]. The buffer effect of proteins is due to their amphoteric character (correspondingly to amino acids). Proteins can act as proton donors and proton acceptors. The ionizable groups of side chains are able to react as a weak acid or a weak base. The mechanism of action of protein buffers can be represented by the next equations:

- excess of acid: $Pt-K + H^+ + Cl^- \rightarrow Pt-H + KCl$
- excess of alkali $Pt-H + K^+ + OH^- \rightarrow Pt-K + H_2O$

Buffer function is performed by the cysteine's sulfhydryl groups and the histidine's imidazole groups.

The protein molecule $COOH-Pt-NH_2$ occurs in the blood and different tissues [3, 4, 16, 21]. The amphoteric molecule of protein neutralizes the acidic and basic metabolic products. This can be expressed as follows:

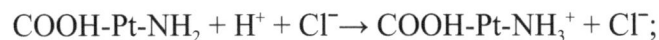

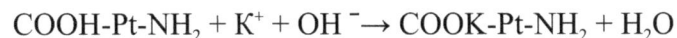

$COOH-Pt-NH_2 + H^+ + Cl^- \rightarrow COOH-Pt-NH_3^+ + Cl^-$;

$COOH-Pt-NH_2 + K^+ + OH^- \rightarrow COOK-Pt-NH_2 + H_2O$

Proteins take part in the preservation of pH in the blood plasma (mostly albumin) and in the intracellular fluids. Thus, the acid-base balance is a vital part of the homeostasis of the inner environment, which ensures normal biochemical processes in the human body. Disorders of acid-alkaline balance can be caused by a variety of reasons - by the production of ketone bodies in diabetes, loss of HCl during vomiting, formation of lactate in hypoxia, increased elimination of HCO_3^- in renal malfunction, *etc.*

Hydrogen Peroxide

Another oxygen compound of hydrogen is hydrogen peroxide H_2O_2. It is the most important of the biological reactive oxygen species, excess of which causes damage to cells and tissues. Hydrogen peroxide is a by-product of respiration, a product of numerous metabolic reactions, predominantly peroxisomal oxidation pathways, and a possible transmitter of cellular signals [22, 23]. H_2O_2 is formed in all cells of the body during various oxidative and reduction metabolic processes and immediately decomposes under the influence of the enzyme catalase:

$$2H_2O_2 \rightarrow 2H_2O + O_2$$

Hydrogen and carbon combine in a vast number of biomolecules involved in life processes - carbohydrates, lipids, proteins, and nucleic acids.

Stomach acid is made up of hydrochloric acid, HCl. Practically, hydrogen is very important for digesting food properly and for absorbing the other elements for organism survival.

Lithium

Lithium is a trace microelement and is a permanent part of living organisms. The lithium-ion, which has the smallest radius among alkali metals, is very strongly hydrated in water solutions (13 water molecules are retained in the composition of the ion hydrate) its size in the hydrated state far exceeds the radius of the hydrated Na^+ ion (holds 8 water molecules) and K^+ ion (holds 4 water molecules). This prevents the penetration of Li^+ ions through the ion channels of the cell membrane.

Lithium is not one of the essential elements for vital functions but has beneficial effects on the nervous system. It is used in medical preparations for the treatment of depressive illness with positive effects [24 - 26]. The lack of lithium in the diet contributes to the incidence of manic-depressive psychosis, schizophrenia, *etc.* For depressed patients, an excess is characteristic, and for those suffering from mania - a lack of sodium in the cells is typical. There are minor ranges between the therapeutic and toxic doses of lithium.

The very small Li^+ ions affect the activity of some enzymes and control the ionic Na^+ - K^+ balance of the cerebral cortex cells. Due to the chemical resemblances between Li^+ and Na^+ ions, the former can affect the messages of nerves transmitted by the second. For many patients, prophylaxis with lithium has led to perfect freedom from mood fluctuations and disturbances [24 - 26]. Additionally, the role of lithium in equalizing the sodium-potassium balance in the organisms of patients is important. Lithium compounds have complex properties when absorbed by the body. Although they are not poisonous, Li salts can disturb the bioprocesses dependent upon salt balance. Lithium intoxication may occur, predominantly in patients with low Na^+ diets. Lithium compounds can be rapidly excreted in the urine.

Lithium as Li^+ cation at low levels is present in certain natural water sources, particularly thermal spa waters and in some kinds of drinking mineral water.

Toxicity: Lithium can be transferred in the food chain from soils through flora and fauna to humans. Li is usually widely spread in trace amounts in rocks, soils, and water, including surface water, groundwater, and seawater. Because of its very low concentration in nature, lithium does not cause serious damage to the environment. Mild Li noxiousness is often difficult to diagnose because its indications are analogous to those of various other complications. Exposure to elevated Li concentrations over days to weeks, known as chronic Li toxicity, is manifested as a significant amount of thirst, worsening lethargy, confusion, tremor, ataxia, and seizures. Resolution of neurotoxic effects may take weeks and can be incomplete. In acute Li toxicity, this metal affects the kidneys, CNS, endocrine system, and gastrointestinal tract. In severe cases, the patients can experience diabetes, as well as neurological and cardiovascular complications [26, 27]. If left untreated, Li toxicity may progress and get worse. Li intoxication can be life-threatening and must be monitored and treated on time.

Sodium and Potassium

Sodium and potassium occur widely in the Earth's crust [27] and are both crucial elements for living organisms. They are existing in the body as free ions. Potassium cations are more concentrated inside than outside the cells, while Na^+ ions are mostly available in extracellular fluids. Despite the similarity in their chemical behavior, these ions demonstrate biological antagonism.

Sodium and potassium exist in high amounts in the biofluids (112 g of Na and 160 g of K). The vital role of these ions in homeostasis is well recognized and they possess many biological functions. Sodium and potassium cations have analogous biochemistry, though these ions have differences in their ionic radii and hydration energy. Sodium and potassium cations are always together in the geosphere and the separation processes are difficult. In contrast, in the biosphere Na^+ and K^+ cations circulate on different sides of cell membranes [28].

Na^+ and K^+ ions are distributed throughout the body, with the former being a part mainly of intercellular fluids, while the latter are found mainly inside cells. The intracellular concentration of sodium ions is less than 10% of its content in the extracellular fluid, while the concentration of potassium ions inside the cells is almost 30 times higher than outside the cells [27 - 29]. Evaluation of the absolute values shows that approximately 95% of the sodium ions involved in metabolism are outside the cells and about the same proportion of potassium ions are inside the cells.

In the body, sodium, as the main extracellular ion, is in the form of soluble salts $NaCl$, Na_3PO_4, and $NaHCO_3$, distributed in the blood, cerebrospinal fluid, eye fluid, digestive juices, bile, kidneys, lungs, and brain. Sodium cations play a key role in the control and maintenance of osmotic pressure of body fluids and acid-base equilibrium (phosphate buffer system: $Na_2HPO_4 + NaH_2PO_4$). Na^+ ions are associated with the maintenance of water by tissues in the organism ($NaCl$ in blood plasma is the chief origin of HCl formation and 15 g of $NaCl$ retains up to two liters of fluid in the human body). Sodium cations are related to the preservation of acid-base balance in organisms ($NaHCO_3$ - alkaline blood reserve - a constituent of the bicarbonate buffer system), with the transfer of amino acids and sugars through the cell membrane and with the maintenance of regular irritability of muscles and the cell permeability [27 - 29]. Sodium ions participate in the establishment of short-term memory.

Potassium cations are the principal cations of the intracellular fluids and are associated with acid-base balance with the cardiac muscle contractions (a suitable plasma K^+ level is vital for regular heart function more exactly for the relaxation of the myocardium), and K^+ ions are connected with the transmission of nerve impulses.

Na^+ and K^+ ions collaborate in a notable way as carriers of nerves' messages. To make this probable, the nerve membrane permeability changes, and Na^+ cations pass in, while K^+ ions move in the opposite direction. Na^+ pump rapidly restores the Na^+ - K^+ balance and the osmotic equilibria [27 - 29]. The most important is the cell membrane function of potassium cations. As mentioned above, the gradients of Na^+ and K^+ ions across the cell membranes are associated with the retention of the membrane potentials of nervous tissues, the vehicle for impulse transmissions. K^+ ions increase the function of the parasympathetic nervous system as well as acetylcholine activity on the muscle nervous terminals. They also decrease the stimulating influence of additional ions on the muscle system. Potassium is also essential in glycogenesis. It is withdrawn from the extracellular fluid leading to hypokalemia. K^+ ions help the protein synthesis by ribosomes. Many enzymes need K^+ for their activity, for instance, pyruvate kinase and dialkylglycine decarboxylase, belonging to pyridoxal phosphate-dependent enzymes and are activated by potassium and inhibited by sodium ions [29].

Most cells keep intracellular potassium ions and extracellular sodium ions at a fairly high amount because of the functions of transmembrane enzymes, such as $(Na^+ + K^+)$-adenosine triphosphatase (Na^+,K^+-ATP-ase). Na^+ and K^+ ions activate Na^+,K^+-ATP-ase of cell membranes, which pumps out Na^+ ions from the cell and provides a conjugate accumulation of K^+ ions in the cell. The precise protein pumps for sodium and potassium ions in cell membranes differentiate the two cations and preserve their concentrations. Diverse amounts of these two ions on different sides of the membrane cause the appearance of a transmembrane potential difference (up to 100 mV), which ensures the existence of an easily accessible source of energy for many processes related to the functioning of membranes. Na^+, K^+-ATP-ase uses the energy produced from adenosine triphosphate to drive the transport of sodium and potassium cations against the concentration gradient [27 - 29]. In non-marine organisms, the kidney precisely controls the concentration of sodium in cells. If the sodium quantity within the cells increases, water enters and the osmotic pressure destroys the membranes of the cells. If the sodium amount is higher, ions are displaced from the cells by means of sodium pumps.

Organometallic compounds of IA group elements contain metal-carbon chemical bonds and tend to be particularly reactive. Na^+ and K^+ salts being natural constituents of body tissues are not toxic in ordinary physiological conditions [3, 4]. The sodium and potassium oxides and hydroxides are caustic and corrosive compounds that harm the exposed tissues. Oxides can be produced by the combustion of organometallic compounds of Na^+ and K^+. Their hydroxides can be produced by the interaction of the organometallics with water:

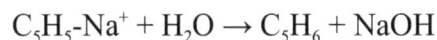

$$C_5H_5\text{-}Na^+ + H_2O \rightarrow C_5H_6 + NaOH$$

Carbonyl compounds of sodium and potassium, NaCO and KCO, are extremely reactive solid compounds likely to detonate once exposed to H_2O or air [3, 4]. Their decomposition produces caustic Na and K oxides and hydroxides, as well as toxic CO.

Sodium and potassium have alkoxides of the type M^+-OR, where R represents a hydrocarbon group:

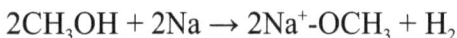

$$2CH_3OH + 2Na \rightarrow 2Na^+\text{-}OCH_3 + H_2$$

These alkoxides are very basic, and caustic, having high reactivity with water leading to the formation of the respective hydroxides:

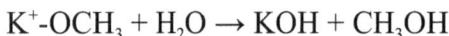

$$K^+\text{-}OCH_3 + H_2O \rightarrow KOH + CH_3OH$$

The increased levels of Na^+ cations in the serum, named hypernatremia, occur in gushing disease, and in diabetes insipidus [30]. Some studies have indicated that adrenocorticotropic hormone (ACTH) can stimulate the salt-regulating function of the adrenal cortex in humans, thus decreasing the Na^+ excretion and increasing that of K^+ in the urine. Patients with an excess of Na^+ are predisposed to peripheral and pulmonary edemas with respiratory failures and raised venous pressure. There is a connection between the salt content and water balance in the body, the low consumption of salt causes loss of water. Considerable amounts of Na^+ are eliminated by sweating by the skin, and substantial amounts are excreted by the urine.

On the contrary, low concentrations of sodium cations in the serum are named hyponatremia. It happens in acute Addison's disease, nephrosis, severe burns, diarrhea, vomiting, intestinal obstruction, active sweating, *etc.* The serious decrease of Na^+ cations in the extracellular environment leads to hypovolemia, hypotension, circulatory collapse, or syncope [31]. Sodium deficiency causes muscle spasms, twitches or cramping, while sodium excess in the diet leads to higher blood pressure. There is a tendency to substitute the common salt in the food with low-sodium alternatives, meaning salt mixtures with KCl and other potassium salts.

Potassium is a vital nutrient and is used by plants. In nature, K from the decomposing plants returns to the soil's clay minerals. Almost all potassium salts are highly soluble in water, but unlike sodium salts, they do not contain crystallization water. With a lack of potassium in the soil, plants are affected by fungal and bacterial diseases, and their leaves turn pale. In cooperation with nitrogen and phosphorus, K is one of the main elements of plant nutrition, in the absence of it they die.

The increased concentration of potassium cations in the serum is named hyperkalemia, which occurs in chronic dehydration and shock, Addison's disease, and advanced chronic renal failure [32]. The main reasons for hyperkaliemia can be some high releases of cellular K^+ ions from muscle tissues by hard traumas, surgical operations, hemolysis, as well as acidosis when H^+ ions displace K^+ cations from the cells. Symptoms of hyperkaliemia manifest themselves mostly in the heart (ECG fluctuations, bradycardia, and arrhythmias) and in the nervous system. The excess potassium can be excreted by the kidneys, allowing serum potassium levels to return to normal.

On the opposite, low concentrations of potassium cations in the serum lead to hypokalemia [33]. It occurs in metabolic alkalosis, diarrhea, and periodic paralysis. Hypokalemia is mostly observed in decreased K^+ intake (in starvation and malnutrition conditions), in excessive renal loss and renal tubular disorders (when using some diuretics), in severe vomiting, *etc.* The mainly detected symptoms of hypokalemia are anorexia, nausea, a fall of blood pressure, muscle weakness, irregular pulse, and mental depression.

The metals sodium and potassium present an inhalation or contact hazard. They react easily with moisture to form hydroxides, which are highly destructive to tissues. Contact of Na with H_2O, together with perspiration, causes the NaOH fumes formation, which is highly irritating to the eyes, nose, skin and throat. This causes coughing and sneezing. Very high exposure can result in breathing difficulties, and bronchitis [32]. Skin interaction causes tingling, itching, thermal, and caustic injuries. Eye contact results in lasting damage and complete vision loss.

In general, potassium reacts similarly to sodium with the exception that K is more reactive. Potassium can affect the human body when inhaled. Breathing of dust or mist results in respiratory manifestations such as inflammation, edema and pneumonitis. Higher exposure may lead to accumulation of fluid in the lungs, which may cause death. Skin and eye contact causes burns or irritations that lead to serious damage.

Rubidium and Cesium

Rubidium is present in almost all body tissues, but is not supposed to be an essential element. In an adult, there is approximately 37 mg of rubidium. It is similar to potassium in its spreading and excretory character. Comparatively high levels of rubidium are found in soft tissues, while the skeletal tissues contain low levels [34]. Rubidium salts have no vital properties, either poisonous or essential. This element, being similar to K, has a mild stimulating effect on metabolic processes. Plants have an affinity for rubidium, but its concentration in soil is very small. As Cs has many resemblances with K, it can be absorbed by plants and transported to the meat and milk products of grazing animals.

Cesium is a typical non-vital and trace metal in the body. Around 1.6 mg of this element is distributed mainly in muscles, bones, and blood [35]. Cesium has no identified biological functions. The amount of cesium is around 0.2 ppm in tea leaves and very low in other plants. Very hazardous is the acceptance of radioactive isotopes of cesium. Cs isotopes are commonly produced during the uranium fission. It has been observed that the most intensive radiation dominates from ^{134}Cs ($T_{1/2}$ = 2 years) and ^{137}Cs ($T_{1/2}$ = 30 years). ^{137}Cs is responsible for the continued radioactive pollution. ^{131}Cs ($T_{1/2}$ = 9.7 d; X-rays) is a potentially interesting Auger electron emitter.

It should be noted that rubidium and cesium ions tend to bind to C=O groups in membranes, allowing them to be used as probes in studying the cell membrane channels [34, 35]. When binding K$^+$ ions, the internal charge of the membrane cavity changes and releases K$^+$ ions from the cells.

s-Elements of the IIA Group

Beryllium

Beryllium is not an essential element and its amount in the body is around 3 μg. The biological role of beryllium is not yet clear. Beryllium compounds are poisonous, especially volatile beryllium compounds and dust containing beryllium and Be compounds. It is well known that Be is a beneficial metal for numerous industrial processes. By means of growing beryllium manufacturing use, industrial contact to this element is a significant problem.

The metal Be is one of the most poisonous elements [36 - 42]. It interacts with vital phosphate-based systems in the organism and creates healthy problems. Because of its very small levels, it does not cause general anxiety. Due to its negligible natural occurrence, biosystems have not developed any defense against this metal. Contacts with Be are much more dangerous at inhalation than at ingestion because Be and its salts are almost not absorbed by the gastrointestinal system.

Beryllium has a pronounced allergic and carcinogenic effect [36]. Inhalation of air containing beryllium and its salts leads to long-term accumulation of beryllium in the lung tissues and leads to serious chronic diseases of the respiratory system - berylliosis and lung cancer. When introduced in the body, this metal is excreted slowly from the organism and is usually located in the bones.

Be^{2+} ions displace Ca^{2+} ions from bone tissue, causing its softening (beryllium rickets). As a lighter homologue of magnesium, Be^{2+} ion inhibits the activity of numerous enzymes triggered by Mg^{2+} ions. Be^{2+} cations can reach easily the cell nucleus, where they exert mutagenic and carcinogenic effects. In case of intoxication with beryllium salts, an excess of magnesium salts can be administered, which results in a restoration of enzyme activity. Beryllium reacts as well with the immune system, that is why beryllium compounds are allergenic contact pollutants. Once the body contacts with metal ions by skin, inhalation, or by metal-based artificial body implants, some allergic occurrences can be observed. Presently, the most extensively considered human hypersensitivities are to Ni and Be, although still poorly understood. Beryllium-peptide coordination interactions seem to play a significant role in these immune responses [37]. Be^{2+} is a small cation and subsequently highly acidic in water, hydrated in aqueous solutions as $[Be(H_2O)_4]^{2+}$ and shows a predisposition to produce polymeric hydroxide-based species. Metal cations and the bioligands work as small biomolecules which can excite the respective immunogenic response when attached to protein molecules [38]. In spite of the many models proposed, the mechanisms of beryllium hypersensitivity and allergic-type responses are still badly understood.

Like beryllium, its oxide and other Be(II) compounds are used progressively in industry, therefore stringent safety measures are needed to avoid exposures to dust and fumes released from the manufacturing processes. Chronic Be disease, sometimes called berylliosis, is a hypersensitivity condition activated by Be workplace exposure. It is manifested by granulomatous inflammation of the lungs (pneumonitis) [39 - 42]. While most commonly associated with lung diseases, Be may also disturb the liver, heart, kidneys, nervous, and lymphatic systems. At present, there is no cure for chronic beryllium disease.

Because of the harmfulness of Be compounds, they cannot be used as drugs in medical practice [41]. Conceivable chelation therapy of Be intoxication is not reasonable, since specific oxygen-based ligands that bind to Be^{2+} are similarly strongly associated with such biologically significant ions as Mg^{2+} and Fe^{3+}.

Magnesium

In the plant kingdom, this element plays a crucial role in photosynthesis. Mg^{2+} cation is the coordination agent of chlorophyll. The activity of numerous enzymes involved in the photosynthetic processes is significantly influenced by slight variations in Mg^{2+} quantity. In plants, magnesium is also involved in the transformation of phosphorus compounds, in the formation of fats, and in the synthesis and breakdown of carbohydrates. The absence of magnesium in soils causes diseases in plants such as chlorosis (destruction of chlorophyll and discoloration of the chloroplast), muscle cramps in animals, *etc.* In fact, in plants, Mg^{2+} is a fragment of coordination centers of the main enzymes that regulate such a significant process as photosynthesis. At the "light" stage of photosynthesis, the enzyme chlorophyll is photochemically excited and reduces CO_2. In photosynthesis, which occurs in the dark (dark phase), Mg is the coordination center of the enzyme holding ribulose-1,5-diphosphatecarboxylate, which is named Rubisco - a key enzyme in the global carbon cycle [43, 44]. The enzyme ribulose-1,--bisphosphate carboxylase-oxygenase is the most abundant enzyme in the biosphere which is responsible for the binding of CO_2. Rubisco is found in all the domains of life: archaea, bacteria, and eukaryotes. It can be considered the most important enzyme because, without it, most life on earth could not exist. In the original structure of the enzyme, the Mg^{2+} ion coordinates with the carboxyl groups of glutamic and aspartic acids, three H_2O molecules, and the residue of lysine carbamate, having coordination number 6. Carbamate is obtained by the reaction of CO_2 portion with the lysine amino groups, so the initially available CO_2 "triggers" the mechanism of the photosynthetic process.

Magnesium is one of the most plentiful elements in the body and Mg^{2+} homeostasis is important [45]. In total, the body contains around 40 g of magnesium, of which more than half is in bone tissue (60%), in tooth enamel, where it takes part in the formation of coordination complexes; 30-40% of Mg is concentrated in skeletal muscle and soft tissues and only 1% of this element is distributed in the extracellular fluids.

Magnesium is a vital constituent of tissues and body fluids, nevertheless little is known concerning its metabolism or necessity. The bulk of the magnesium, which is outside the bone, is concentrated inside the cells. Mg^{2+} ions are the second most abundant intracellular cations after K^+ ions. Therefore, Mg^{2+} ions play an important role in maintaining osmotic pressure inside cells [45, 46]. Mg is needed for the production of energy, oxidative phosphorylation and glycolysis. It contributes to the structural formation of bones and is needed for the synthesis of DNA, RNA and the antioxidant glutathione. It has been reported that this element also plays a role in the active transport of Ca^{2+} and K^+ ions across cell membranes, a process that is important to nerve impulse transmissions, muscle contractions and regular heart rhythm.

In humans and animals, Mg^{2+} ions are among the main activators of enzymatic processes acting as a cofactor. Mg^{2+} ions activate important enzymes, including peptidase, phosphorylases, phosphoglucomutase, alkaline phosphatase, enolase, RNA polymerase, DNA polymerase and many others. Magnesium cation is an important cofactor in the mechanism of replication, transcription, and translation of genomic information [46, 47]. It is also associated with the maintenance of lipid membranes, DNA, RNA, ribosomes, *etc.* [48 - 50]. Magnesium, which has a crucial role in the metabolism of phosphates, catalyzes the vital hydrolysis of ATP

(Fig. **2**). The magnesium complex with ATP is contained within the substrate of the enzyme kinase, which controls the transfer of phosphate groups. Despite its influence on human health, the exact mechanisms of the regulation of magnesium transport and storage are still unknown.

Magnesium ions, injected subcutaneously or into the blood, cause depression of the CNS and lead to a narcotic state, lowering blood pressure and cholesterol. Magnesium ion exerts an effect on neuromuscular irritability like that of Ca^{2+} ion, where high levels induce depression and low levels - tetanus [45, 46]. The biochemistry of Mg^{2+} and Ca^{2+} ions is similar, although Mg^{2+} has a smaller radius and exchanges its coordinated water ligands more slowly. Mg^{2+} and Ca^{2+} ions act as antagonists to each other counteracting certain effects. For example, the central peripheral nervous system depression, connected with hyper-magnesium conditions is reversed very well by intravenous injection of an equivalent amount of Ca^{2+} ions.

The minimal optional requirements for the magnesium diet are 300-350 mg/day for men. Some substances (calcium, protein, vitamin D, alcohol, *etc.*), which interfere with magnesium retention, may rise the necessity to 700-800 mg/day. Magnesium, in contrast to calcium, shows predispositions to remain inside the blood cells [45, 46]. About 70 to 85% of the serum magnesium is diffusible, the rest being bound to plasma proteins. The increased level of Mg^{2+} cations in the serum (about 8 mmol/L) leads to fast and deep anesthesia and paralysis and rises renal failure.

Low levels of Mg^{2+} cations in the serum might occur in malabsorptive syndrome, chronic alcoholism, diabetic acidosis, cirrhosis of the liver, higher renal loss (ingestion of diuretics, gentamycin *etc.*) and primary renal disease, continued and serious loss of body fluid as well as continued magnesium intravenous administration [51]. The mainly observed symptoms of hypomagnesemia are neuromuscular disorders manifested by weakness, tremors, and muscle fasciculations as well as disorders of the CNS like delirium and psychosis. Despite that magnesium deficiency is not common, it can occur principally due to low dietary consumption or in patients who use certain diuretic medications. It has been found that serious Mg deficiency may result in hypocalcemia or hypokalemia (low serum Ca^{2+} or K^+ levels). In certain respects, there are reciprocal connections between Mg^{2+} and Ca^{2+}, and Mg^{2+} and PO_4^{3-} concentrations in the serum. For instance, in oxalate intoxication, Ca^{2+} decrease in serum is accompanied by an Mg^{2+} increase. Acute Mg deficiency can be treated with intravenous $MgSO_4$. It has been suggested that taking supplemental magnesium is beneficial for patients suffering from fatigue and for treating some medical indications. A great range of oral magnesium drugs are on the market that are beneficial to deal with any deficiency. It can be injected intravenously in emergency situations like acute heart and asthma attacks. Magnesium relaxes the muscles along the air route to the lungs, allowing easier breathing.

Higher levels of magnesium in serum (hypermagnesemia) cause dropping of the blood pressure (hypotension) [52]. Certain of the future effects of Mg toxicity, like confusion, lethargy, disorders in standard cardiac rhythm, and weakening of kidney functions, are associated with hypotension. If this condition progresses, difficulty breathing, and muscle problems may occur. In some cases, hypermagnesemia may lead to cardiac arrests.

Calcium

Calcium is a crucial biogenic element for all living organisms [53]. It is one of the five (O, C, H, N, Ca) most common elements in the body (Ca comprises 1.5% of body weight). Calcium is existing in the body in major quantities in all mineral compounds present in the human body in the form of phosphates and carbonates. The bulk of calcium is concentrated in the skeleton and teeth. Calcium is an extremely significant macronutrient for the construction and maintenance of strong bones and teeth. The skeleton calcium is regularly exchanged with Ca^{2+} from interstitial fluid and this is controlled principally by the parathyroid hormone - calcitonin. Its absorption depends on the content of vitamin D.

The composition of the dense bone matrix includes a thermodynamically and kinetically stable at pH 7.40 form of calcium phosphate - calcium hydroxy phosphate $Ca_{10}(PO_4)_6(OH)_2$.

Two categories of cells are the main constituents of bone, *viz.*, osteoclasts and osteoblasts. Osteoclasts are responsible for aged bone resorption whereas osteoblasts are responsible for new bone formation. These cells must be well synchronized; otherwise, pathologies can arise. They maintain stable Ca^{2+} levels in the blood [53]. As with calcium, the main amount of body phosphates (around 85%) occupies the mineral segment of bone. The rest of the body phosphate is in the form of organic and inorganic compounds dispersed within the intra- and extracellular compartments. The phosphate concentration in normal blood is similar to that of calcium.

There are three main Ca^{2+} pools in the body - intracellular Ca^{2+}, calcium in extracellular fluids and blood, bound to proteins and bone calcium - the vast reservoir of calcium, which is physiologically inert. The fraction of extraosseous calcium (calcium in tissues outside of bone), although it is only 1% of its total content in the body, is essential because of its effects on blood clotting, the normal transmission of nerve impulses, neuromuscular excitability and heart muscle contraction [54]. By regulating the cell membrane permeability Ca^{2+} cations are responsible for the nerve's excitability. Calcium ions play a role in initiating contractions in vascular and additional smooth muscles. Calcium is important for hormonal activity, fertilization, and cell division. This element also regulates the mechanical stability of cell walls and membranes, and stimulates muscular contraction.

The Ca^{2+} ions are abundant in extracellular fluids and exist in three forms: ionized Ca^{2+}, bound to plasma albumin, and coordinated with citrate, malate, *etc.* On the contrary, the intracellular quantity of Ca^{2+} ions is very low. This unequal spreading of Ca^{2+} has a vital signal role. The regulated opening of specific ion channels in the cell membrane rises the intracellular concentration of Ca^{2+} ions. This signal may initiate several cell processes such as the contraction of muscles, secretory action, and the release of neurotransmitters from nerve terminals [55].

Calcium is required to keep the blood pressure. It is essential for maintaining the integrity of the capillary walls, which leads to its anti-inflammatory and antiallergic effects [55]. Calcium participates in blood coagulation and influences the secretion of insulin. It also allows other molecules to make energy and digest food. Properly increased calcium intake is supposed to lower high blood pressure and prevent heart disease. It is also used in the treatment of arthritis.

Certain hormones are influenced by Ca^{2+} ions. For instance, the adrenaline effect on liver cells is partially due to increased Ca^{2+} ions within these cells [55]. The hormones parathyrin (in the parathyroid gland), calcitonin (in the thyroid gland), and calcitriol (produced by the transformation of calcium and vitamin D) efficiently control plasma Ca^{2+} amounts.

Calcium ions act as a cofactor of many enzymes [53 - 55]. The best-known Ca-based enzyme calmodulin activates the protein kinase, catalyzes the phosphorylation of proteins, and stimulates Fe-based enzyme NO-synthase (NOS). In calmodulin Ca^{2+} ion with a coordination number of 6 is surrounded by 3 carboxylic groups of asparagine acid with monodentate coordination, one bidentate molecule of glutamine acid and one water molecule. The release of NO from the enzyme NO-synthase is controlled by calcium-dependent calmodulin, which tolerates electron transport in NOS. The Ca-calmodulin complex attaches to several enzymes: adenylate cyclase, Ca^{2+}-ATPase, phosphorylase kinase, myosin kinase, phospholipase and phosphodiesterase. Calcium also affects the activity of many enzymes, for instance, adenosine triphosphatase, succinic dehydrogenase, lipase, *etc.*

Deficient amount of calcium (hypocalcemia) leads to demineralization of bones with typical symptoms like muscle spasms, leg cramps, osteoporosis, and brittle bone. When the organism does not get enough calcium, it will use the calcium deposited in bones, that makes the bone thinner and more brittle [56]. Chronical calcium deficiency may contribute to osteoporosis. Lack of calcium is a result of its deficient consumption, malabsorption of fats, and extreme urinary loss of calcium in chronic renal circumstances.

High amounts of serum calcium (hypercalcemia) lead to hyperparathyroidism or malignancies [57]. Hypercalcemia can be connected with large amounts of calcium supplements in combination with antacids. Minor hypercalcemia may have no indications or may result in loss of appetite, vomiting, abdominal pain, nausea, fatigue, and hypertension. More serious hypercalcemia may result in delirium and coma. Ca^{2+} cations take part in human metabolism, and serious disturbance of normal metabolism results in deposits of various calcium salts in organs, for example, formation of stones, atherosclerotic changes in blood vessels, glaucoma, *etc.*

The organometallic chemistry of the IIA group metals is analogous to that of the IA group metals with predominantly ionic bonds [3,4,53]. The magnesium organometallic chemistry has been of greatest importance for many years as useful in organic chemical synthesis Grignard reagents:

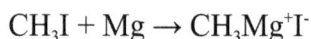

$$CH_3I + Mg \rightarrow CH_3Mg^+I^-$$

Grignard reagents are very reactive and particularly hazardous. Unlike the basic oxides and hydroxides of IA group, $Mg(OH)_2$ is a comparatively benign compound which is used as a food additive and constituent of magnesia milk.

It is rather difficult to obtain organometallic compounds of calcium. Whereas magnesium organometallic compounds have Mg-C covalent bonds, the calcium organometallics have typical ionic bonds which makes them extremely reactive and not as convenient for synthetic purposes as the corresponding Mg organometallics.

Strontium

Although there is approximately 0.4 g of Sr in the body, it is not supposed to be biogenic. This most abundant element has no identified function in the human organism. In the bodies of animals and humans, Sr accumulates in large amounts in bone and affects the bone formation processes. Sr^{2+} is able to replace Ca^{2+} in many bioprocesses. Strontium is processed in the organism in a similar way to its analog Ca. Its excess causes brittle bone, so called "strontium rickets". The reason is the replacement of the similar calcium bone matter with strontium: the strontium ion is easily washed out of the bones and their destruction occurs. It is almost not possible to extract Sr from the bones. Strontium compounds are used in the treatment of osteoporosis as a fractional substitute for Ca, interfering with the biological mineralization and degradation processes of human bones [58].

Some marine organisms use $SrSO_4$ in the formation of skeletal materials. Strontium can be added to aquariums water as the corals need it.

An increase in the radioactive background of the biosphere can cause the appearance in the atmosphere of the fission product of the heavy elements - ^{90}Sr (half-life 29 years). As a highly radioactive isotope, settling in the bone, ^{90}Sr irradiates and disrupts bone marrow hematopoiesis.

Barium

For biological functions in human body, barium is not required, but there are species for which this element is essential. Some algae use $BaSO_4$ as a sensor for the orientation of their location in the sea water. If Ba is not present, their growth stops.

The biogenic role of barium has not yet been studied much. There is around 24 mg of Ba in the body. It is often linked with its toxic activity. The metabolism is activated by Ba, but in high amounts it causes ventricular fibrillation.

All soluble in water and acids, barium salts are very poisonous [59]. Barium ions seriously damage the myocardium and CNS. They block potassium channels. The manifestations of barium intoxication are diarrhea, colic, vomiting, and paralysis. As a rule, the barium content in food plants is very low (in ppm).

Ba(II) salts are noxious to humans, but insoluble in water and acids, barium sulfate absorbs X-rays well, and therefore it is used in the study of the human gastrointestinal tract [59].

GENERAL CHARACTERISTICS OF P-ELEMENTS AND THEIR COMPOUNDS

The p-elements include elements of IIIA-VIIIA groups of the periodic table. If the hydroxides of the s-elements have basic properties, then amphoteric properties are characteristic of the hydroxides of the p-elements. In groups of the periodic table, with an increase in the atomic number of the element (with an increase in the metallic properties of the elements), the basic function of oxides and hydroxides increases [6 - 10]. If the same element forms several hydroxides of different composition, then the basic properties are more pronounced in hydroxides, in which the oxidation state of the element is lower; for example, $Pb(OH)_2$ is a stronger base than $Pb(OH)_4$. $Pb(OH)_2$ exhibits amphoteric properties:

$Pb(OH)_2 + 2HCl \rightleftarrows PbCl_2 + 2H_2O$

$Pb(OH)_2 + 2NaOH \rightleftarrows Na_2[Pb(OH)_4]$

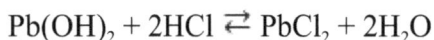

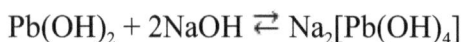

p-Elements (except Al) form cations of various oxidation states. Aluminum in all of its stable compounds exhibits an oxidation state of +3. For antimony and bismuth, for example, the possible oxidation states are +5, +3; for tin and lead, +2 and +4. In the group with an increase in the atomic number, the stability of the compounds with the maximum oxidation state of the p metal, decreases; for example, Bi is most characterized by an oxidation state of +3.

Cations of p-elements have a strong polarizing effect due to an increase in the charge of the nucleus and a decrease in radius. The high polarizing effect of p-element cations causes the formation of many compounds with covalent bonds and low solubility in water (sulfides, phosphates, hydroxides, *etc.*). Their salts with strong acids are highly soluble in water, except for lead sulfate and chloride, which was the reason for the assignment of Pb^{2+} in analytical group V of cations precipitated by HCl (according to the classification of cations). Cations of p-elements are colorless, but due to their high polarizing ability they can form colored compounds with a number of colorless anions (sulfides, iodides). The salts of p-elements have a high ability to hydrolyze by cations [6 - 10]. The degree of hydrolysis of salts increases with a decrease in the oxidation state of the elements.

Cations of p-elements are predisposed to the formation of complex compounds due to the presence of free p-orbitals and high polarizing properties [60]. They form complex compounds with both inorganic (iodide, bromide, chloride ions) and organic ligands. Possessing variable oxidation states, p-elements easily enter into oxidation-reduction reactions.

Due to the amphoteric character, the hydroxides of p-elements pass into anions of oxoacids in an alkaline environment. In the form of cations, they exist mainly in an acidic environment, so the detection of p-element cations should be carried out in an acidic or neutral environment.

The p-elements located in the upper right corner of the periodic table have a high ability to form anions. Since p-elements have variable oxidation states, they are capable of forming various acids, and the strength of the acids increases with increasing the oxidation state of the element. Most p-elements form oxoacids (H_2SO_4, HNO_3, *etc.*), and only the elements of VIA and VIIA groups can form binary acids (HF, HBr, HCl, H_2S *etc.*).

According to the oxidation-reduction properties, anions are divided into oxidizing anions, in which the element has the highest oxidation state (NO_3^-), reducing anions with a lower oxidation state (Cl^-, Br^-, S^{2-}) and anions that show neither oxidative nor reducing properties (CO_3^{2-}, PO_4^{3-}, SO_4^{2-}) [6 - 10]. Sulfuric acid in concentrated form can exhibit the properties of an oxidizing agent. The oxidation-reduction properties of some anions (SO_3^{2-}, NO_2^-) depend on the reaction conditions and may vary.

p-Elements of the second period, *viz.,* nitrogen, oxygen, and fluorine, have exposed a strong capability to participate in hydrogen bond formation. It is not typical for the other p elements. The resemblance between p elements of the third and subsequent periods is typically expressed by the external shell structures and the valences due to the unpaired electrons of atoms in their excited state [60]. Especially B, C, and N show differences from the other elements in their groups. When passing from elements of the second to third and next periods, all characteristic bond types of the second period elements are preserved and additionally more various chemical bond types appear. This rises the capacity for the formation of coordination complexes and the value of their coordination numbers. Consequently, if elements of the II period have coordination numbers of 2, 3, 4, the elements of the subsequent periods show higher coordination numbers of 5, 6, 7, 8 to 12.

Therefore, the alterations in the chemical properties of p-elements both in the group and in the period are much greater than those of the elements of IA and IIA groups [6 - 10]. All p-elements and particularly these of the second and third periods form many chemical bonds with s-, d-and f-elements. Most of the known bonds in nature are the chemical bonds formed by p-elements.

BIOLOGICAL ROLE OF P-ELEMENTS

p-Elements of the IIIA Group

Boron

Boron refers to impurity trace elements, its mass fraction in the human body is only $10^{-5}\%$. More than half of the total amount of boron is concentrated in the skeleton, possibly as insoluble salts of H_3BO_3. About 10% falls on soft tissues. Boron is required by the body in very small quantities to enable Ca, Mg, and P to function properly and is necessary for healthy bones and joints [61]. Without minor quantities of B, the bones would become brittle. As a nutritional additive, boron may be effective in avoiding or in the treatment of arthritis [62]. This element stabilizes vitamin D and estrogen, vital for bone health [63]. There is a relationship between the boron quantity in soil/drinking water and the incidences of arthritis in inhabitants. In the driest world areas, with the highest concentrations of boron in the drinking water and soil, the arthritis incidences tend to be intensely lower than in humid zones.

In terms of biological properties, boron differs from aluminum and next analogues of the group due to the difference in the structure and bonding of its atoms. Boron is not characterized by the formation of cations, in the body, it is in the form of oxygen-containing anions, which are included in complex compounds as ligands [60].

The biological role of boron is not well understood. Boron plays an important role in the carbohydrate and fat metabolism. Numerous vitamins and hormones affect the activity of certain enzymes [61 - 63]. This element is also required to allow the brain to function properly by increasing the mental alertness. According to recently published information, low boron consumption by humans causes reduced brain activity. Boron excess is also detrimental for human. A large excess of this element inhibits proteinase, amylase, and decreases adrenaline activity. The weakening of the adrenalin activity is associated with its interaction with H_3BO_3. Of the boron inorganic compounds, halides and hydrides (boranes) are highly toxic.

Although boron is not so essential for humans, it is supposed to be important for the growth of some plants, marine algae, and cyanobacteria [64]. It is known that higher plants need B, but information on its biological functions is controversial. Some recent investigations have revealed that boron is necessary for certain animals. Boron participates in carbohydrate-phosphate exchange and acts with many bioactive compounds including proteins, carbohydrates, vitamins and hormones. Nevertheless, for animals, ingesting food with high boron concentration disturbs the carbohydrate and protein exchange, which causes enteritis.

The isotopes of boron ^{10}B and ^{11}B are used in nuclear medicine. The isotope ^{10}B (20% of natural boron) is a very strong absorber of neutrons and is useful in controlling rods of nuclear reactors. It is more effective than Pb as a shield for nuclear radioactivity. The pure B isotopes are very expensive, that is why in many cases instead of isotopes elemental boron is utilized. Boron isotope ^{10}B is clinically used in boron neutron capture therapy [65].

Aluminum

Aluminum, like boron, belongs to impurity microelements and is not in the group of essential elements. For humans, the everyday dose of foods and drinks is limited to 3-5 mg. It is excreted through the urine and only 10 µg can be absorbed by the body.

Consistent with the content in the body (10^{-5}%), aluminum is classified as an impurity trace element, although it is the most plentiful element of the Earth's crust after O_2 and Si. It is concentrated in the lungs, liver, and bones. It is also a part of the structure of the nerve membranes in the human brain. Al disturbs the epithelial and connective tissue development, skeletal regeneration, phosphorus exchange and some enzyme processes.

Toxicity: Aluminum is the most plentiful environmental agent in the Earth's crust. Air emissions from Al production process, waste incineration, coal combustion, mining and motor vehicles exhaust, all contribute to progressive Al concentration in the air [67 - 70]. Owing to its predominant existence, humans are often exposed to various Al compounds in daily life. Toxicokinetic studies have demonstrated that Al additives are more easily absorbed and therefore have larger bioavailability than naturally occurring Al compounds. Aluminum in the form of Al^{3+} ions, to which people are unavoidably exposed, is often discussed relating to its toxic effects which are not well understood [67 - 70].

Even if aluminum is necessary for some life functions, the excess of Al^{3+} in the human body leads to a violation of the mineral metabolism, which is associated with the similar properties of Mg^{2+}, Ca^{2+}, and Al^{3+} cations. For instance, Mg^{2+} and Al^{3+} cations have similar radii and coordination numbers and Ca^{2+} and Al^{3+} cations have equal ionization energy. Aluminum has no identified role in humans, but there is an indication that it is connected with some acute and chronic human conditions [66]. Aluminum excess in the organisms inhibits the hemoglobin synthesis, due to the Al^{3+} complexing capability which blocks the active enzyme centers responsible for blood formation. Problems appear to arise in kidney failure cases when absorption of Al into the blood leads to its accumulation in the brain and to dementia. Aluminum can damage mitochondrial bioenergetic processes by generating ROS, which in sequence results in oxidative stress - the main factor for some neurodegenerative conditions, for instance Parkinson's and Alzheimer's diseases [67 - 69].

$Al(OH)_3$ is low soluble at neutral pH, but its solubility increases at acidic and basic pH values. Acidic rains leach Al from soil minerals, which rises the Al^{3+} concentration in rivers and lakes. Water, which dissolves more Al from the ground causes ecological damages because of the increased consumption of Al^{3+} by the organisms. A harmful effect of excess Al^{3+} is that the accessibility of PO_4^{3-} is limited because of the formation of slightly soluble $AlPO_4$, which leads to weaker assimilation of vital phosphorus in living organisms. Another consequence of acid rain and dissolved Al^{3+} from the soil, leads to precipitation of $Al(OH)_3$ at neutral pH of water and its deposition in fish, leading to problems with oxygen uptakes. Aluminum cation also is able to form chelate complexes with biological ligands, such as organic acids, carbohydrates, polyphenols and lipids. Typically, the bonding with bioorganic ligands occurs through oxygen donor atoms [70].

Unfortunately, the needed amount of Al is greatly exceeded by human consumption through the food, drinking water, deodorants, and certain antacids. This element is existing in many marketable products, especially cosmetics, and contact with Al is increasing [71]. Inhalation of finely separated Al and Al_2O_3 powders has been described as a source for pulmonary fibrosis and lung damages. This effect, known as Shaver's disease, is complicated by the presence of silicon and iron oxides in the air.

Gallium

Gallium and indium are not vital elements for life functions and do not have a significant biological role. Though gallium has no known biological function in humans, some of its properties enable it to stimulate metabolism and to interact with biological proteins in certain cellular processes, particularly those of Fe metabolism.

Gallium ion is an abiogenic ion, identified as an anticancer, antibacterial, and anti-inflammatory agent. The basis of its therapeutic effect lies in its close mimicry of the ferric ion. Iron is important for the growth of pathogenic microbes. Gallium mimics Fe and interferes with Fe-dependent cellular functions. Gallium is an interesting element to be used in medicine [72]. Gallium nitrate is used in the treatment of hypercalcemia. This condition occurs secondary to some types of cancer. Ga-containing compounds have therapeutic potential as anticancer and antiinfection agents.

Gallium compounds appear not to be particularly toxic. Although they are not dangerous, these compounds must not be inhaled or consumed. Gallium is a corrosive element and its contact can severely irritate and burn the skin and eyes. Breathing Ga(III) compounds can irritate the nose and throat causing coughing and wheezing. Gallium is harmful for the liver and kidneys.

Gallium is one of the four non-radioactive metals (with cesium, rubidium and mercury) that are known as liquids at room temperature.

Indium

Indium has no known biological functions in humans but is poisonous when breathed or ingested. In low doses, it stimulates metabolic processes [73]. This metal is toxic to some range, but due to its low amounts, its influence on the biosystems is not significant.

Indium(III) compounds should be regarded as very toxic to the body if ingested, but further research is required to assess their effects. In(III) ion damages the kidney functions and is a more poisonous in water solutions compared to direct injection of elemental In. Human can develop symptoms of toxicity through ingestion, eye contact, inhalation, and contact with skin. Indium compounds are encountered rarely by humans. Indium is typically stored in the skin, muscles, and bones, but it is excreted within around two weeks.

Thirty-nine isotopes of indium are known, which range in mass number from 97 to 135. There are only two naturally occurring isotopes, indium-113 and indium-115 [74]. Indium-115 is an abundant radioisotope with a long half-life of 4.41 x 10^{14} years. Among the synthetic isotopes, ^{111}In is the most stable ($T_{1/2}$ = 2.8 days). Radioactive isotope indium-111 is used as a radiotracer in nuclear medical studies for labeling white blood cells and proteins in the body.

Thallium

Thallium has no known biological use and does not appear to be essential for life. It has been considered one of the most toxic heavy metals [75]. It is absorbed through skin contact and rapidly by ingestion or inhalation. Tl(I) and Tl(III) compounds are extensively dispersed in the body, the maximum concentration being collected in kidneys. They are excreted through the urine and feces, but the excretion is slow and some amounts can be detected months after exposure. Excretion happens additionally through hair, which usually contains the highest thallium concentration. The acute hair loss is caused by thallium's capability to bind to cysteine -SH groups found in hair. Tl exposure leads to mitochondrial damage and weakens energy production. It causes progressive oxidative stress, changes in the properties of cell membranes, and deactivation of antioxidant mechanisms. Thallium produces a stable, highly poisonous Tl^+ cation under physiological conditions. Due to the chemical similarity, the monovalent thallium ion can interfere with K^+ pathways in the transmission of nerve impulses. Tl^{3+} cation can be easily reduced to Tl^+. The ionic radii of Tl^+ and K^+ ions are relatively comparable and Tl^+ enters membranes through K^+ ion channels and pumps reaching almost all areas of the body thus causing disorders. Enzymes necessitating K^+ for their functions, for instance Na^+/K^+-ATPase and pyruvate kinase, are inhibited by thallium. That is why thallium is a very toxic metal.

Actually, an increased potassium consumption counteracts to some range the effects of thallium intoxication. Thallium also crosses the placental barrier freely.

Toxicity: Thallium is a toxic rare heavy metal which is dispersed in nature at very low levels. Thallium is hazardous, such as Hg and Pb, but causes much less ecological problems because it has not been used in manufacturing so far [75, 76]. Its chemical behavior resembles the heavy metals (Pb, Au, and Ag) on the one hand and the alkali metals (K, Rb, and Cs) on the other. Despite its high toxicity (more toxic than Hg, Cd, and Pb), thallium has been studied to a much lesser extent than other toxic metals such as Hg, Cd and Pb because the standard analytical methods have lesser sensitivity for thallium than for other toxic metals. That is why the exact mechanism of Tl toxicity still remains unidentified.

Thallium compounds have been used until recently as rodenticides and insecticides. Thallium sulfate is very toxic like arsenic salts. Thallium sulfate is tasteless and odorless, with no warning of its occurrence. Thallium compounds are broadly utilized as rodenticides and ant killers. The use of thallium sulfate as an insecticide and a rodenticide has been forbidden [76]. Acute Tl intoxication is manifested by gastroenteritis, nausea, vomiting, and abdominal pain. A consumption of 1 g has lethal effect, but several milligrams are sufficient to generate psychosis and neurological disorders. By interfering with potassium and sulfhydryl-containing enzymes, thallium interrupts normal energy production. The tendency of thallium to easily form sulfides is a significant reason for its toxicity as it can replace other biogenic metals in vital enzymes. Although it is toxic to all organs, the peripheral nervous system and integumentary system are the most sensitive. Involvement of the CNS becomes obvious in a few days. The earliest clinical sign of thallium poisoning is a rapidly progressive, painful sensory polyneuropathy, mental confusion, delirium, convulsions, respiratory complica-tions, *etc.* Within 2-3 weeks, alopecia can be developed. Neurological symptoms (paresthesia) prevail with chronic contacts. They tend to progress, in spite of the decrease in Tl levels in blood.

Chelation therapy is not recommended in the treatment of thallium intoxication as the formed Tl complexes are extremely lipophilic and can increase Tl levels in brain. Suitable treatments of thallium intoxication include dialysis and high supplementation with potassium and iron cyanide complex compounds to shift the equilibria of tissue-bonded thallium(I) [75, 76]. The use of potassium iron(III) hexacyanoferrate(II), $K[FeFe(CN)_6]$ (Prussian Blue) can be explained by the fact that Tl(I) is chemically similar to Ag(I). That is why Tl(I) produces an insoluble coordination compound with the complex ion $[Fe^{3+}Fe^{2+}(CN^-)_6]^-$:

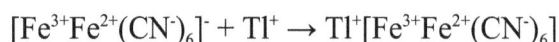

$$[Fe^{3+}Fe^{2+}(CN^-)_6]^- + Tl^+ \rightarrow Tl^+[Fe^{3+}Fe^{2+}(CN^-)_6]$$

In that way, any Tl(I) in the gastrointestinal tract can be precipitated and evacuated. The particles of the antidote Prussian Blue in colloidal form can function as harmless ion exchangers. They easily bind monovalent cations like Tl(I) and Cs(I) instead of K(I) removing them from the living organism.

p-Elements of the IVA Group

Carbon

Carbon is essential to life on Earth and biological processes. It is a component of all bioorganic compounds and living beings on earth. Carbonate CO_3^{2-} and hydrogen carbonate HCO_3^- anions react with metal cations to form carbonate natural sediments. Atmospheric CO_2 is in constant equilibria with the dissolved CO_2 in water pools and therefore with the content of CO_3^{2-} and HCO_3^- anions. The equilibrium of the carbon cycle is changed by industrial production, which generates vast quantities of CO_2 that it supplies to the air. A substantial environmental disturbance occurs, which is called "greenhouse effect" [5, 77]. Carbon also exists on many planets in the form of carbon dioxide. The planet Venus has a pure CO_2 atmosphere and its temperature in the surface is around 430°C. Therefore, liquid H_2O cannot exist on the surface of this planet. Mars has a thin atmosphere and a low surface temperature (-53°C) thus producing a very small greenhouse effect.

Carbon occurs in nature in an uncombined state (graphite, diamond) and in its naturally occurring compounds (calcium, magnesium, and other metals' carbonates) and CO_2, a small but critically significant component of the air.

From a biological viewpoint, carbon is perhaps the single most important organogen [5 - 7]. It is a part of all tissues and cells in the form of proteins, carbohydrates, nucleic acids, lipids, vitamins, hormones, and metabolites. The carbon content in the human body is around 21.15% (15 kg per 70 kg of total body weight). In cooperation with H_2, O_2 and N_2 these biogenic elements constitute about 99% of the cells' mass.

Carbon, the second most abundant element in humans, forms different kinds of chemical bonds (single, double, and triple) with other C atoms and with many other elements to make a range of biochemical compounds. In humans, the oxidation states of carbon vary from +4 in many compounds like CO_2, bicarbonates, *etc.*, to −4 in hydrocarbons. The C atom can be assumed of as a basic building block. Carbon, having an exceptional ability to form long chains of atoms together with other elements, gives numerous diverse organic compounds and biomolecules and determines their structural features [5 - 7]. Thanks to carbon, all richness and variety of plant and animal species arose. The very stable carbon-carbon single and multiple bonds are of greatest importance in biology. Covalently connected carbon atoms in biological molecules can form different carbon skeletons with linear chains, branched chains, and cyclic structures along with additional functional groups, that confer the specific biological and chemical properties of the biomolecules.

With its intermediate electronegativity, C can form less polar chemical bonds with the vital elements (H_2, O_2, N_2, S, *etc.*). The analogous elements of the IVA group form chemical bonds mainly through the O atoms. The carbon analogue lead binds through S atoms, which is the reason for its toxicity by blocking protein -SH groups. Carbon is the only element that forms compounds with so many different shapes and sizes with numerous functional groups [5 - 7, 9, 10]. The most important feature of carbon atoms is its capability to form multiple bonds. It is pertinent to note that this ability to form multiple bonds is inherent almost exclusively in carbon, nitrogen, and oxygen. In those rare cases, when we encounter multiple bonds in addition to this trio of elements, they are most often formed by sulfur and phosphorus.

In its free form, carbon is not toxic, but many of its compounds have significant toxicity. Prolonged inhalation of coal dust can lead to anthracosis, a disease accompanied by the deposition of coal dust in the lung tissue and lymph nodes, sclerotic changes in the lung tissue.

Carbon in the nature consists of ^{12}C (99%) and ^{13}C (1%). In the upper atmospheric levels, the radioactive isotope ^{14}C is constantly produced by the influence of cosmic rays [5 - 7, 77]. ^{14}C is directly oxidized to ^{14}C-based carbon dioxide $^{14}CO_2$. The content of ^{14}C is very small, around 10^{-12}. The radioactive $^{14}CO_2$, mixed with the other molecules, is consumed by green plants during photosynthesis. In this way, the radioactive ^{14}C is incorporated in the living cells. When the organism dies, the ^{14}C radioactivity decreases. ^{14}C decay is used in the method for age determination, referred to as radiocarbon dating or carbon-14 dating. This method provides reliable results on samples up to 5000 years old.

Carbon Monoxide

The colorless and odorless gas carbon monoxide CO is extremely toxic to aerobic organisms. When inhaled, carbon(II) monoxide enters the blood and forms a stable compound with hemoglobin - carboxyhemoglobin (HbCO), ineffective for oxygen delivery. Simultaneously, hemoglobin loses its ability to bind O_2, which is the cause of death in severe carbon monoxide poisoning [13 - 15]. The binding of CO to hemoglobin is 200 times stronger than that of oxygen, which explains its high toxicity.

In lungs, carbon monoxide moves easily through the alveolar capillary membrane, dissolves and diffuses in blood. CO interacts in opposite reactions with HbO_2 and Hb:

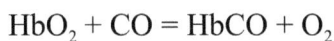

$$HbO_2 + CO = HbCO + O_2$$

$$Hb + CO = HbCO$$

The primary symptoms of CO poisoning are analogous to flu, fatigue, nausea, shortness of breath, and dizziness, observed at low concentrations of CO. High concentrations of poisonous CO result in increasingly more serious symptoms, like loss of muscular coordination, mental confusion, vomiting, loss of awareness, and finally death. The intoxication with CO can be treated with O_2 at high pressure (hyperbaric oxygen therapy). This method enables the dissociation of carbon monoxide from carboxyhemoglobin [13 - 15]. The toxic pollutant CO is produced in nature by the partial burning of different fuels.

On the other hand, the release of CO, controlled *in vivo*, seems to have some vital biological effects. Cells and tissues produce minor quantities of carbon monoxide as a metabolic product by heme degradation through the enzyme heme oxygenase. The body produces around 3-6 ml of carbon monoxide per day. This compound acts in the CNS as a signaling molecule. It participates in the control of neurotransmitters, as well as a vasodilative agent. Since CO represents a natural metabolite having signaling body function, this oxide could be of interest as a medication [78]. Particularly, metal complexes with carbonyl ligands like $[Ru(CO)_3Cl(glycinate)]$ (CORM-3) exhibit the capacity as CO releasing compounds for transportation and distribution of carbon monoxide to target locations [79]. Such usage may be protective against inflammation, transplant organ rejection, oxidative damage, and possibly afford antibiotics to combat infection [80].

Carbon Dioxide

Throughout photosynthesis, CO_2 combines with H_2O molecules to produce glucose $(C_6H_{12}O_6)$ and O_2, which are vital components for the life survival on earth [5]. Carbon dioxide CO_2 is the final product of cell respiration. In the human body, the oxidation of saccharides, lipids, and proteins produces large quantities of CO_2. Carbon dioxide is converted in erythrocytes by carbonic anhydrase to carbonic acid, which is almost completely dissociated under physiological pH values (≈ 7.4). The obtained hydrogen carbonate (bicarbonate) HCO_3^- ion is transported to lungs where it is converted back to CO_2 and removed through ventilation. Thus, most of the carbon dioxide obtained in metabolism is transported in the form of HCO_3^- ion in the blood and the rest is passed as carbamate connected to the nitrogen-terminal amino groups of Hb, producing carbaminohemoglobin. Very minor portions of CO_2 remain unaffected and passes dissolved in blood.

Carbon dioxide regulates breathing and is not directly toxic [6 - 10]. In lower amounts, CO_2 stimulates the breathing center. At a concentration of more than 10%, carbon dioxide causes acidosis (a decrease in blood pH), shortness of breath, and paralysis of the respiratory center. Concentrations above 30% are lethal even if the quantity of O_2 is sufficient.

The issues of pollution of the biosphere with carbon(IV) oxide coming from the products of fuel combustion are widely discussed. It is worrying that with an increase in air temperature by several degrees, the continental ice of Antarctica and Greenland will melt, which can cause a rise in the level of the World Ocean from 0.5 to 1.5 m. As a result, low-lying cities in the mouths of rivers, as well as vast agricultural areas, may be flooded. The whole reason is that CO_2 has strong absorption bands in the IR region of the spectrum. For this reason, CO_2 in the atmosphere, passing solar radiation, does not pass back thermal infrared radiation, which causes the "greenhouse effect" [81].

Water solution of CO_2 is the carbonic acid H_2CO_3, which is a weak acid. The most of CO_2 molecules do not change in water solution, they are just dissolved. Only a very small part of CO_2 is transformed to the weak H_2CO_3.

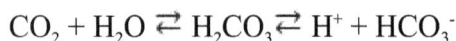

$$CO_2 + H_2O \rightleftarrows H_2CO_3 \rightleftarrows H^+ + HCO_3^-$$

Water solutions of the salts of carbonic acid possess alkaline reaction (pH>7):

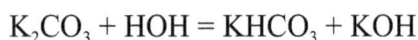

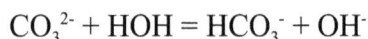

$$K_2CO_3 + HOH = KHCO_3 + KOH$$

$$CO_3^{2-} + HOH = HCO_3^- + OH^-$$

Hydrogen carbonates or bicarbonates of all the cations are soluble salts in water. Because of hydrolysis, their water solutions have weakly alkaline reaction. The hydrogen carbonates of calcium and magnesium occur only in solutions, and at evaporation or heating they are transformed into low soluble carbonates $CaCO_3$ and $MgCO_3$. A minor amount of low soluble carbonates of calcium and magnesium, occurs in bone.

Sodium and potassium carbonates are soluble giving strong basic solutions, whereas the other carbonates are almost insoluble. Introducing CO_2 into the suspension of an insoluble carbonate produces the corresponding hydrogen carbonate. The excess of strong acids causes the whole decomposition of the carbonate, for instance:

$$CaCO_3 + 2HCl \rightarrow CaCl_2 + H_2O + CO_2\uparrow$$

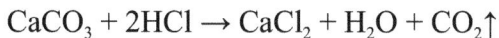

Carbonate buffer system ($H_2CO_3 + HCO_3^-$) is the main buffer system of extracellular liquids (blood plasma), which has a chief role in acid-base homeostasis [6 - 10].

HCN, cyanides and cyanogen compounds are highly toxic, which represent protoplasmic toxins at inhibition.

CCl_4 and all the chlorinated hydrocarbon substances are harmful for the CNS.

Between the diverse organic substances, the most poisonous are the compounds which contain halogens (F, Cl, Br, and I), S, Se, Te, N, P, As. The most toxic are Pb- and Hg- based organo metallic compounds [14 - 15]. Oxygen -based hydro carbons have generally less toxicity.

Silicon

Silicon, a widespread mineral, is a microelement which occurs at high levels in the human body, around 21 g. Some plants have a specific silicon uptake mechanism. It is vital for bone growth and development of higher animals. The increased silicon content is characterized by tissues in which nerve fibers are poorly developed or absent. Its maximum amount is contained in skin, cartilage, tendons, in place of active calcification of bone, and in some tissues of the eye (iris and cornea). This element, along with calcium, is essential for bone formation, matrix mineralization, and the synthesis and stabilization of collagen [82]. Silicon increases bone mineral density. Thus, Si supplementations have a direct beneficial effect on the density and strength of bones in animals and humans. Silicon is correspondingly vital to the formation of connective tissues like ligaments and tendons, for hair, skin, and fingernail growth [83]. There is relatively little being done to understand its importance for human health. It is probable that Si is significant in avoiding veins and arteries from hardening and stiffness, however, there is no information about the mechanism of this action. It has been identified that Si reduces effectiveness of aluminum in the body. Silicon may also postpone or prevent the degenerative Alzheimer's disease of the brain. Normally, it is fairly easy to get a sufficient amount of silicon in a standard diet and deficiency is very rare.

Elemental silicon and most Si-based compounds seem to be non-toxic but still very dangerous. Elemental Si is an inert material, which seems to lack the property of causing fibrosis in lung tissues. Silicon dust has little adverse effects on the lungs and does not produce substantial toxic effects when exposures are kept below the corresponding limits.

Silicon inorganic compounds cause chronic effects on the respiratory system [82, 83]. Different from carbon, Si in the strictures of biological molecules is bound only to O atoms forming Si-O bonds. The energy of the Si-O bond is higher than that of silicon bonds with other nonmetals such as Si-H, Si-C, Si-S, *etc.* Silicon dioxide SiO_2 is a powerful respiratory toxin. Since Si(IV) oxide in nature has low solubility in water, Si gets into the organism not by ingestion, but by inhalation through the lung as powdered SiO_2. The inhalation of dust holding SiO_2 causes silicosis disease. The symptoms of this metabolic disorder are rheumatism, hypertension, ulcers, and anemia. Silicon is typically located in cartilages and skin, where the metal is strongly bound with the OH groups of carbohydrate compounds. Continued and extensive exposures to some solid silicates such as quartz, tridymite, cristobalite, asbestos, *etc.* are problematic and represent a strong health hazard [82, 83]. With a high content of insoluble silicon compounds (silica, silicates) in the inhaled air, serious professional diseases can be developed - pneumoconiosis (silicosis, asbestosis, talcosis), particularly in workers in mining, coal, cement, faience and other industries. In the case of silicosis, difficult breathing and a high risk of tuberculosis are the main symptoms. Inhaled asbestos remains in the lung and causes serious health complications including lung cancer.

Germanium

Germanium is a trace microelement. Its biological role is not definitively established. This element is not vital for living organisms. It is not a danger to ecosystems. Most of germanium compounds are low soluble and produce low Ge amounts in nature [84].

Over the past years, much studies have gone into discovering the functions of germanium in human bodies. Germanium compounds prevent the development of acute oxygen starvation of body tissues, increase immunity, reduce the manifestation of pain, and show antitumor activity [85]. Widely used in medicine, ginseng absorbs germanium from the soil and accumulates it up to 0.2%. Germanium is also found in garlic and aloe, traditionally used to prevent and treat various human diseases. It is also found in certain therapeutic plants, recognized by the East traditional medicine. Consequently, it has been expected that there is a connection between the germanium content in plants and their biological profiles. Actually, germanium has many vital medicinal properties. A wide variety of bioactivities of germanium compounds has been observed, including neurotropic, hypotensive, anesthetic, bactericidal, antiviral, antifungal, antiradiation and antitumor properties.

The metabolic processes of germanium and silicon in the living body are connected, because of the resemblance in their physicochemical properties [86]. Germanium interacts with oxygen molecules in the body and subsequently, it is effective for getting oxygen to the tissues which helps to improve the immune system. It also supports the human body to eliminate harmful toxins and to control pain. There are commercial germanium supplements that can be used for treating arthritis, and food allergies, helping in reducing cholesterol levels, and preventing high blood pressure, and even cancer. In fact, many investigations have been devoted to the antitumor activity of newly synthesized germanium complexes and more recent research has gone into determining the importance of germanium-based compounds in coronavirus infection [87].

The toxic effects of Ge and its inorganic, metalloorganic and complex compounds are still poorly defined and clarified.

Tin

Although many years ago, this element was believed to be vital for animals growth and projected to be an important element for humans, nowadays there is little suggestion about the biological role of tin. By its low content in the body ($\approx$ 10^{-4}%) tin is a typical trace microelement [88]. Tin is probably essential for animals, but no precise role for this element in human health has been recognized. It has been found that very small amounts of tin are required for some animals species, providing a stimulating effect on their growth in small amounts.

Humans are extensively exposed to tin by using dinnerware and cans for food packaging, thus there are trace quantities of tin in the human body (around 16 mg). Tin can be ingested from an acidic food conserved in cans, covered with tin layers [88]. Sn dissolves easily in acid medium and passes into the bloodstream possessing a poisonous effect:

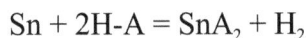

$$Sn + 2H\text{-}A = SnA_2 + H_2$$

Some investigations have shown that tin deficiency causes baldness in humans, but that is not confirmed and requires further study [88].

Tin oxide is less soluble in water and subsequently the Sn content in rivers and seawater is very low. Tin differs from its periodic table neighbors, cadmium and lead, in relation to its affinity for S. that is why, elemental tin is considered a non-toxic metal, and is therefore, safely used in the body.

The organotin compounds are different, however [89]. Organic compounds of tin, commonly used as fungicides, are poisonous to human beings. The toxic tributyltin $(C_4H_9)_3SnOCO·CH_3$ (TBT), used as sea paint, is harmful to algae preventing their growth on ship hulls [90]. That is why the use of paints containing TBT was prohibited.

Lead

The biological functions of lead have not been established. Lead is a comparatively unreactive element. It possesses a weak metallic character with an amphoteric nature, thus lead as well as Pb(II) and Pb(IV) oxides interact with acids and bases.

Toxicity: Lead is the first metal recognized as toxic to humans [91, 92]. It is a non-biodegradable metal, a multiorgan poisonous substance and one of the most ubiquitous environmental pollutants which can be harmful even in low quantities due to its ability to accumulate in different parts of the organisms. Contrary to toxic metals such as Hg and Cd, lead is not principally rare in the earth's crust. Pb is used in the production of storage batteries, plumbing, ammunition, cable coverings, production of tetraethyllead, sound absorbers, paints, radiation shields for X-ray equipment, and nuclear reactors. If proper precautions are not taken, the industrial workers may be overexposed to Pb.

Pb(II) and Pb(IV) compounds, extensively spread into the environment by humans, are very poisonous. The harmfulness of lead and cadmium, chemical elements occurring in nature mainly as sulfides, can be explained by their chalcophilic character, whereas the toxicity of some metals like tin and iron, that occur in nature as oxides, is due to their lithophilic character. Chalcophilic nature of lead and its predisposition to bind S is the main reason for its extreme toxic effects.

By inhalation or ingestion, lead can disturb the CNS, and lasting exposures can lead to many side effects such as anemia, nephropathy, brain damage and abdominal pain [91]. In humans, lead is transported by blood and nearly 99% of the captivated lead collects in erythrocytes, letting it be dispersed from blood to soft tissues of other organs like the liver, brain, lung, aorta, and spleen [92]. In the human body, lead accumulates mostly in the skeleton (up to 90%), teeth, liver, and kidneys which keep the highest lead amounts. Scientists believe that lead is a synergist of metals, *i.e.,* contributes to the toxicity of other metals. Symptoms of lead poisoning are a sulfur border on the gums ("lead border"), pallor of the face and lips, constipation, and loss of appetite. The phenomenon of acute and chronic poisoning (saturnism) can occur in workers of various industries associated with the production and use of lead. In the case of saturnism, there are numerous symptoms of CNS damage (headache, insomnia, convulsions, hallucinations, atrophy of the optic nerve), as well as impaired function of the kidneys (albuminuria) and gastrointestinal tract ("lead colic").

Lead is displaced from the organism primarily through urine and feces and its half-life is strongly dependent on the body's location. For instance, in blood and soft tissue, its half-life is approximately 30 days. Lead interacts with the metabolic processes of vital metal cations, predominantly those of the biogenic Ca, Cu, Fe, Zn. The main portion of the accumulated lead is deposited in bones because of the analogous chemical properties of Pb^{2+} and Ca^{2+} ions. Approximately 95% of the absorbed Pb can substitute Ca in the hydroxyapatite of bone. The disorder of calcium metabolism is the most significant mechanism identified for Pb-induced neurotoxicity. The half-life of lead in bone might reach more than 30 years, so lead intoxication is a very long-term problem, influencing the development of degenerative processes, for instance, osteoporosis. Oxidative stress has been also concerned as a pathological syndrome in Pb poisonousness [93].

In fact, there are no known health benefits of Pb for humans. On the contrary, lead has side deleterious effects that harm the human body. It affects almost all organs and systems in the human body (brain, kidneys, nervous system, reproductive system, *etc.*). Environmental lead pollution has found tremendous attention due to its public health concerns [94].

Pb^{2+} ions participate in the porphyrin synthesis which controls hemoglobin synthesis. Pb^{2+} ions dislocate many biogenic ions Met^{2+} and inhibit the enzyme functions [91 - 93]. Lead poisonousness arises not only as a result of its capability to displace other identical ions as Ca^{2+} and Zn^{2+} but also because of its high attraction to sulfhydryl groups of protein molecules, disturbing numerous essential bioprocesses of the body:

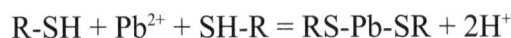

$$R\text{-}SH + Pb^{2+} + SH\text{-}R = RS\text{-}Pb\text{-}SR + 2H^+$$

Lead in the body interacts with the sulfhydryl and amide groups in enzymes, competing with crucial metals such as Ca, Zn, Fe and Cu, which interrupt the vital functions of enzymes. Additionally, lead accumulates in the body for a long time. Lead poisoning can be treated with ethylenediaminetetraacetic acid (EDTA), which produces a very stable complex with lead that can be excreted in the urine. The most frequently used chelators for the lead intoxication treatment represent a combination of $CaNa_2EDTA$ and dimercaprol [95].

Though lead and low soluble Pb(II) and Pb(IV) compounds cannot be absorbed by human tissues and are therefore quite innocuous, all of the soluble lead compounds are toxic, with toxicity increasing as solubility rises [91 - 93].

Significantly more serious is the hazard caused by PbO, ingested with food or cigarettes. Intoxication with inorganic Pb compounds mostly causes gastrointestinal and hematological symptoms, especially anemia, because of the heme synthesis inhibition (quite low amounts of Pb^{2+} constrain Zn^{2+}-dependent enzyme which is responsible for the catalysis of porphyrin reactions and consequently the heme synthesis). Furthermore, the noxious effects of Pb(II) intoxication involve reproductive conditions like sterility and miscarriage. Substantial lead contact can result in renal dysfunction and renal chronic diseases. Acute intoxication leads to classical symptoms, involving nausea and vomiting, abdominal and muscle pain, and seizures.

Basic lead carbonate $Pb_3(CO_3)_2(OH)_2$ has until recently been used as a paint pigment and in cosmetics but nowadays has been replaced. Predominantly, organic lead compounds are very poisonous. Lead cations form viscous albuminates by the reaction with the cytoplasm of bacterial cells and tissues. The most toxic are organolead compounds, particularly tetraethyl lead, which is used as a fuel additive. Low-level atmospheric pollution and water contamination, due to the use of tetraethyllead $Pb(C_2H_5)_4$ (a constituent of the motor fuels), is a great concern. Organolead compounds, like alkyl-lead compounds of Pb(IV), metabolize into neurotoxic products. The formation of these metabolic compounds is catalyzed by cytochrome p450-dependent monooxygenases in the liver [96]. Organolead compounds can cause serious conditions of the CNS and PNS (cramps, paralysis, loss of coordination). Additionally, lead can pass the placenta and can influence the fetus nervous system.

In low amounts, lead(II) salts display astringent effects, causing the jellification of proteins [91 - 93, 96]. These processes prevent the penetration of germs into the cells and reduce the inflammatory responses. The effects of tin wash are based on the same action. With a rise of Pb^{2+} concentration, the formation of albuminates becomes an irreversible process and albuminates of proteins accumulate in superficial tissues:

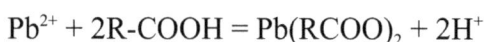

$$Pb^{2+} + 2R\text{-}COOH = Pb(RCOO)_2 + 2H^+$$

Therefore, medications of lead(II) are designated solely for external usage, because in case of their absorption by the gastrointestinal and respiratory systems, they show high toxic activity. Compounds of lead affect the protein synthesis and the energetic balance of cells. It was observed that lead is one of the elements whose occurrence in food stimulates the caries development.

It can be concluded that the elements of the IVA group differ significantly from each other in terms of their content in the body and in their bioactivity. From the brief overview of the biological properties of the elements of the IVA group, their inconsistency is visible (from the first organogen carbon, which plays a central role in the organisms life, through the vital biological role of microelements silicon and germanium to the toxicity of tin and lead). As a rule, the toxicity of elements and their inorganic and organometallic compounds rises with an increase in the atomic mass of the elements.

p-Elements of the VA Group

Nitrogen

Nitrogen is one of the most important biogenic macroelements for humans and the fourth most common among the elements in the living body [3, 4, 6-10]. Its content in the human body per dry matter is approximately 3%. Together with O_2, H_2, and C, nitrogen forms vital amino acids, which serve as building blocks for the construction of proteins - the basic of life. Consequently, nitrogen is a part of many biologically active molecules - amino acids, proteins, nucleotides, hormones, RNA and DNA, biogenic amines, *etc.* The bases which form the DNA genetic code (guanine, adenine, thymine, and cytosine) contain N atoms in their molecules. The wide variety of oxidation states is significant in nitrogen biochemistry, extending from −3 (in NH_3) to +5 (in nitrates) [14, 15].

In the body, nitrogen is typically in -3 oxidation state, being part of a wide range of compounds such as amino acids, imido acids, vitamins (primary amines), polypeptides (secondary amines), adenine, guanine, vitamin B_6, vitamin PP (tertiary amines), choline, acetylcholine, vitamin B_i (quaternary amines). Essential (in biological terms) are nitrogen-containing macrocycles - porphyrins, which are part of complex compounds in the form of bioligands. The porphyrin ring represents a tetradentate ligand. In this organic molecule, the alternating double bonds hold the structure in a rigid plane with four N atoms oriented in the direction of the center. The space in the center is the perfect size for numerous metal ions to form vital porphyrin units (chlorophyll, hemoglobin, *etc.*). The porphyrin metal complexes are among the most common in the living world [3, 4].

Nitrogen is involved in the digestion of food and growth. The degradation of proteins and deamination of amino acids, primarily glutamate, lead to the formation of NH_3:

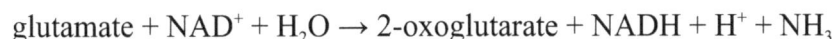

$$glutamate + NAD^+ + H_2O \rightarrow 2\text{-}oxoglutarate + NADH + H^+ + NH_3$$

The released ammonia in high concentrations is toxic to the CNS. In the organism, the detoxication of NH_3 takes place in the liver. NH_3 is converted into innocuous urea $CO(NH_2)_2$, which is excreted by the kidneys into urine.

Humans live in a nitrogen atmosphere [5]. The volume fraction of nitrogen in the air is 78% in the form of nitrogen gas N_2, moderately enriched with oxygen and in very small quantities with other chemical elements. The atmospheric nitrogen is inert, because the triple bond in N_2 molecule has a high bond energy barrier of (945 kJ/mol). That is why N_2 is unobtainable for direct usage by most organisms. Humans cannot absorb gaseous N_2 in the breath of air, it has to be taken in a different form from the food. There are some prokaryotes (nitrogen-fixing bacteria of the *Azotobacter strain* or *Rhizobium bacteria*) that are capable of adapting or fixing enormously stable atmospheric nitrogen and converting it into ammonia by utilizing the enzyme nitrogenase.

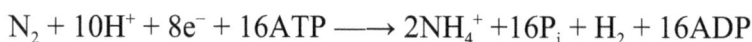

$$N_2 + 10H^+ + 8e^- + 16ATP \longrightarrow 2NH_4^+ + 16P_i + H_2 + 16ADP$$

The enzyme nitrogenase represents the only natural substance that reduces the "inert" dinitrogen molecule N_2 to NH_3 under mild conditions, compared to the industrial synthesis of NH_3 [3 - 5]. In addition to N_2, nitrogenase reduces various small unsaturated molecules, for instance, $C_2H_2 \rightarrow C_2H_4$; $N_2O \rightarrow N_2$; HCN $\rightarrow$ CH_3NH_2 *etc.* The enzyme nitrogenase, which contains proteins, as well as Mo and Fe, is active only under anaerobic conditions. Studies have shown that the reduction of N_2 to NH_3 or NH_4^+ does not produce NH=NH and NH_2-NH_2. Only some special leguminous plants possess bacteria that transform molecular N_2 from the atmosphere into compounds that the plants can use for producing proteins. NH_3 and nitrates are taken up readily and are preferred, as, for example, in fertilizers. There is also another kind of bacteria, the so-called nitrifying bacteria, which oxidize NH_3 to NO_2, nitrites, nitrates, *etc.* It has to be mentioned that in the plant kingdom, nitrogen is one of the 3 chief biogenic elements along with potassium and phosphorus, the so-called key plant nutrients. Plants can commonly use either NH_3 or nitrate as a source of nitrogen, nonetheless, vertebrates have to get nitrogen in the form of organic compounds like amino acids.

Molecular nitrogen does not take part in metabolism. The natural metabolic products in plants are nitrates, which then enter our body with food and water [3 - 5]. Nitrates have been proven to be low-toxic. For an adult, the lethal dose of nitrates is from 8 to 14 g with a single dose. Eating such an amount of nitrates is almost impossible. Nitrates dissolved in drinking water cause problems for children. In addition, in the human body on the reduction of nitrates to bioorganic compounds, noxious nitrites can be produced as intermediate ions, which with amines form carcinogenic nitrosamines in an acidic environment. Such transformations occur in a living organism. This has been proven experimentally, when animals were injected with pure nitrates, nitrites, and amines necessary for the above reactions. In fact, these reactions in humans do not occur in the gastrointestinal tract. Fruits and vegetables contain antioxidants that block such reactions.

Human body produces 25-50% of nitrates from the composition of the products and drinks consumed. Almost all sausages and ready-made meat products contain nitrates and nitrites (food additives E249 - E252), which give them a pink color and protect against spoilage. Already in the mouth, under the action of bacteria, nitrates turn into nitrites and with saliva, enter the stomach. It is believed that the main part of nitrites reacts with iron in hemoglobin, oxidizing the ferrous iron of hemoglobin to trivalent and methemoglobin is formed. Toxic effects of nitrites are exhibited because of transforming Hb into methemoglobin, which is not able to bind and transport O_2 in the blood [97]. Thus, moving into the blood, nitrites generate oxygen deficiency:

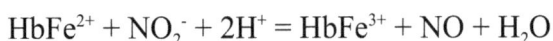

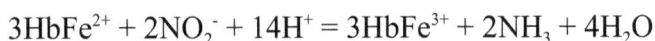

$$HbFe^{2+} + NO_2^- + 2H^+ = HbFe^{3+} + NO + H_2O$$

$$3HbFe^{2+} + 2NO_2^- + 14H^+ = 3HbFe^{3+} + 2NH_3 + 4H_2O$$

Methemoglobin is commonly obtained under the action of different oxidizing agents: nitrogen oxides, nitrates, aniline. Blood methemoglobin content can also rise in case of some hemoglobin-based pathologies connected with a hereditary absence of the enzyme reductase, which converts methemoglobin to hemoglobin. Additionally, methemoglobin can be formed when taking high dosages of some drugs as sulfonamides. Methemoglobinemia condition can be treated by using methylene blue or ascorbic acid [98].

From the other part of the nitrites, not so much carcinogenic nitrosamines are formed, such as nitric(II) oxide, which is useful for the body. Nitric(II) oxide is considered as a factor regulating vascular tone from the moment of its detection in the human body and animals. Nitric(II) oxide binds to hemoglobin and nitrosothiols (Hb-SNO) are formed. Hb-SNO dilates blood vessels and increases blood flow. In general, nitric(II) oxide in humans and animals is not only a universal physiological regulator of the cardiovascular system, but also the immune and nervous system. The biochemistry of N(II) oxide attracted a lot of attention. It plays a vital role in nitrogen metabolic processes as a natural free radical molecule. This reactive free radical (with one unpaired electron: $\cdot N=O$) is an essential signaling molecule in the cardiovascular system of the organism, accountable for the regulation of many bioprocesses like muscle contractions, neurotransmissions and immune reactions [99]. It is formed throughout the oxidation of all N-based compounds with an oxidation state of -3, as well as in reduction of compounds with oxidation states from +3 to +5.

As a radical, NO is readily penetrable through the cell membranes and shows some additional functions such as vasodilation, cell proliferation, neurotransmission, wound healing, antibacterial and antifungal activity. NO is synthesized at physiological conditions in blood vessel endothelium, phagocytosing cells and neurons by the translation of L-arginine to L-citrulline by means of the enzyme nitric oxide synthase (NOS) with NADPH and O_2 [100], which is illustrated by the reaction:

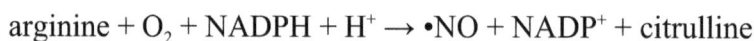

$$arginine + O_2 + NADPH + H^+ \rightarrow \bullet NO + NADP^+ + citrulline$$

Three isoforms of NOS are established: endothelial (eNOS), neuronal (nNOS), and inducible (iNOS) [101]. eNOS produces NO in the blood and contributes to vasodilation. As an endothelium-resulting factor, NO leads to vasodilation by relaxing vascular muscles and consequently reduces the blood pressure. Neuronal NOS participates in the formation of NO in nervous tissues and in the cell communication, thus NO also acts as a neurotransmitter, plays an essential role in macrophage function and prevents platelet aggregation. iNOS is situated in the cardiovascular and immune systems and upon stimulation by proinflammatory cytokines produces great amounts of NO.

NO-induced cardiac muscle relaxation is the same response induced by nitroglycerin and additional nitro-vasodilators against angina pectoris, caused by the contraction of the heart deprived of oxygen due to the blocked coronary arteries [101]. The half-life of nitric oxide is very short in tissues (only 3-10 s) because it interacts with oxygen and superoxide, and then converts into nitrate and nitrite, as well as peroxynitrite ($ONOO^-$) - a reactive nitrogen species.

Along with nitrates in high concentrations, nitrous acid is also very toxic. Nitrous acid HNO_2 can be formed from nitrites and nitrates. It is a powerful activator of the nucleobases' deamination, for instance, cytosine $\rightarrow$ uracil, adenine $\rightarrow$ hypoxanthine, and guanine $\rightarrow$ xanthine.

Reactive Nitrogen Species

Reactive nitrogen species (RNS) are various NO-derived compounds, involving nitrosonium cation, nitroxyl anion, nitrogen oxides, S-nitroso-thiols, and dinitrosyl Fe complexes. Radical and nonradical reactive species are produced mainly from nitrogen and the most important are NO or nitroxide radical ($NO\bullet$), nitrogen dioxide ($NOO\bullet$) and peroxynitrite anion ($ONOO^-$). Between the nitrogen containing species, indicated as RNS, relatively unreactive is nitric oxide $NO\bullet$, while its derivative the peroxynitrite anion ($ONOO^-$) is a powerful oxidizing agent, which damages many biomolecules [102, 103]. RNS act jointly with ROS, producing nitrosative stress [104].

Nitroxide radical ($NO\bullet$) belongs to the fundamental signals participating in intercellular regulation and cellular functions [102 - 104]. It is synthesized from arginine by many cells, including macrophages, endothelial cells, Kupffer cells and hepatocytes, kidney's epithelial cells, cells of the adrenal glands, heart and frontal brain. NO• radical is not stable and rapidly interacts with hemoglobin, myoglobin, O_2 or $•O_2^-$. In nonenzymatic processes in aqueous environment NO• reacts with O_2 producing other nitrogen oxides, nitrates, and nitrites:

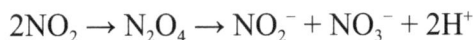

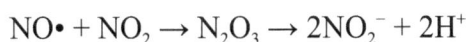

$$2NO• + O_2 \rightarrow 2NO_2$$

$$2NO_2 \rightarrow N_2O_4 \rightarrow NO_2^- + NO_3^- + 2H^+$$

$$NO• + NO_2 \rightarrow N_2O_3 \rightarrow 2NO_2^- + 2H^+$$

Subsequent interactions of the nitrogen oxides with secondary amines cause the production of oncogenic nitrosamines.

Superoxide anion radical ($•O_2^-$) interacts rapidly with nitroxide radical NO• in the vasculature to form peroxynitrite anion:

$$NO• + •O_2^- \rightarrow ONOO^-$$

Both initial radicals contain unpaired electrons. Thus, the rate of the reaction is relatively high. The produced peroxynitrite diminishes the bioactivity of NO [102 - 105].

Peroxynitrite itself is an extremely active species which can directly and selectively interact with many biotargets involving amino acid residues, lipids, thiols, DNA bases, and low-molecular antioxidant agents. Peroxynitrite can also interact directly with proteins containing transition metal centers, for instance, hemoglobin, myoglobin, and cytochrome c by the oxidation of Fe^{2+} heme to its Fe^{3+} form. Peroxynitrite can modify protein structure by reactions with many amino acids in peptides, for instance, cysteine oxidation, tyrosine nitration. These reactions affect the structure and function of the corresponding proteins and cause changes in the enzymes' catalytic activity [105]. Peroxynitrite ($ONOO^-$), contrasting NO• or $•O_2^-$, is a very strong oxidizing and nitrating agent. In addition, peroxynitrite anion can interact with other biomolecules to form different chemically reactive types of RNS such as $•NO_2$, N_2O_3, ONOOH, *etc*. By protonation of peroxynitrite anion, peroxynitrous acid ONOOH can be formed. ONOOH decomposes quickly and yields a reactive hydroxyl radical:

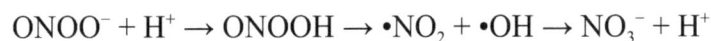

$$ONOO^- + H^+ \rightarrow ONOOH \rightarrow •NO_2 + •OH \rightarrow NO_3^- + H^+$$

Other important reactions involving RNS include the production of additional types of free radicals (nitrosoperoxycarbonate, carbonate radicals, and nitrogen oxides):

$$ONOO^- + CO_2 \rightarrow ONOOCO_2^-$$

$$ONOOCO_2^- \rightarrow \cdot NO_2 + O{=}C(O\cdot)O^-$$

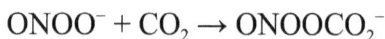

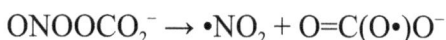

All above reactions make a connection between the reactive metabolites of RNS and ROS in macrophages and neutrophils [102 - 105]. The final result is the production of the most active antimicrobic and cytotoxic hydroxyl radical •OH.

Nitrogen Compounds

Nitrogen, as an inert gas, is innocuous except when breathed under pressure, when it dissolves in the blood fluid in high concentrations, producing a narcotic effect.

Some nitrogen compounds with oxygen and hydrogen are toxic. Ammonia NH_3 is a toxic gas, which is regularly formed by the catabolism of amino acids in the human body. It is a typical weak base:

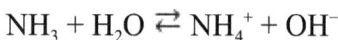

$$NH_3 + H_2O \rightleftarrows NH_4^+ + OH^-$$

Inhalation of ammonia NH_3 vapor in large quantities is harmful, since ammonia creates a strongly alkaline environment on the surface of the mucous membranes of the larynx and lungs, which causes their irritation and swelling. In addition, small molecules of NH_3 easily penetrate cell membranes and become competitors to many bioligands in coordination with metal ions.

Dinitrogen monoxide N_2O (nitrous oxide, laughing gas) is a colorless gas with weak anesthetic activity. It is used in surgery as an inhalation anesthetic. The combination of N_2O and O_2 affords good oxygenation with a reduced risk of excessive sedation.

The synthesis of HNO_3 and other inorganic compounds produces N-based gases which represent a mixture of toxic oxides of nitrogen: NO, NO_2, N_2O_4, N_2O_3 [97, 99 - 101]. These oxides can contact with the wet surface of the lungs, forming HNO_3 and HNO_3, and thus leading to edema and additional respiratory conditions. Nitrogen intoxication of blood by N-based gases can also form nitrates and nitrites.

Nitrogen oxide NO, despite the difficulty of its formation from N_2 and O_2, is present in the atmosphere in large quantities. In the human body, NO is formed from arginine by the enzyme NO synthetase by the reaction:

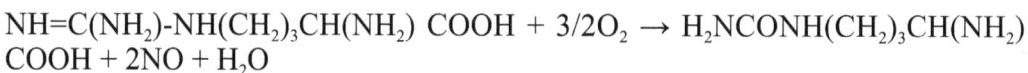

$$NH{=}C(NH_2)\text{-}NH(CH_2)_3CH(NH_2)\ COOH + 3/2O_2 \rightarrow H_2NCONH(CH_2)_3CH(NH_2)$$
$$COOH + 2NO + H_2O$$

NO molecules are able to penetrate into the cells of the walls of blood vessels and regulate blood flow. One of the functions of nitric monoxide NO is the relaxation of smooth muscle cells of arterial walls [97, 99 - 101, 103]. In addition, NO controls insulin secretion, renal filtration, reparative processes in tissues, *etc.* The vasodilatation activity of NO on the coronary vessels is used in the therapy of ischemic heart disease. Thus, NO is a molecule with a dual function that exhibits both toxic and undoubtedly beneficial effects. For instance, when taking the common cardiological drug nitroglycerin, it is hydrolyzed to form a nitrate ion, which is restored by the hemoglobin gland to NO, and then NO causes the smooth muscles relaxation.

Nitrogen dioxide NO_2 is synthesized by the interaction of NO with oxygen. Nitrogen dioxide in water undergoes dismutation:

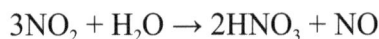

$$3NO_2 + H_2O \rightarrow 2HNO_3 + NO$$

This oxide is the main constituent of irritating and poisonous nitrous fumes, formed during the industrial reduction of nitric acid and nitrates. The amount of nitrogen oxides NO_x in the atmosphere is the main indication for the air pollution. Nitrogen oxides contribute to the acidity of rainfall and soil [5].

Nitrous acid HNO_2 (HO-N=O) is present only in diluted solutions as a weak and very unstable acid, which decomposes by disproportionation:

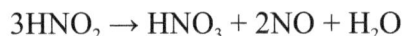

$$3HNO_2 \rightarrow HNO_3 + 2NO + H_2O$$

The salts of HNO_2 (nitrites) are stable in the solid state. They are water-soluble, and quite toxic. Along with their contribution in the oxidation of Fe(II) to Fe(III) in hemoglobin, they form such carcinogens as nitrosamines R^1R^2N-N=O by the reaction of secondary amines R^1R^2NH with HNO_2 in strongly acidic stomach environment [97, 99 - 101, 103]. The formation of nitrosamines can be inhibited by vitamin C. $NaNO_2$ was previously used as a vasodilator for angina pectoris and spasms of cerebral vessels. Recently, $NaNO_2$ has been abandoned due to its undoubted toxicity, replacing it with nitroglycerin $C_3H_5N_3O_9$ or nitrosorbitol $C_6H_{13}NO_8$, which do not have such side effects.

Nitric acid HNO_3 (HO-NO_2) is a strong acid with strong oxidation properties. All of its salts, nitrates, are water soluble and are used as oxidizing agents. The so-called saltpeter, $NaNO_3$, KNO_3, and ammonium nitrate, are used as industrial fertilizers. Nitrates are comparatively not very toxic and can be rapidly excreted in urine. Although a high consumption of nitrates poses a danger because part of them in the body can be reduced to poisonous nitrites, particularly in the case of some intestinal infections [97,101,103]. Nevertheless, in low amounts, certain inorganic and organic nitrites R-O-N=O and nitrates R-O-NO$_2$ help coronary circulation and are useful in prevention of the coronary heart disorders and to stop strokes, for example glycerol trinitrate.

Many synthetic fertilizers are N-containing compounds (nitrates, ammonia, ammonium salts, or urea) [106]. Because of their water solubility, nitrates move readily to the soil. The anhydrous NH$_3$ gas, when used directly as a fertilizer, it can interact with H$_2$O in the soil and convert to NH$_4^+$ ion. Ammonium phosphates, such as (NH$_4$)$_3$PO$_4$, NH$_4$H$_2$PO$_4$, and (NH$_4$)$_2$HPO$_4$, are perfect fertilizers as they contain two essential nutrients - nitrogen and phosphorus. Soil microbes convert the ammonium cation to nitrates, which represent the key N-based forms consumed by the plants. Urea CO(NH$_3$)$_2$ can be produced from NH$_3$ and CO$_2$:

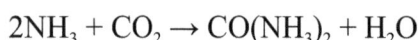

$$2NH_3 + CO_2 \rightarrow CO(NH_3)_2 + H_2O$$

Urea is a good fertilizer, used in solid state or in concentrated water solutions, containing additionally NH$_4$NO$_3$ and ammonia. Enzymes of soil microorganisms naturally convert urea nitrogen to nitrate.

Phosphorus

Phosphorus is the fifth most important element in biology after carbon, hydrogen, oxygen, and nitrogen, which is vital for all living organisms. Phosphorus along with Ca is essential for skeletons and teeth. There is around 0.9 kg of this crucial element in the body, 90% of P is in the composition of apatite (in bone and teeth), and the rest is located in extracellular fluids (hydrogen phosphate and dihydrogen phosphate ions) and soft tissue, mainly in muscle and blood [107].

The significance of this element is that sugars and fatty acids cannot be used by cells as energy sources unless they are pre-phosphorylated. Many compounds (fatty acids, proteins, *etc.*) form biologically active complex compounds with phosphorus (nucleoproteins, phosphoproteins, phosphorus esters of carbohydrates, *etc.*). The intracellular matrix contains many types of biologically significant inorganic phosphates and phosphate esters - phospholipids in cell membranes, phosphorylated proteins that regulate protein function, nucleic acids, and high energy phosphate esters of sugars. In cooperation with proteins, they are the key intracellular buffer bases [107]. As a constituent of these important bioactive compounds, P plays a fundamental role in energy formation.

All living organisms require a constant source of energy to function properly. Phosphorus participates in the formation of high energy compounds and is a part of the energy storage system in the body. Exchange of P in the organism is closely connected to the exchange of Ca because of their biological antagonism, meaning that the decrease of one leads to the increase of another element in the blood. Cells contain special compounds with high energy in which phosphates are linked by anhydride bonds. The bioinorganic derivatives of diphosphorus acid $H_4P_2O_7$ and not contained in free form triphosphoric acid $H_5P_3O_{10}$, the so-called adenosine diphosphate acid (ADP) and adenosine triphosphate acid (ATP), respectively, are essential [3, 4]. At physiological pH, they exist practically ionized in the form of ATP^{4-} and ADP^{3-} anions. The most significant in the human body is ATP, adenosine triphosphate. Similar to polyphosphate anions, ATP^{4-} and ADP^{3-} anions can hydrolyze. As a result of hydrolysis with H_2O molecule ATP^{4-} hydrolyzes into ADP^{3-} and hydrogen phosphate anion HPO_4^{2-}:

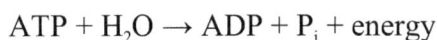

$$ATP + H_2O \rightarrow ADP + P_i + energy$$

ATP acts through losing the endmost phosphate group with the help of enzymes. This hydrolysis interaction releases lots of energy, which can be used for building proteins and to influence energy-requiring bioprocesses (cell growth, muscle movements, regular heart contractions, *etc.*). Numerous biosynthetic interactions occur because of the transmission of the phosphate groups from a high-energy to a low-energy acceptor. Adenosine diphosphate and adenosine triphosphate form complexes with metal ions, mainly magnesium ones ($MgATP^{2-}$ and $MgADP^-$), which are active forms in enzymatic phosphorylation reactions [3, 4]. When the body rests and energy is not needed immediately, the phosphate group re-attaches to the molecule using energy derived from food or sunlight. This way, the ATP molecule acts as a chemical battery, storing energy when it's not needed, but being able to instantly release it when the body requests it. Phosphorus, which stands in the middle part of the periodic table, has a moderate affinity for electrons (in contrast to F, O, Cl, S). In this connection, phosphorus and phosphoric acid are assigned the role of depot and biocatalytic use of energy. Carbon and nitrogen cannot participate in these processes, as they do not have the ability to use d-orbitals. Arsenic is poisonous, and silicon produces low-soluble acids. From an evolutionary point of view, this is a perfect example of individuality in chemistry, typical for phosphorus.

Phosphorus supports maintaining healthy blood sugar levels. It is also found in significant quantities in the nervous system. Phosphorus takes part in the synthesis of RNA and DNA; of phospholipids and phosphoproteins. It also participates in phosphate buffer ($H_2PO_4^- + HPO_4^{2-}$) which buffering action is essential for the regulation of the acid-base balance and the maintenance of pH in the blood as well as in the cells [3,4,107]. Phosphorus is an essential component of some nucleotide coenzymes, *e.g.,* NAD, NADP, ADP, AMP, pyridoxal phosphate. Numerous proteins and enzymes are activated by phosphorylation.

In the plant kingdom, P is one of the three chief elements that make plant life possible, the other two are K and nitrogen [5 - 10]. They are referred as key plant nutrients (N-P-K). Such designations as 5:10:5 for fertilizers denote the corresponding weight percent composition of materials with regard to N-, P-, and K-based oxides, containing the key elements required for the plant growth. Nitrogen in fertilizers is in the form of $NaNO_3$ or KNO_3, NH_3, ammonium salts, or some organic mixtures. Phosphorus is supplied mainly in the form of inorganic phosphates. Plants which are deficient in phosphorus are stunted with dark green or bluish-violet leaf color and need P-based fertilizers. Inorganic phosphate is present as HPO_4^{2-} and $H_2PO_4^-$ ions in soils. This equilibrium can be shifted in the presence of highly charged metal cations which force the equilibrium to insoluble salts. Particularly important is Ca^{2+} which forms insoluble $Ca_3(PO_4)_2$. Increasing the pH leads to the formation of the corresponding low soluble compound:

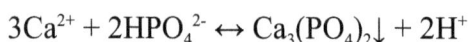

$$3Ca^{2+} + 2HPO_4^{2-} \leftrightarrow Ca_3(PO_4)_2\downarrow + 2H^+$$

The availability of phosphate in the form of solution is also limited at low values of pH, because aluminum cation becomes more soluble when pH decreases [5]. The solubilized Al^{3+} structures interact with the phosphate species to give low soluble alumino-phosphates:

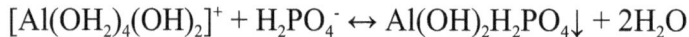

$$[Al(OH_2)_4(OH)_2]^+ + H_2PO_4^- \leftrightarrow Al(OH)_2H_2PO_4\downarrow + 2H_2O$$

As a result, the amount of inorganic phosphates in soil becomes very low excepting the narrow range of pH from 6 to 7.

Organophosphates are the most soluble in soil [3 - 5]. These are phosphates with covalent bonds such as phospholipids, phosphates of nucleic acids, phosphates of inositol $C_6H_6(OH)_6$ *etc*. Some organic esters of H_3PO_4, used as lubricating oil additives, have been observed to cause lasting paralysis upon ingestion.

Phosphorus Compounds

Phosphorus(V) has a chief role in biomolecules, predominantly in phosphate diester linkages in the structures of DNA and RNA [3, 4]. Polyphosphate diesters are responsible for the transport of cellular energy, particularly ATP.

Phosphoric acid H_3PO_4, which is a weak triprotic acid, in the third step of dissociation, is a very weak acid:

$$H_3PO_4 \rightleftarrows H^+ + H_2PO_4^-$$

$$H_2PO_4^- \rightleftarrows H^+ + HPO_4^{2-}$$

$$HPO_4^{2-} \rightleftarrows H^+ + PO_4^{3-}$$

An anhydride produced from phosphoric acid is pyrophosphoric or diphosphoric acid with salts diphosphates that are found in assemblies of many nucleotides (ADP) and cofactors (NAD^+, FAD). Diphosphoric acid is the first condensation product of phosphoric acid:

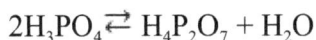

$$2H_3PO_4 \rightleftarrows H_4P_2O_7 + H_2O$$

Breaking the anhydride bond in diphosphate results in the release of energy, so diphosphate belongs to high-energy compounds (ADP, ATP).

Phosphoric acid has three types of salts - dihydrogen phosphates ($H_2PO_4^-$), hydrogen phosphates (HPO_4^{2-}) and phosphates (PO_4^{3-}). All dihydrogen phosphate salts are water-soluble and their solutions show a weak acid reaction because $H_2PO_4^-$ releases H^+ quite readily [3,4,108]. Sodium, potassium, and ammonium hydrogen phosphates (HPO_4^{2-}) and phosphates (PO_4^{3-}) are water-soluble, but their solutions display a basic reaction due to hydrolysis. Phosphates play two key roles in biology. First, they serve as structural elements of a number of biological components; for instance, the sugar phosphate backbone of nucleic acids or the deposition of calcium phosphate of bone and teeth $Ca_{10}(PO_4)_6(OH)_2$ - hydro xyapatite and $Ca_{10}(PO_4)_6 F_2$ - fluorapatite. The second role of orthophosphate ion derivatives in the body is related to the transfer of energy. The specific role of phosphorus as an energy transfer agent is determined by several factors. First of all, phosphorus forms weaker bonds than oxygen and nitrogen. Additionally, due to the presence of 3d-orbitals, phosphorus atoms can form more covalent bonds. Along with this, among the elements of the third period, only phosphorus and sulfur retain the ability to form multiple bonds. That is why the phosphoric acid derivatives in living organisms are numerous (ATP, ADP, AMP, creatine phosphate, guanosine-5'-triphosphate (GTP), *etc.*).

Phosphorus is a constituent of plant cells, essential for cell division and plant cultivation. For this reason, phosphate fertilizers are vital for plants. Rock phosphate is the raw material used in the production of most of the phosphate fertilizers. Synthetic phosphate fertilizers are obtained by treating apatite with H_2SO_4. The products are monocalcium phosphate $Ca(H_2PO_4)_2 \cdot 2H_2O$ and calcium sulphate $CaSO_4$. Superphosphate is the most common phosphate fertilizer, containing around 20% of P_2O_5, suitable for soil assimilation [108]. The triple phosphate fertilizer, which contains 48% of absorbable P_2O_5, can be synthesized by the decomposition of apatite with H_3PO_4:

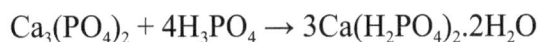

$$Ca_3(PO_4)_2 + 4H_3PO_4 \rightarrow 3Ca(H_2PO_4)_2.2H_2O$$

Elemental phosphorus forms P_2O_5 on the surface of the skin, which hydrolyzes to release a large amount of heat that aggravates the burn. White phosphorus is the most hazardous allotropic form of phosphorus to human health which is known [6 - 10]. It is extremely toxic, because of its reactivity and high fat solubility, and therefore the ability to enter through the cell membranes. In many cases, exposure to white P could be fatal. The symptoms of its exposure are stomach cramps, skin and liver burns, as well as heart and kidneys damages. The other phosphorus allotropic modifications due to their low solubility are considered non-toxic.

P(III) with a well-known chemistry is a very strong reducing agent for living organisms. Phosphine PH_3 is highly toxic, as are its organic derivatives. The most noxious substances identified, together, named nerve gas, are phosphorus organic derivatives [3, 4]. Organophosphorus compounds containing C-P bonds are powerful toxins, which include chemical warfare agents and pesticides.

The disruption of phosphorus homeostasis in the body leads to many detrimental conditions such as cardiac problems, chronic kidney disease, hemolysis, respiratory failure, *etc.* [109, 110].

Hypophosphatemia, which characterizes with low amounts of serum phosphate, leads to respiratory failure, hemolysis, and cardiac failure [109]. Since phosphorus can be found in many foods, a deficiency of this element is not often observed. Phosphorus deficiency occurs mainly in people taking antacids for a long time. Many of these drugs, commonly used in the therapy of gastritis, peptic ulcer disease, and acid reflux, hold Mg and Al, which have affinity to phosphate, stopping its absorption into the body.

Hyperphosphatemia, associated with increased amounts of serum phosphate, is usually connected with chronic kidney disease [110]. It is also worth noting that the role of vitamins and hormones in the regulation of phosphorus metabolism is important. Hormones like calcitriol, calcitonin and parathyroid hormone are the main factors that control the plasma P within a narrow interval. Calcitriol is a bioactive form of vitamin D which acts at intestine, bone, and kidney levels. It increases the intestinal Ca and phosphate absorption and the mobilization of Ca and P from the bone. Calcitriol also reduces the excretion of Ca and P through the kidney.

Arsenic

Arsenic is a trace microelement in the human body. The normal levels of As in human blood (4-30 nM) have a half-life of around 2 hours [111]. The biogenic role of arsenic and the forms of its content in the body are still unknown. However, there is reliable evidence according to which a deficiency of arsenic leads to a reduction in fertility and inhibition of growth. The addition of sodium arsenite to food leads to an increase in the growth rate in humans.

The semimetallic arsenic is distributed in soil, air, surface and groundwater, and in certain foods. As in nature occurs in the form of compounds in +3 or +5 oxidation states. In spite of its status as a highly poisonous element, arsenic may really be required for good health. Current *in vivo* experiments demonstrate that As possesses positive biological functions and is necessary for their proper growth and reproduction, probably connected with protein synthesis. Therefore, As is a vital element for some organisms, maybe also for human, which is supposed, but still not identified. Arsenic has a positive effect on the processes of hematopoiesis, it is concentrated in erythrocytes and participates in the synthesis of hemoglobin [14,15,111]. It is believed that the anti-anemia effect of arsenic is determined by its direct effect on the bone marrow. In addition, arsenic takes an active part in oxidative reduction processes, as well as in nucleic exchange processes. It is believed to be necessary for the CNS functioning and for proper growth. Since As is present in food and water, human bodies contain some As, thus arsenic deficiency in humans has almost never been detected. A low necessary intake can be obtained from drinking water.

Toxicity: Arsenic has many technical applications, including: manufacture of glass, pyrotechnics, semiconductor devices, light-emitting diodes, solar cells, lasers, and integrated circuits; in the production of paints, enamels, and bronze; in galvanizing, soldering, etching, lead plating, and smelting; in wood preservation; and as a constituent of varieties of pesticides, herbicides, insecticides, fungicides, and rodenticides, whose ingestion may cause As toxic conditions. Arsenic environmental pollution is a serious concern of human health. Inorganic As compounds accumulate in the spleen, kidneys, liver, lungs, and digestive tract [112]. It passes through these locations nevertheless leaves a residue in tissues such as hair, skin, and nails. As is associated with cardiovascular diseases, peripheral vascular diseases, and diabetes mellitus (type II), hearing problems, hypertension, hepatic damage, *etc.,* as well as blood and CNS abnormalities. There is a relationship between the severe inorganic As poisoning and the serious health complications [112].

Arsenic compounds in large doses are very toxic and belong to the accumulating poisons [112]. As compounds slowly penetrate the skin. They are rapidly absorbed by the lungs or by the gastrointestinal tract. After absorption, As is spread *via* the bloodstream to other organs. Arsenic accumulates at maximum levels in the bones, nails, skin, and hair and cannot be completely removed from them for several years. The toxicity of arsenic can be different in the various As-based compounds. Arsenic sulfides were used in ancient times. Like metallic arsenic, the sulfides have low toxicity. As(III) oxide and As(III) hydride are very toxic inorganic compounds.

The mechanism of toxic action of arsenic in the cell is still not completely clear. However, it is known that arsenic combines with sulfhydryl groups of proteins and blocks them. It is possible that arsenic can inactivate enzymes that contain -SH groups and thus be an inhibitor of respiratory enzymes [113, 114]. Arsenic can inhibit about 200 enzymes involved in cellular energy routes through the reaction of As(III) with -SH groups. This binding of the soft acid As(III) to the soft base sulfide of thio-amino acids of the respective protein could modify its conformation and damage its function. Additionally, arsenic replaces selenium, iodine, and phosphorus. Breaking the metabolic bioprocesses, As is a typical antimetabolite of these vital elements.

Arsenic is poisonous in the range to +5 oxidation state, contrasting P, which is toxic only in +3 oxidation state. This is caused because the body readily reduces As(V) to As(III) [112 - 114]. Arsenic(III) compounds are commonly more poisonous than As(V) compounds. In methylated form, As substances are less poisonous and widespread, predominantly in aquatic organisms like fish and crustaceans. The main route of excretion is by the kidneys in the urine within 1-2 days and only a low amount is eliminated in feces.

As(V) as inorganic hydrogen-arsenate ($HAsO_4^{2-}$) is an analogue of hydrogen-phosphate (HPO_4^{2-}) and therefore can compete for phosphate ion transporters and replace phosphates in some bioreactions [111 - 114]. For instance, arsenate can replace phosphate in ATP, thus forming ADP-arsenate and additional phosphate intermediate compounds concerned with glucose metabolic processes, which may reduce the normal glucose metabolism, and disturb the energy production.

Organoarsenic compounds do not cause cancer or DNA damage. Nevertheless, exposure to high concentrations causes some effects on human health, such as nerve injury and stomachache [112].

Acute As exposure leads to gastrointestinal and neurological effects on the CNS and PNS [114]. Indications of acute arsenic intoxication include diarrhea, blood in the urine, vomiting, thirst, abdominal pain, headaches, dizziness, and finally death.

Chronic As exposure is connected with adverse health effects on more than a few body systems, involving the dermal, hepatic, nervous, renal, hematological, and cardiovascular systems. In chronic intoxication, arsenic accumulates in the hair, nails, epidermis (hyperpigmentation, skin cancer) and can be detected there [115]. When raised arsenic concentrations are taken up, it converts to monomethyl- and dimethyl-As compounds by the enzyme arsenite methyltransferase mainly in the liver and then is quickly excreted by the kidney [116]. Arsenate ions lower the levels of ATP by disrupting its formation *via* the biochemical process recognized as arsenolysis, thus producing As(III) ions. Arsenic(III) ions have a strong affinity towards thiol compounds and inhibit enzymes like pyruvate dehydrogenase which leads to the decrease of ATP in the cell cytoplasm [117].

As is one of the most extensively studied metals which induces ROS production and leads to OS. The exposure to As and its compounds produces superoxide radical ions and hydrogen peroxide in cellular systems as well as dimethylarsinic radical $(CH_3)_2As\bullet$, dimethylarsinic peroxyl radical $(CH_3)_2AsOO\bullet$, nitric oxide $NO\bullet$ and hydroxyl $\bullet OH$ radicals [118]. Arsenic is a known human carcinogenic element and inhaled or ingested As is involved in progress of some cancers (kidneys, skin, bladder, lungs, and liver) however, the exact mechanism by which As causes human cancer diseases is not clear. For the treatment of arsenic intoxication, some effective chelating agents like dimercaprol, DMPS, and DMSA have been recognized [119].

Antimony

The total mass fraction of antimony and bismuth in the human body is $1 \cdot 10^{-6}\%$. The biological role of Sb, apparently, is comparable to that of As. Arsenic As^{3+} cations, antimony Sb^{3+} cations, and in smaller degree Bi^{3+} cations are synergistic. It is identified that in regions with arsenic excess, there is a growth of not only As, but also Sb concentration in the body. If these two metals are accumulated in the thyroid, they inhibit the function of the thyroid gland which leads to goiter [120]. This synergism, typical for As and Sb, is dependent on by their ability to form bonds with sulfur-containing bioligands.

The water-soluble compounds of antimony, entering the body, exhibit a poisonous effect, comparable to the toxic impact of As compounds. Continued exposure to Sb is a serious risk for persons occupied in refuse incineration, smelting, refining, metal mining, coal-fired power plants, which leads to respiratory irritation, pneumoconiosis, Sb skin spots, and gastric indications [120]. The poisonous adverse effects of antimony compounds are pancreatitis and cardiotoxicity, usually detected in patients with HIV and leishmaniasis infection diseases [121].

Antimony compounds have previously played some medical role and have been applied in antiseptic treatments and as emetics. Currently, this element is considered toxic [120, 121], with an environmentally tolerable minimum value in the air around 0.5 mg/m^3 for the metallic antimony and its oxides.

Bismuth

Bismuth has no known biological role, and is not toxic. In nature, Bi occurs as a native metal and in some minerals. The main source of Bi is as a byproduct of refining Pb, Cu, Sn, Au, and Ag ores [3 - 5].

Although the metal is not toxic, possessing minimal threat to the ecosystems and up to 15 g can be tolerated by the adults, continuing use of Bi can lead to adverse effects and even harmfulness to humans [122, 123]. Bismuth crystals are safe to handle as they have a very low level of toxicity. Unlike Pb, Hg, Ni, or other metals, there is no significant health risk from fumes or from touching bismuth or ingesting small amounts. Bismuth at high levels taken by ingestion is poisonous. 90% of the ingested bismuth is excreted by urine, so the maximum amount of bismuth is observed in the kidneys. It has been confirmed that bismuth crosses the blood-brain barrier. Bismuth excess may cause nausea, weight and appetite loss, stomatitis, diarrhea, fever, headache, malaise, albuminuria, depression, sleeplessness, skin reactions, rheumatic pains and black lines may be formed on the gums in the mouth because of the bismuth sulfide deposition.

There are only limited statistics on the properties and fate of Bi compounds in living organisms and environment. They commonly have low solubility. Nevertheless, bismuth compounds must be handled with caution. Due to their low solubility, they are commonly poorly absorbed, around 0.2%, but soluble bismuth nitrate can be lethal at elevated serum levels. Bismuth, due to the enhancement of metallic properties, is more difficult to interact with sulfur-containing compounds. It reacts preferably with ligands that contain NH_2 groups. Therefore, Bi compounds inhibit the amino- and carboxypolipeptidaze enzymes, which may explain the toxicity of bismuth salts. Though generally harmless and well tolerated, with long-lasting use, Bi salts can lead to bismuth toxicity established as the cause of the reversible condition categorized by subacute development of myoclonus, encephalopathy, dysarthria, seizures, absence of coordination, parkinsonism indications, neuropsychiatric manifestations (psychosis, ataxia, delirium, myoclonus, and dementia) and acute renal failure by causing tubular necrosis. Many cases of nephrotoxicity have been reported [122]. Getting into the gastrointestinal tract, most Sb and Bi compounds almost do not demonstrate toxic effects. The main reason is that the salts of Sb(III) and Bi(III) in the gastrointestinal system are exposed to hydrolysis with the production of soluble substances which cannot be absorbed through the digestive tract.

Bismuth toxicity is reversible over several weeks or months, when bismuth intake is stopped. Bismuth is accumulated in membrane-bound vesicles in cell nuclei as "Bi inclusion bodies," but the biochemical character of these deposits is not known. The most severe adverse effects of Bi-containing medications were noted in the '60s and '70s, XX century, when outbreaks of encephalopathy were described [122]. The most effective antidotes used in the case of bismuth intoxication are compounds comprising sulfhydryl groups, aromatic hydroxyl groups, or suitably situated phosphonate groups. Of the compounds presently permitted for therapy, the chelators 2,3-dimercapto-1-propanesulfonic acid (DMPS) and D-penicillamine were proved to be the most effective antidotes for acute Bi intoxication. Bismuth(III) can interfere with the chemistry of Fe(III). Bi(III) binding constants for a wide range of oxygen and nitrogen donor ligands correlate with the values of similar constants in the case of Fe(III). Bismuth(III) binds strongly to transferrin, which transports Fe(III) ions.

Bi(III) compounds have been applied in the treatment of bacteria-related diseases in traditional Chinese medicine for more than two centuries [123]. Bi compounds are found in certain medicinal herbs that accumulate Bi. Some of Bi compounds are used to treat syphilis and some cancers. The most important use of Bi-containing substances is in the treatment of digestive syndromes. They not only have antimicrobial activity (against the bacterium *Helicobacter pylori*) but also seem to strengthen the gastric mucus and activate cytoprotective processes [124, 125].

When comparing the biological and chemical properties of the elements of the VA group, some conclusions can be drawn. Nitrogen binds to C and H atoms in biological molecules. Phosphorus is bonded preferably *via* O atoms. Arsenic, antimony, and bismuth usually bind to O and S donor groups. This results in the absence of mutual substitution of N and P, as well as the absence of replacement of these biogenic elements with arsenic, antimony, and bismuth. The first two elements of the group are vital for all the living organisms. Possibly arsenic can be a necessary element, simultaneously, the need of antimony and bismuth for living organisms is unidentified. The last three elements of the group are typically synergistic, blocking the -SH groups of biological ligands, and in huge amounts they may be very toxic. The observed positive biological role of As in micro amounts proposes that Sb and Bi may be also useful for living organisms.

p-Elements of the VIA Group

Oxygen

Oxygen, the single most important substance to life, enters almost all vital molecules. Oxygen is the most abundant nonmetal of the Earth by weight and the third most plentiful element in the universe (next to H and He) [3 - 5]. Oxygen is vital occurring in elemental state as dioxygen O_2 to support cell respiration. It is present in nature also in the form of ozone O_3, or in combined state in numerous minerals (oxides, aluminosilicates, carbonates). Oxygen reacts and forms compounds with practically all the other elements and displaces them from the compounds by chemical interactions. It is also a component of H_2O and a key constituent of almost all biomolecules (proteins, carbohydrates, *etc.*). Only a few anaerobic microorganisms can live lacking oxygen.

The volume fraction of oxygen in the air is 21%. Atmospheric O_2 comes practically entirely from photosynthesis [5]. Photosynthetic cells of green plants absorb sunny energy and use this energy to transfer electrons from H_2O to CO_2, producing carbohydrates (glucose) and releasing free O_2 into the atmosphere:

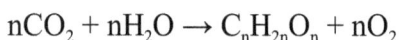

$$nCO_2 + nH_2O \rightarrow C_nH_{2n}O_n + nO_2$$

Oxygenic photosynthesis has formed the oxygen we breathe and most of the biomass. The oxygen content was enlarged throughout geological periods and became a hazard to green plants [5]. But, in contrast, the growing O_2 amounts formed the desirable environment for a novel type of living beings, animals. They exploited O_2 for their bioprocesses. Thus, an equilibrium has arisen with an atmosphere suitable for animals and plants, based on photosynthesis. The human behavior nowadays may disturb this balance. O_2 is crucial for life on the Earth and for the fate of humanity. Many life processes are associated with the oxygen content in the air. For example, "altitude sickness" is caused by a lack of oxygen in high-altitude conditions. A reduction of the partial pressure of oxygen in the air by 1/3 causes oxygen starvation and by 2/3 - death.

Oxygen is an essential biogenic macroelement and over half of the body mass consists of oxygen [6 - 10]. Its content in living organisms per dry matter is approximately 70%. In cells and tissues, oxygen is combined with C and H_2 in the bioorganic compounds which possess structural and metabolic functions. Oxygen is also a significant substrate for the construction or breakdown of numerous cellular constituents. Oxygen is the key center for the biologically active functional groups, such as hydroxyl, carbonyl, and carboxylate groups, essential in almost all biomolecules responsible for life. To supply oxygen from the atmosphere to the body, specific biomolecules namely Fe-containing proteins have been developed. Myoglobin serves as a carrier and store for O_2 in the muscle cells, and the Fe-containing protein hemoglobin transports it from the lungs to the blood and peripheral tissues.

Oxidation of nutrients (carbohydrates, proteins, fats) is a source of energy required for the work of organs and tissues of the living body [3 - 5]. Oxygen provides the body with the ability to recover and strengthen its immune system. Most of the oxygen introduced into the body is released in the form of CO_2, mainly through the lungs.

Oxygen is a nearly universal oxidizing agent (critical electron acceptor) in the biosystems. It is vital for the organisms that get energy by aerobic oxidation of H-rich nutrients. O_2 is crucial for cellular respiration in all aerobic organisms. In oxidation-reduction reactions, O_2 accepts electrons, which leads to the formation of ATP, the energy source for cell functions. In the inside mitochondrial membrane, electrons derived from diverse body fuels move *via* cascades of oxidation-reduction processes with O_2, reducing it to H_2O (respiratory chain) [3 - 5]. The reduction of O_2 catalyzed by cytochrome-*c*-oxidase forms O^{2-} anions and H_2O by accepting H^+ cations:

$$O_2 + 4e^- \rightarrow 2O^{2-}$$

$$2O^{2-} + 4H^+ \rightarrow 2H_2O$$

Simultaneously, a proton gradient is created that drives the ATP generation force, the direct source of energy required for cell functions.

In pathological conditions, an incomplete reduction occurs:

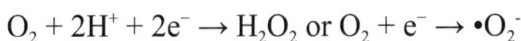

$$O_2 + 2H^+ + 2e^- \rightarrow H_2O_2 \text{ or } O_2 + e^- \rightarrow \cdot O_2^-$$

The obtained products (H_2O_2 and $\cdot O_2^-$) can be useful when they destroy uncontrollably growing cells, but they can also be very toxic when destroying the cell membranes of healthy cells in the body.

The homeostasis of oxygen is vital for the organism's survival. The human body has evolved to guarantee optimum oxygenation of the cells and tissues, starting with the O_2 entrance through the lung and continuing with the oxygen circulation and distribution inside the living body [126]. In organisms, oxygen enters the blood and binds to hemoglobin Hb, producing oxyhemoglobin HbO_2, that is readily dissociated. In blood, oxyhemoglobin passes into the capillaries of different organs. The bond between Hb and O_2 is not stable and is performed by donor-acceptor interaction with Fe^{2+} forming a complex $Hb(Fe^{2+})O_2$, where oxygen acts as a donor. The same kind of complexes can be formed by Cu^{2+} ions with hemocyanin, $He(Cu^{2+})O_2$, Cu-containing oxygen transport metalloproteins found in arthropods and mollusks. In the tissues, HbO_2 is transformed into hemoglobin and oxygen, used for the oxidation of various biologically active compounds. These bioreactions finally lead to the formation of the main metabolic products: CO_2, H_2O and energy.

Oxygen uses its oxidation capacity in many other metabolic processes, catalyzed by oxygenase or oxidase enzymes, such as hydroxylation, degradation of aromatic rings of amino acids, oxidative deamination of amines and amino acids.

The typical oxidation states of oxygen in biosystems range from 0 (in the O_2 molecule) to -2 (in H_2O) [3 - 10]. Oxygen takes part in different metabolic interactions in the organisms and throughout these processes it may form reactive oxygen species (ROS): singlet oxygen ($^1O_2$), hydroxyl radical (HO•), hydrogen peroxide (H_2O_2) and superoxide anion radical ($•O_2^-$). The ground stable state of dioxygen O_2 is a relatively unreactive triplet state ($^3O_2$), even though it is a strong oxidant. The excited and unstable state is a singlet oxygen $^1O_2$ and in contrast is very reactive and highly harmful killing cells, which is the base of photodynamic therapy. The decrease of O_2 amounts reduces the protective phagocytic functions of the body against the foreign pathogenic bacteria, fungi, malignant cells *etc*. In phagocytes, O_2 reduces to superoxide anion radical ($•O_2^-$):

$$O_2 + e^- = •O_2^-$$

Oxygen initiates the oxidation radical-chain reactions of foreign bioorganic compounds RH, captured by phagocytosis:

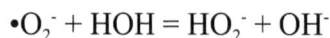

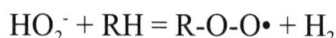

$$•O_2^- + HOH = HO_2^- + OH^-$$

$$HO_2^- + RH = R\text{-}O\text{-}O• + H_2$$

In the absence of O_2, these processes are delayed. As a result, the body's resistance to infection is reduced. Studying the role of reactive oxygen species for signaling functions is a significant research area [127].

The excess supply of O_2 (hyperoxia) leads to many unfavorable consequences, especially to the production of high concentrations of ROS (superoxide anion O_2^-, singlet oxygen $^1O_2$, hydrogen peroxide H_2O_2, hydroxyl radical HO•), causing damage to the organism [128]. Excess supplies of oxygen induce OS by disordering the equilibrium between antioxidants and oxidants. This OS results in damages to molecules such as proteins, DNA, and lipids, leading to numerous pathologies including cardiovascular diseases, HIV activation, cancer, neurodegenerative disorders, ageing, *etc*.

The deficiency of oxygen (hypoxia) is a chief factor for serious pathological conditions including myocardial and cerebral complications and cancer [129]. Tissue hypoxia and all severe consequences occur within a short time when breathing is stopped. In medical practice, inhalation of O_2-enriched air is used when either respiratory ventilation is limited or tissue hypoxia originates because of scarce blood circulation, anemia, *etc*.

Ozone

The allotropic form of oxygen is ozone O_3. The triatomic molecule of ozone is not stable and highly reactive. Ozone is a diamagnetic gas with a blue color and a typical pungent odor. Ozone is $1 \times 10^{-6}\%$ of the volume of air. 90% of its content is concentrated at an altitude of 10-50 km. The total ozone content in the atmosphere is 3-4 billion tons. The ozone layer thickness is on average 2-3 mm (at the equator about 2 mm, at the poles about 3 mm). With the distance from the Earth's surface, the concentration of ozone increases and reaches a maximum at an altitude of 20-25 km. Ozone as a component of the upper atmospheric layers, plays a significant role as an absorbing agent of UV radiation. Without the O_3 layer, the ultraviolet radiation would reach the surface of the Earth [5 - 10, 130].

Oxygen in atomic state can be released by the photochemical decomposition of NO_2. It combines with O_2 and forms O_3. At higher altitude in the stratosphere, some O_2 molecules are split into O atoms [5, 130]. Ozone formation in the atmosphere occurs as a result of electrostatic discharge (*hv*) in the presence of molecular O_2, illustrated by the reactions:

$$NO_2 \rightarrow \bullet NO + \bullet O$$

$$O_2 \rightarrow O + O$$

$$O + O_2 \rightarrow O_3$$

Ozone ensures the preservation of life on Earth, because the ozone layer delays the most detrimental to living organisms and plants part of the UV radiation of the Sun with a wavelength of less than 300 nm. Mass release of nitrogen oxides into the atmosphere as a result of flights of jet aircraft and the use of chlorofluorocarbons (CCl_3F, CCl_2F_2), so-called freons, can lead to a decrease in ozone content in the atmosphere. Affected by the UV sunlight rays, freons decompose and Cl atoms are released [3 - 5, 130]. They catalyze the breakdown of O_3, creating the so-called ozone holes, a phenomenon observed particularly over the Antarctic. O_3 is a summertime contaminant and a major constituent of summer smog. Ozone absorbs not only UV but also IR radiation contributing to the greenhouse effect. Increased intensity of UV light, as a consequence of the "ozone holes", influences negatively the Earth's biosystems and is in close connection with the frequency of malignant melanoma, a form of human skin cancer, and eye disease.

Ozone is a very toxic and harmful substance to human organisms, animals, and plants. The maximum permissible ozone concentration in the air of the working places is 0.1 mg/m^3. Inhalation of air with ozone concentration of 0.002 - 0.02

mg/l causes irritation of the respiratory system, cough, vomiting, asthma, emphysema, bronchitis, dizziness and fatigue. It can be also neurotoxic. Sources of ozone are working copiers and laser printers, as well as sources of ultraviolet and X-ray radiation [130]. High-level ozone is a serious air pollutant with damaging effects. Ground-level O_3 also accelerates the aging of plants and causes fragility in plastic and rubber materials.

In the human body, O_3 can be hazardous or beneficial, which depends on the route of exposition and on its quantity. Ozone is a strong oxidizing agent and at low concentrations it eliminates microbes in air and water [131]. This is the base of O_3 usage in the sterilization of drinking water. It can be used also for air purification, for degradation of toxins in food, *etc.* [132]. Low concentrations of ozone in the air create a feeling of freshness. Small doses of ozone are used in the surface caries treatment, in the treatment of chronic wounds, and epithelization. Inhalation exposure to continued high levels of ozone damages the respiratory tract.

Being the strongest oxidizing agent (second after fluorine), ozone intensively oxidizes amino acids and enzymes containing sulfur (cysteine $HSCH_2$ $CH(NH_2)COOH$, methionine CH_3 SCH_2CH_2CH $(NH_2)COOH$, as well as tryptophan $C_8H_6NCH_2CH(NH_2)$ $COOH$, histidine C_3 H_3N_2 $CH(NH_2)$ $COOH$, tyrosine HOC_6 H_4CH_2CH $(NH_2)COOH$ [130 - 132]. The oxidizing and toxic effect of O_3 on bioorganic substances is connected with the free radicals' formation:

$$RH + O_3 = RO_2 + HO\bullet$$

The obtained radicals initiate radical-chain processes in biomolecules, including proteins, DNA, and lipids. These processes lead to cells damage and death. Drugs against ozone and free radicals' intoxication are effective antioxidants, for instance, vitamins C and E [3 - 5, 130].

Accordingly, molecular oxygen O_2 is not toxic to living organisms unlike other forms such as ozone, excited molecule $O_2\bullet$, radical $OH\bullet$, atomic O, radicals $\bullet O_2^-$ and $HO_2\bullet$.

Compounds of Oxygen and Hydrogen

Water

It is worth mentioning that H_2O is the major molecule found in living systems, constituting over 50-60% of the organisms' weight [3, 4].

Hydrogen bonds (H-bonds) provide many of the critical life-sustaining properties of water [20, 133]. They strongly affect its properties. The melting point (0°C) and boiling point (100°C) of water are significantly higher than expected. If no H-bonds were acting among H_2O molecules, the water is expected to crystallize at around -100 °C and boil at -80 °C. One H_2O molecule binds to four neighboring H_2O molecules through H-bonds forming a tetrahedral arrangement with a rigid, open, and less dense structure in the solid state of water. This is the reason for the greater viscosity of liquid water. These properties explain why ice floats on water, and how fish can survive at the bottom of a frozen pond over the winter. This allows water to dissolve various molecules. These facts are of paramount importance for the survival of life. The biomolecules of living matter (proteins, DNA, lipids, *etc.*) have complex structures. In the interactions, some bonds in biomolecules must be readily broken and changed. The H-bonds energy is of a magnitude which allows such interactions [134]. Hydrogen bonds are important for the formation of the secondary structure of proteins, holding the biological macromolecules in a specific three-dimensional arrangement that determine the particular biological functions.

The exceptional physical properties of water, including its ability to dissolve numerous low and high molecular weight life-supporting substances, originate from the dipolar H_2O molecule and its excellent capacity to form H-bonds [20, 134]. These features influence the structures and functions of vital biomolecules. H_2O is a universal solvent for inorganic and organic compounds. Being a weak electrolyte H_2O can act as an ampholyte. It ionizes to a small degree (as a weak acid or a weak base) to form H_3O^+ cation and OH^- anion:

$$2H_2O \rightleftarrows H_3O^+ + OH^-$$

Water is essential to acid-base balance of the organisms with a stabilizing buffering capacity which keeps the stability of the internal environment of cells. In the form of hydration water, it is a structural constituent of biomacromolecules. Water is also an activator of many biochemical reactions [133 - 135]. It is a substratum or product of bioreactions like photosynthesis, cellular respiration, *etc.* Water helps to regulate temperature of the organism. Water balance (intake and excretion) is regulated by hormones, such as antidiuretic hormone (ADH, vasopressin), the steroid hormone aldosterone, and atrial natriuretic peptide ANP.

The H-bonds in H_2O molecules reproduce freezing and boiling temperature changes, determining the unique features in its solid, liquid and gaseous state. A small heating (up to 50-60 °C) results to the denaturation of proteins and stops the functioning of living systems. Meanwhile, cooling to complete freezing and even to absolute zero does not lead to denaturation and does not violate the configuration of the biomolecule system, so that the vital function is preserved. This position is essential for the preservation of organs and tissues intended for transplantation. Water in the solid state has a different ordering of molecules than in the liquid and after freezing and melting acquires slightly different biological properties, which is the reason for the use of melt water for therapeutic purposes [135]. After melting, water has a more ordered structure, with the nuclei of clathrates of ice, which allows it to interact with biological components and dissolved substances at a different rate. When using melt water, small centers of an ice-like structure enter the organism, which in the future can grow and transfer the water to an ice-like state and thereby produce a healing effect.

Hydrogen Peroxide

Hydrogen peroxide (H-O-O-H) is almost colorless or pale blue in the liquid state. It is less volatile than H_2O and to some extent denser and more viscous. Mixes of H_2O_2 with organic readily oxidized materials are hazardously explosive. In hydrogen peroxide molecule, the oxidation state of oxygen is -1. This oxidation state is intermediate between 0 for O_2 and -2 for H_2O. This means that H_2O_2 can act either as an oxidant or a reducer [22]. It decomposes spontaneously to H_2O and O_2. This is a reaction of disproportionation:

$$2H_2O_2 \rightarrow 2H_2O + O_2$$

This decomposition is accelerated by peroxidases, predominantly by catalase, abundant in the blood. The organism produces H_2O_2 as a byproduct of oxidation-reduction metabolic processes. As H_2O_2 belongs to ROS, playing an imperative role in Fenton reaction, it can be rapidly transformed into less hazardous compounds [136]. Consequently, the organism has evolved different enzymes to avoid OS produced by H_2O_2 and further ROS.

Hydrogen peroxide exposes broad-spectrum activity against various microorganisms. In addition to the role of H_2O_2 as a destructive oxidant to protect the body from pathogens, it serves as a "secondary messenger" [137].

Reactive Oxygen Species (ROS)

ROS are a subcategory of free radicals containing oxygen [138]. They can be produced by a range of bioprocesses involving aerobic metabolism and pathogenic defense mechanisms. They occur as a result of outside exposure (radiation, contaminants, cigarette smoke). The ROS include superoxide anion radical $\cdot O_2^-$, singlet oxygen $^1O_2$, hydroxyl radical $\cdot OH$, and perhydroxyl radical $HO_2\cdot$. Partially reduced anions ($\cdot O_2^-$ and O_2^{2-}) are produced by numerous bioreactions in cells. Other ROS ($\cdot OH$ and $^1O_2$) arise from these anions by unfavorable oxidation. The most aggressive of ROS are $\cdot OH$ and $^1O_2$. They cause peroxidation of polyunsaturated fatty acids (PUFAs), changing the cell membranes functions. In proteins, they oxidize sulfhydryl groups of amino acids. In DNA, ROS can attack the nucleotide bases or alter the sugar constituent following DNA fragmentation thus changing the genetic information. The antibacterial and cytotoxic properties are among the positive effects of ROS.

Superoxide anion-radical ($\cdot O_2^-$) is a result of one-electron reduction of O_2:

$$O_2 + e^- \rightarrow \cdot O_2^-$$

Superoxide anion radical is stable and not reactive, but its production generates subsequent processes of O_2^- to other ROS, *viz.* $\cdot OH$, H_2O_2 and $^1O_2$. In living organisms, this radical is produced from oxygen molecules by NADPH oxidase, xanthine oxidase, nitric oxide synthase (NOS), lipoxygenase enzymes and mitochondrial electron transfer systems [139]. Superoxide is generated from various sources. It is commonly produced throughout nonenzymatic oxidation reactions of certain compounds by O_2, for example, oxidation of ubiquinone, hydroquinones, semiquinones, thiols, flavines, hemo- and glycated proteins:

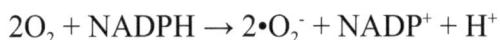

$$2O_2 + NADPH \rightarrow 2\cdot O_2^- + NADP^+ + H^+$$

NOS enzymes convert L-arginine to L-citrulline [100] by the same reaction of NADPH (Fig. **4**) and oxygen and thus produce NO, as shown above:

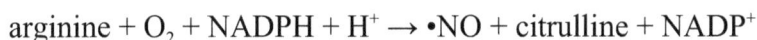

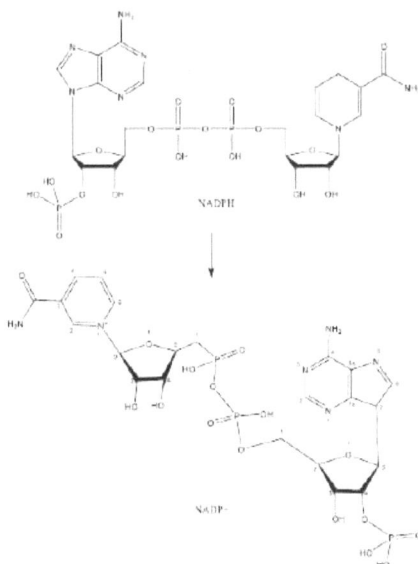

$$arginine + O_2 + NADPH + H^+ \rightarrow \cdot NO + citrulline + NADP^+$$

Fig. (4). Reaction NADPH $\rightarrow$ NADP$^+$.

Alternatively, in the bioreaction catalyzed by xanthine oxidase, the superoxide anion radical is formed in cells with ischemic reperfusion conditions, that is an illustration of the negative effects of $\cdot O_2^-$ production [138].

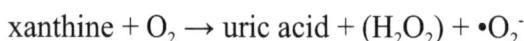

xanthine + O_2 → uric acid + (H_2O_2) + $\cdot O_2^-$

Nevertheless, the production of $\cdot O_2^-$ is necessary through phagocytosis, which leads to favorable antibacterial or cytotoxic effect.

The protonated form ($HO_2\cdot$) is more reactive than non-protonated form ($\cdot O_2^-$) and causes DNA damage [138].

The most significant protection against $\cdot O_2^-$ is its dismutation to O_2 and H_2O_2 catalyzed by the enzyme superoxide dismutase (SOD) [138, 139]:

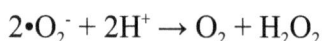

$2\cdot O_2^- + 2H^+ \rightarrow O_2 + H_2O_2$

However, in the presence of NO, which is produced by activated NO-synthase, $\cdot O_2^-$ forms peroxynitrite, one of the highly reactive RNS.

Hydroxyl radical ($\cdot OH$) is typically formed in the Fenton reaction in cells from hydrogen peroxide and free Fe^{2+} or Cu^+ cations [138 - 140]:

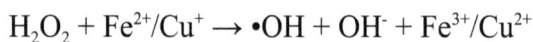

$H_2O_2 + Fe^{2+}/Cu^+ \rightarrow \cdot OH + OH^- + Fe^{3+}/Cu^{2+}$

Frequently, the toxicity of $\cdot O_2^-$ is attributed to its capability to reduce metal cations and subsequent re-oxidation of the metal by H_2O_2 yields harmful oxidizing species [138 - 140]. Superoxide promotes hydroxyl radicals' formation and consequent DNA damage in cells of all types. $\cdot OH$ is produced from $\cdot O_2^-$ and H_2O_2 in the availability of reduced metal cations M^{n+}, like Fe^{2+} and Cu^+:

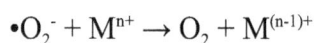

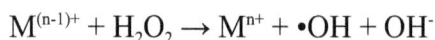

$\cdot O_2^- + M^{n+} \rightarrow O_2 + M^{(n-1)+}$

$M^{(n-1)+} + H_2O_2 \rightarrow M^{n+} + \cdot OH + OH^-$

In phagocytes, $\cdot OH$ is formed at respiratory bursts even in the lack of metal cations, if $\cdot O_2^-$ reacts with NO or with ClO^-.

The $\cdot OH$ radical is highly reactive and its damaging effects can be observed near the place of its origin [140]. It eliminates H atoms from many biomolecules or binds to them. In these cases, secondary reactive free radicals (peroxyl $ROO\cdot$, alkoxyl $RO\cdot$, alkanyl $R\cdot$) are formed. Additional reactions initiate new radicals' production or terminate their formation, if radicals with free electrons bind to each other by covalent bonds in biomolecules. The hydroxyl radical is carcinogenic and reacts extensively with nearly every type of molecules existing in living cells, like lipids, amino acids, nucleotides, and sugars. Hydroxyl radical is the most toxic ROS because of its high reactivity. There are no endogenous antioxidants which could remove it.

Singlet oxygen ($^1O_2$) is the lowest excited state of the dioxygen molecule [138 - 141]. The highly reactive singlet oxygen is produced in the body at excitation of the normal triplet dioxygen $^3O_2$. *In vitro*, $^1O_2$ can be produced through photosensitization processes. The photosensitizer absorbs H^+ to form excitation state with a following energy transfer to O_2 leading to the formation of $^1O_2$. Such phenomenon is successfully used in the photodynamic therapy of tumors. Singlet oxygen can be formed in the reaction of $\cdot O_2^-$ anion radical with $\cdot OH$:

$$\cdot O_2^- + \cdot OH + H^+ \rightarrow H_2O + {}^1O_2$$

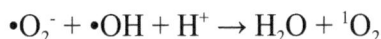

$^1O_2$ is also produced in the interaction of ClO^- anion with H_2O_2, significant in leukocytes in the myeloperoxidase microbicidal system:

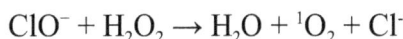

$$ClO^- + H_2O_2 \rightarrow H_2O + {}^1O_2 + Cl^-$$

$^1O_2$ can be formed in the troposphere by the photolysis of O_3 by rays of short wavelength. At excessive quantities, singlet oxygen induces OS and displays carcinogenic effect owing to the oxidation of fatty acids in lipids, cholesterol, nucleic acids, and proteins reacting mostly with unsaturated biomolecules with double bonds [141].

Hydrogen peroxide is also included in the group of ROS although it is not a radical. In the cells, H_2O_2 is a product of two-electron reduction of O_2 in dehydrogenation processes catalyzed by oxidases. The coenzyme flavin adenine dinucleotide (FAD) transfers H atoms of the substrate to O_2 producing H_2O_2. SOD as an antioxidant protein catalyzes the dismutation of O_2^- to H_2O_2, that is further detoxified to H_2O and O_2 by the enzymes catalase, glutathione peroxidase (GPx), and peroxiredoxins (Prx) [22, 137].

Hydrogen peroxide is less reactive than other ROS. It can diffuse through phospholipid membranes and oxidize -SH groups of enzymes, thus inhibiting their activity [22]. H_2O_2 can readily interact with free Fe or Cu by Fenton reaction to form $\cdot OH$, which is an extremely reactive radical with a short half-life:

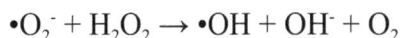

$$\cdot O_2^- + H_2O_2 \rightarrow \cdot OH + OH^- + O_2$$

In phagocytosis, H_2O_2 oxidizes chloride anions to hypochlorite anions in the reaction catalyzed by myeloperoxidase:

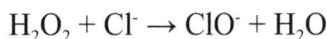

$$H_2O_2 + Cl^- \rightarrow ClO^- + H_2O$$

Hypochlorite ions thus produced exhibit bactericidal properties [142].

Oxidative Stress

Oxidative stress is a phenomenon that arises as a result of the imbalance between the free radicals and antioxidants. This disorder is either due to the increase of the production and accumulation of ROS caused by external factors or some pathologies (primarily inflammation), or due to the lower ability of the biological system to detoxify and eliminate ROS [143]. OS is associated with altered redox regulation of cell signaling pathways and the formation of cancerous cells. There are numerous external inducing factors as pollution, extreme exposure to ionizing radiation, xenobiotics taken up with processed food, high in fat and sugar, insufficient amounts of antioxidants in the diet, *etc.* However, under physiological conditions, there is a balance between the ROS formation and the defensive antioxidant mechanisms, which retain low ROS concentrations.

Protective Antioxidant Systems

Inhibiting oxidative harm by adding antioxidants is a therapeutic strategy for reducing the risk of oxidative stress [136 - 143]. The antioxidant molecules are sufficiently stable to donate electrons to the raging free radicals and neutralize them, to delay or stop the chain processes, thus reducing the damaging capacity of the free radicals. The antioxidants work principally thanks to their free radical scavenging capacity. So, they are often good reducers like polyphenols, thiols *etc.* The evolution and development of organisms, comprising their adaptation to take advantage of the antioxidant mechanisms, have protected aerobic organisms against the ROS toxicity. There are certain antioxidant systems and approaches in the organism which act in various ways: antioxidant enzymes, nonenzymatic high-molecular weight compounds, low-molecular antioxidant agents, and compounds binding metal cations.

High-molecular weight antioxidant agents include enzymes like superoxide dismutase, catalase, peroxidases, and nonenzymatic proteinaceous antioxidant compounds such as ceruloplasmin, transferrin, albumin.

Enzyme antioxidant agents are essential in the intracellular space [136 - 143]. In the protective way, antioxidant enzymes (superoxide dismutase, catalase, and glutathione peroxidase) hinder the ROS production and prevent oxidation processes by lowering the rate of chain reactions. This can be done by scavenging ROS or by binding radicals with transition metal cations (Cu, Fe). Enzymes with antioxidant properties are the primary systems in the organism which directly eliminate radicals. The summary of ROS eliminated by these enzymes is presented in Table **4**.

Table 4. Antioxidant enzymes.

Enzyme antioxidants	ROS eliminated
Superoxide dismutases (SOD)	$\cdot O_2^-$
Glutathione peroxidases (GPX)	H_2O_2, hydroperoxides of lipids
Catalase	H_2O_2
Glutathione-S-transferases (GST)	H_2O_2, peroxides, organic hydroperoxides

Three isoforms of SOD are available in mammals, *viz.,* mitochondrial Mn-SOD, cytosolic Cu,Zn-SOD and extracellular SOD (EC-SOD). The role of SOD is to scavenge superoxide radicals. This enzyme catalyzes the decomposition of $\cdot O_2^-$ into O_2 and H_2O_2. In the absence of SOD, the dismutation reaction turns out to be very slow [144].

Glutathione system includes glutathione peroxidase (GPX), glutathione S-transferase (GST), and glutathione reductase (GR). The role of glutathione peroxidases is realized through the reduction of H_2O_2, lipid hydroperoxide, and additional organic hydroperoxides. GPX cooperate with tripeptide glutathione (GSH) existing at comparatively high mM concentration in cells [136 - 145]. The substrates for GPX reactions are hydrogen peroxide or organic peroxides. GPX breaks down peroxides to H_2O or alcohol and simultaneously it is oxidized from GSH to GSSG.

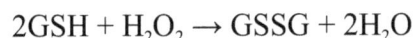

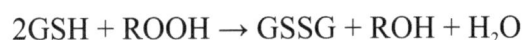

$$2GSH + H_2O_2 \rightarrow GSSG + 2H_2O$$

$$2GSH + ROOH \rightarrow GSSG + ROH + H_2O$$

Glutathione reductase activates the reduction of GSSG to GSH which enables the cell to tolerate right levels of GSH.

Glutathione-S-transferases are a key enzyme group, that take part in the detoxification of xenobiotic, cytotoxic, genotoxic compounds in cells and in the tissue protection against oxidative damaging [145]. Certain GST iso-enzymes can exhibit GPX action and catalyze the organic hydroperoxides reduction to the corresponding alcohols.

Catalase (H_2O_2 oxidoreductase) reduces the accumulation of hydrogen peroxide. This enzyme contains four polypeptide chains with four porphyrin heme (Fe) groups which allow this enzyme to interact with H_2O_2.

For optimum catalytic activity, the trace metals, like Cu, Fe, Mn, Se, Zn, work as cofactors of antioxidant enzymes to defend the body from ROS produced throughout OS [136 - 144], for example Cu/Zn superoxide dismutase, Se-independent glutathione-peroxidase, Se-dependent glutathione-peroxidase *etc.*

Non-enzymatic high-molecular weight anti oxidant compounds include ceruloplasmin, transferrin, and albumin [146 - 152]. Ceruloplasmin eliminates superoxide radicals $\bullet O_2^-$, and is active in the oxidation of Fe^{2+} and inactivation of Cu^{2+}. Transferrin is a chelator of Fe^{3+}. Albumin has a detoxifying effect on hydroperoxides of fatty acids.

Table 5. Low-molecular lipophilic antioxidants and the main detoxifying effects.

Lipophilic antioxidants	ROS eliminated
Tocopherol (vitamin E)	$\bullet OH$, $ROO\bullet$
β-Carotene (provitamin A), lycopene, *etc.* carotenoids	$\bullet OH$, $^1O_2$
Xanthophyl	$\bullet O_2^-$, H_2O_2, $\bullet OH$
Ubiquinol (coenzyme Q)	Peroxyl radical

Low-molecular antioxidant agents reduce ROS quantities [146 - 152]. Some of them could be regenerated to the active reducing forms. Consistent with their structures and polarity, these antioxidants can be classified into two groups - lipophilic and hydrophilic. The natural low-molecular antioxidant agents are given in Tables **5** and **6**.

The most active low molecular lipophilic antioxidant agents are alpha-tocopherols. Vitamin E can terminate radical chain reactions with peroxyl radicals $ROO\bullet$ or to capture directly some ROS like $HO\bullet$. Vitamin E acts in synergy with vitamin C. It has been reported to protect cell membrane from oxidation by eliminating ROS intermediates and by interacting with lipid radicals [146].

Carotenoids, pigments of vegetal or microbial origin, can interact with $^1O_2$ and return the excited O_2 molecule to the basic energy state. Carotenoids may also directly capture ROS. Between the naturally occurring carotenoids, the most biologically effective agent is lycopene. The antioxidative ability of Vitamin A is negligible. Carotenoids exist in the liver, milk, butter, egg yolk, carrots, spinach, tomato, and grains [146 - 152].

Xanthophylls have the ability to act as chain-breaking antioxidants in the peroxidation of membranous phospholipids.

Coenzyme Q (CoQ), a 1,4-benzoquinone, is related with the production of free radicals in mitochondria (as a prooxidant) and with their elimination (as an antioxidant). CoQ inhibits the initiation and distribution of protein and lipid oxidation. It is able to regenerate other antioxidants like vitamin E. CoQ prevents the oxidation of low-density lipoprotein (LDL), known as "bad cholesterol", providing a beneficial effect in cardiovascular disease. The best-known coenzyme Q in the human mitochondria is CoQ10 [146 - 152].

Table 6. Low-molecular hydrophilic antioxidants and the main detoxifying effects.

Hydrophilic antioxidants	ROS eliminated
L-Ascorbate (vitamin C)	$\bullet O_2^-$, $\bullet OH$, $^1O_2$, organic radicals
Flavonoids	H_2O_2, $\bullet OH$, $^1O_2$
Uric acid	$\bullet O_2^-$, $\bullet OH$, $^1O_2$, chelator of metal ions
Glutathione (GSH)	$\bullet OH$, $^1O_2$
Lipoate	$\bullet O_2^-$, $\bullet OH$
Thiols (cysteine)	$\bullet O_2^-$, $^1O_2$
Bilirubin (bound to proteins)	Peroxyl radical

Ascorbic acid has numerous antioxidant properties in human plasma. Its antioxidant effect is firmly limited by the existence of transition metal ions [147]. In the existence of metal ions, ascorbate behaves as a prooxidant. Ascorbic acid occurs in plants and animals, nonetheless it should be obtained from the food since it cannot be produced in humans.

Natural flavonoids (quercetin, catechin) or other phenolic and polyphenolic compounds (ferulic acid, caffeic acid, resveratrol), which are widespread in the plant realm, also contribute to the body antioxidant capacity. They show activity in hydrophilic and lipophilic locations. Their antioxidant action depends on the number and positions of the phenolic -OH groups in their molecules. The beneficial effect of flavonoids on the body is revealed in several ways - along with the antioxidant effect *via* stimulation of SOD and GPX antioxidant enzymes, flavonoids possess also a vasodilating, anti-inflammatory, antithrombotic, antiapoptotic and antimutagenic effects [148]. Flavonoids are found widely in beverages and foods, such as vegetables, fruit, cocoas, red wine and tea. The antioxidant activity of phenolic compounds is related to numerous different mechanisms, for instance free radical scavenging, singlet oxygen quenching, H-donation, metal cation chelating and acting as substrates for ROS such as $\bullet O_2^-$ and $\bullet OH$ radicals.

Uric acid, found in human plasma at mM concentrations, is a significant trapper of $\bullet O_2^-$ and $\bullet OH$, quencher of $^1O_2$ and chelator of transition metal ions [149]. It stabilizes ascorbate in human serum at physiological conditions, attributed to its good chelating ability.

The cellular antioxidant glutathione (GSH) plays a substantial role in the protection against OS, being a cofactor of some enzymes, such as glutathione peroxidases, glutathione transferases, dehydroascorbate reductases. GSH directly captures •OH and $^1O_2$, reduces the tocopheryl radical, detoxifies hydrogen peroxide and lipoperoxides through the catalytic effect of glutathione peroxidase [150].

The redox potential of alpha-lipoic acid and its reduced form, dihydrolipoic acid suggests their potent antioxidant potential as direct scavengers of ROS (•O_2^-, •OH) and RNS species.

Thiols can act as electron acceptors, reducing unstable free radicals (•O_2^-, $^1O_2$) by oxidizing, consequently they are powerful antioxidants [151]. Protein- and nonprotein-thiols are working as cellular reducing and protecting agents against many inorganic toxins through -SH groups.

Bilirubin, the end product of heme catabolism in mammals, has been reported to cause powerful antioxidant and cytoprotective effect which regulates cellular redox reactions, decreases ROS and reduces the NADPH oxidase activity [152]. It efficiently scavenges peroxyl radicals. In humans, bilirubin is found in plasma at micromolar concentration and helps prevent the progression of cardiovascular disease. It plays an antioxidant role in newborns.

The above shown soluble in water antioxidants carry out their actions inside and outside the cellular fluids, while fat-soluble antioxidants act mainly in the cell membranes [146 - 152].

Substances decreasing the availability of Fe^{2+} and Cu^+ cations. The reduced cations of Fe and Cu participate in the Fenton reaction and in the formation of •OH radicals [136]. The examples of substances decreasing the amount of reduced ions are low-molecular (some chelating agents) and high-molecular (proteins like ceruloplasmin) compounds.

Sulfur

Sulfur is one of the six essential organogens (C, H, N, O, S, and P) whose atoms make up the bulk of many important organic biomolecules and inorganic compounds [3 - 5]. It is chemically active and reacts with all metals of the periodic table except Au and Pt, producing sulfides and forming compounds with some of the nonmetals. Sulfur is around 0.2% ($\approx$ 160 g) of the total weight of the body, like K. Connective tissue, hair, skin, and nails are specifically rich in S. In the body, sulfur, similar to phosphorus, acts as an agent for the transfer of groups and energy. In biological systems, almost all group and energy transfer reactions are carried out not only by organic phosphates, but also by organic sulfur-containing compounds.

Plants are able to synthesize S-containing amino acids, but animals are not. Animals absorb S-containing proteins stored in plants [3 - 5]. Inorganic sulfur compounds do not compensate the need for sulfur when eating. Interestingly, some photosynthetic bacteria like green sulfur bacteria emit S, an oxidation product of H_2S, by the reaction of H_2S and CO_2, thus forming carbohydrates $C_x(H_2O)_y$:

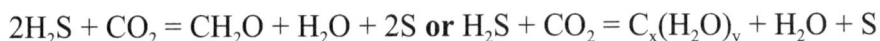

$$2H_2S + CO_2 = CH_2O + H_2O + 2S \text{ or } H_2S + CO_2 = C_x(H_2O)_y + H_2O + S$$

Some bacteria form organic substances from CO_2 without solar energy supply. As an alternative, the energy is obtained by the oxidation of S, H_2S, or H_2. Some bacteria are capable of oxidizing sulfides and polysulfides, for example, *Thiobacillus ferrooxidans*, growing by oxidizing iron pyrite FeS_2, not only to free sulfur, but also to thiosulfate ions at a noticeable rate. Another species is *Thiotrix*, a S-oxidizing bacterium. These microorganism types are called lithotrophs. They are rather independent of the sunlight and are adapted to live on the ocean floor, in rocks, *etc.* [153].

Sulfur is involved in many oxidation reduction processes having oxidation states extending from -2 (in sulfide) to +6 (in sulfate). Hence, S compounds act as donors or acceptors in metabolic processes [3,4,154]. Just as there are C, N, and P cycles, so there is a S cycle in nature. Under the normal pH, SO_4^{2-} ion is thermodynamically preferred:

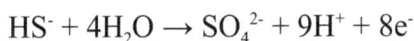

$$HS^- + 4H_2O \rightarrow SO_4^{2-} + 9H^+ + 8e^-$$

If sulfur(VI) is thermodynamically favored, the question is - why S^{2-} is such a common ion? The living organisms achieve the reduction by combining it with a strong thermodynamically preferred oxidation to produce a net negative ΔG value. A characteristic example is the carbohydrates oxidation to CO_2:

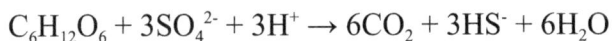

$$C_6H_{12}O_6 + 3SO_4^{2-} + 3H^+ \rightarrow 6CO_2 + 3HS^- + 6H_2O$$

Sulfur-based organic compounds with an oxidation state of -2, mostly thiols, forming disulfides by oxidation, have a critical biological role. Compounds with S^{-2} ions are catabolized to SO_4^{2-} anions existing in all biological fluids. Cellularly, SO_4^{2-} is activated to 3'-phosphoadenosine-5'-phosphosulfate (PAPS), useful in sulphatation reactions for the production of sulpho esters. The rest of the SO_4^{2-} anions are excreted through the kidney. Chemical properties, variety of oxidation states, redox potentials, and multifunctional reactivity make sulphur ideal for oxidation-reduction biological reactions and electron transfer processes [154].

Sulfur is a constituent of many important biomolecules. The -SH group actively participates in the construction of proteins and forms S-bonds or bridges between the peptide residues. In the biosphere, sulfur forms compounds close to natural inorganic polysulfides [3,4,6-10,154]. These are various proteins with bridged S-S, for example, methionine, lipoic acid, glutathione, thiamine, coenzyme A, *etc.* In the body of animals and humans, sulfur is present mainly in proteins in the composition of S-based amino acids - cysteine (Cys) and methionine (Met). Cysteine ($HSCH_2CH(NH_3^+)COO^-$) is essential for the structures and enzymatic activity of proteins. The presence of paired cysteine residues causes the formation of disulfide (-S-S-) bonds that determine the spatial structure of proteins. Disulfide bonds between Cys residues are also essential for protein stability. For illustration, -S-S-bonds (sulfur bridges) are primarily responsible for the mechanical strength and low solubility of keratins, which promote the formation of tissues of hair, nails, and skin. Cysteine is biosynthesized in humans and takes part in enzyme processes as a nucleophile. The sulfhydryl (thiol) groups (-SH) of cysteine are an integral part of the active sites of many enzymes. Sulfhydryl groups react with free radicals like OH• formed as a result of the action of ionizing radiation on water and aqueous solutions:

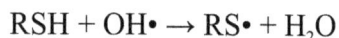

$$RSH + OH• \rightarrow RS• + H_2O$$

The produced RS• radicals are inactive. Therefore, substances containing sulfhydryl groups or disulfide bonds (for example, cysteamine, cystamine) are used as radioprotective substances.

Methionine ($HO_2CCHCH_2CH_2SCH_3$), the thioether amino acid, is the principal CH_3-group donor. It plays a critical role in regulating metabolic processes, initiating protein synthesis and in redox reactions that protect proteins integrity, as well as in immune system and digestive functioning in mammals [155]. Methionine can convert into several sulfur-containing molecules critical for the normal functions of the cells, such as glutathione, taurine, S-adenosylmethionine (SAM) and creatine. Although S and O belong to the same group, Met and Cys analogues with the S-atom replaced by O-atom do not perform equal functions. Sulfur possesses unique properties, different from those of its chemical analogue oxygen.

Glutathione, a significant intracellular S-containing tripeptide (γ-glutamyl cysteinyl-glycine), is in the group of low-molecular weight antioxidant agents against toxic xenobiotics - drugs, pollutants, and carcinogens. GSH is a cofactor of the cellular enzymes glutathione peroxidases (GPX) [156]. As an antioxidant, GSH is easily oxidized by ROS and RNS species to glutathione disulfide. The pair GSH/GSSG is the main redox couple which regulates the antioxidant capability of cells. Many proteins and enzymes like glutathione reductase, peroxiredoxin, thioredoxin, and thioredoxin reductase contain S and take part in redox signaling.

Sulphur is one of the key constituents in Fe/S cluster proteins (Rieske proteins, ferredoxins, and rubredoxins) that participate in electron transfers in biosystems [3,4,6-10]. Hydrogen sulfide is omnipresent in ferredoxins (Fe/S redox proteins). The iron/sulfur clusters are collected in mitochondria, transferred and incorporated in ferredoxins.

Sulfur is existing in α-lipoic acid and coenzyme A (used for the synthesis of S-acetyl lipoate and acetyl-CoA) and in the structure of two B vitamins (thiamine and biotin). Other sulfur-containing biological molecules include many antibiotics, such as penicillin, cephalosporins, and sulfanilamide [3,4,6-10]. Sulfur is also a component of mucopolysaccharides, taurocholic acid, sulfocyanides, indoxyl sulfate, chondroitin sulfate, keratan sulfate, heparin, insulin, melanin, anterior pituitary hormone and many others.

In the body, the sulfur of the SH-group under the action of oxidative enzymes passes into groups SO_4^{2-}, $S_2O_3^{2-}$, $S_4O_6^{2-}$, S_8. Of these oxidation processes of sulfhydryl groups, the most important is the synthesis of endogenous sulfuric acid, which takes part in the neutralization of toxic compounds formed in the intestines from amino acids (poisonous phenol, cresol, skatole, indole), as well as foreign compounds, for example, drugs, *etc.* Sulfuric acid also binds xenobiotics (foreign proteins) due to the formation of conjugate - esters of sulfuric acid [3,6-10]. It is noteworthy that in the analysis of urine the content of H_2SO_4 is significant, which characterizes the process of decay of proteins in the intestine under the action of microbes.

Sulfur is a crucial coordination site in proteins for metal cations. The toxicity of heavy metals Pb, Cd, and Hg can be explained by the interaction of these metals with S in proteins. They occupy places where there is usually no metal or can remove and substitute the vital metals (iron) from their positions. In the liver, specifically rich in Cys groups, metallothionein, which may be produced as a scavenging agent for toxicants [4,6-10]. Sulfur of any amino acid functional group has affinity and binds to the widest range of metal ions, such as Zn(II), Cu(I), Cu(II), Fe(II), Fe(III), Mo(IV)-(VI) and Ni(I)-(III).

Sulfur deficiency in the body can cause a variety of conditions including acne, rashes, brittle nails, depressions, memory loss, arthritis, digestive problems, *etc.*

Constant high sulfur exposure leads to asthma-like allergenic complications. Longer exposure causes asthma attacks, breath shortness, coughing, wheezing, *etc.* [3, 4].

Elemental S is not poisonous, but many inorganic sulfur compounds, like SO_2 and H_2S, are toxic [3,4,6]. Sulfur poisonousness is mostly associated with high levels of the element and its toxic volatile compounds in the environment. Some disorders of sulfur metabolism can also affect people.

The radioactive sulfur nuclide ^{35}S finds practical application in scientific research [3, 4]. Various substances can be labeled by radioactive sulfur, involving drugs (vitamin B_1, penicillin, sulfa drugs, *etc.*), with subsequent introduction into the body and study of their transformations and mechanism of action.

Sulfur Dioxide

Sulfur dioxide is one of the main air contaminants. It is a damaging constituent of fumes from fossil fuels burning and from other S-containing substances. SO_2 is strongly irritating to the mucous membranes, skin, eyes, and respiratory system. At inhalation of low concentration of SO_2 chronic pulmonary diseases (asthma, emphysema) can be caused [3,4,154,155]. The atmosphere amount of SO_2 is constantly monitored as an indicator of the air quality because SO_2 along with nitrogen oxides NO_x influence the acidity of rainfall. Water solutions of sulfur dioxide contain small quantities of the weak and not stable H_2SO_3. The salts of H_2SO_3 are hydrogen sulfites (HSO_3^-) and sulfites (SO_3^{2-}). Solutions of sulfur dioxide and sulfites are good reducers. Sulfites can be gradually oxidized to sulfates even by O_2 from the air.

Sulfur Trioxide

Sulfur trioxide SO_3 can be obtained by oxidation of sulfur dioxide and with water it produces sulfuric acid H_2SO_4. Dissolving SO_3 or concentrated sulfuric acid in water is a very exothermic reaction. Concentrated H_2SO_4 is a strong oxidizing agent. Its salts are hydrogen sulfates (HSO_4^-) and sulfates (SO_4^{2-}). Most of the known sulfates are easily soluble in water. $CaSO_4$ and $PbSO_4$ are not soluble. Barium sulfate is almost insoluble and as such is used in X-ray inspection of the digestive tract as a contrast agent. Soluble sulfates possess low absorption after ingesting and they bind H_2O in the intestine acting as osmotic laxatives.

Thiosulphuric acid $H_2S_2O_3$ is another oxoacid of sulfur with salts thiosulfates ($S_2O_3^{2-}$) [3,4,154,155]. Sodium thiosulfate $Na_2S_2O_3$ is used intravenously as an antidote to cyanide poisoning (converting cyanide to harmless thiocyanate) and as a neutralizing agent capable of binding to reactive chemicals or metabolites:

$$CN^- + S_2O_3^{2-} \rightarrow SCN^- + SO_3^{2-}$$

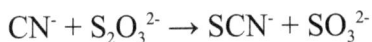

The complex sulfur cycle in nature includes SO_2 and SO_3 [3 - 5]. From the hot springs and volcanoes, large quantities of S are periodically produced and transferred to the atmosphere, mostly as SO_2. The decomposition of dead organisms causes H_2S release, obtained from sulfates with the help of bacteria. The gaseous S-based substances can be oxidized to SO_3 in the air, where with water it produces H_2SO_4. S is transported back to the earth crust by acidic rains, and thus the cycle closes. The S-cycle is the most man-influenced among the natural cycles. Many industrial processes emit SO_2 to the atmosphere, which content in the air has enlarged substantially damaging plant and animal life as well as the global climate on the Earth.

Hydrogen Sulfide

Hydrogen sulfide (H_2S) is an extremely toxic gas [3 - 5]. H_2S is constantly formed at the bottom of large water bodies by the reaction of dissolved sulfates with organic substances, *e.g.,* methane:

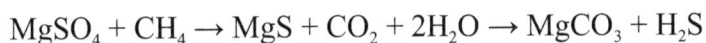

$$MgSO_4 + CH_4 \rightarrow MgS + CO_2 + 2H_2O \rightarrow MgCO_3 + H_2S$$

The resulting gas rises from the bottom of the reservoir to a depth of around 150 m, since there it interacts with O_2 penetrating from above. Furthermore, up to a depth of 200 m, there are bacteria that oxidize H_2S to S.

H_2S, dissolved in H_2O, is a weak diprotic hydro-sulfuric acid. Its salts are hydrogen sulfides HS^- and sulfides S^{2-}. Sulfides of heavy metals are insoluble. In the last years, the role of H_2S as a mammalian messenger for controlling the inflammation and endoplasmic reticulum stress signaling has been discovered [157]. The action of hydrogen sulfide is that it inhibits the enzyme cytochrome oxidase, which is important for the transfer of electrons in the respiratory system.

H_2S is mainly synthesized from cysteine or its derivates. The two key enzymes, cystathionine β-synthase and cystathionine γ-lyase (CSE), are important for the formation of H_2S. The suggested mechanism of hydrogen sulfide signaling is the sulphhydration of active Cys residues in target proteins, which is essential for the control of inflammation and endoplasmic reticulum stress signaling and vascular tension. Numerous additional pharmacologic targets for hydrogen sulfide have been recognized, such as K(ATP), NF-κB, *etc.* Production of endogenous H_2S is advantageous in preventing and treating atherosclerosis (a chronic disease, considered the principal reason of cardiovascular morbidity), since reduced concentrations of endogenous hydrogen sulfide induced by genetic removal of CSE accelerates the disease [158, 159].

Selenium

Selenium is a trace microelement (approximately 90 ppb of the Earth crust) that is vital in small quantities for the normal metabolism. Similar to all essential trace elements, Se is poisonous at higher levels. The body contains around 4 mg of selenium. It has been recognized as one of the significant trace elements, which arouses the synthesis of S-containing amino acids. Se is a constituent of a number of enzymes including glutathione peroxidase, which oxidizes lipids and S-containing amino acids, as well as enzymes for de-iodation of thyroid hormones. In cooperation with vitamin E, Se supports the immune system in producing antibodies. This element helps in keeping pancreas and heart to function properly and make the tissues elastic. The nonmetal Se is chemically associated with sulfur, being found in selenoproteins such as selenocysteine, which is a Se analogue of sulfur-containing amino acid cysteine [160]. While selenium, being a precondition for the production of selenocysteine (SeCys), one of the crucial amino acids, is also identified as a micronutrient for bacteria and animals, it is supposed to be a toxic element in biosystems. Se-based proteins and their actions are listed in Table 7.

Table 7. Selenium-based proteins and their functions.

Protein	Functions
Glutathione peroxidases	Decomposition of lipid hydroperoxides and H_2O_2
Thioredoxin reductases	Reduction of thioredoxin and glutaredoxin, regulation of intracellular redox balance
Methionine-R-sulfoxide reductases	Reduction of methionine residues, melanin metabolism
Iodothyronine deiodinases	Thyroid hormone synthesis and metabolism
Selenoprotein H	Mitochondrial biogenesis and respiratory capacities
Selenoprotein P	Selenium transport and homeostasis
Selenoprotein N, W	Muscle function and metabolism, Ca^{2+} homeostasis
Selenoprotein S, K	ER-associated degradation, immune responses
Selenoprotein O	Kinase action and regulation of signaling cascades
Selenium binding proteins	Intracellular transport
Selenophosphate synthetase	Selenoprotein biosynthesis
Selenocysteine lyase	Selenium recirculation

Organisms need Se for the function of numerous Se-dependent enzymes (glutathione peroxidases GSH-Pxs, iodothyronine deiodinase DIOs, thioredoxin reductase TrxR, selenophosphate synthetase), where selenium is an important component [161]. Se possesses an antioxidant activity as SeCys in glutathione peroxidase (GSH-Px). GSH-Px decreases potentially harmful ROS like H_2O_2 and lipid hydroperoxides, to innocuous products such as H_2O and alcohol. GSH-Px arises in two forms: Se-independent and Se-dependent glutathione peroxidases, which differ in the number of sub-units, in the Se bonds at the active center and in the enzymatic mechanism. Se-independent glutathione peroxidase (glutathione-S-transferase, GST) catalyzes decontamination of numerous xenobiotics. Se(II) ion does not contribute in the enzyme mechanism. Se-dependent glutathione-peroxidase contains four subunits and each of them contains in the active center one Se atom connected to the modified amino acid SeCys. The importance of these Se-based enzymes is in the elimination of peroxides – potential substrates in Fenton reactions. Thioredoxin reductase (TrxR) along with GSH-Pxs act as the most important cellular antioxidants against ROS and RNS such as hydroperoxides, peroxynitrite and lipid peroxides, controlling the redox signaling. Selenium is also present in other selenium-containing proteins (Table **7**). It participates in thyroxine conversion to triiodothyronine, significant in the stimulation and inactivation of thyroid hormones. Most amount of biologically active triiodothyronine is produced by the removal of one I-atom from thyroxine in an interaction activated by Se-dependent iodothyronine deiodinase. This enzyme plays a significant role in the control of thyroid hormones in the human body. Most of the selenium-containing proteins and enzymes contain selenocysteine in their active sites. Being a part of the enzymes, selenium prevents the oxidation of lipid and protein biomolecules of the cell membrane and as a typical antioxidant, it protects organisms from numerous diseases [160, 161]. Nevertheless, the activity of most of selenoproteins and other Se-based biologically available molecules remains uncertain and not clear.

Selenium compounds protect against poisoning with human carcinogens arsenic, mercury, and cadmium, which is a result of competitive binding to proteins [162, 163]. It reduces metal-induced harmfulness in the most important organs.

Selenium deficiency (decrease in the concentration of glutathione peroxidase), although rare in nature, increases the development of cardiovascular and oncological diseases (selenium is found in meat, cereals, seafood and cottage cheese - about 0.2 - 0.3mg/kg) [164]. Deficiency in selenium refers to compounds of selenium. In normal conditions, the most frequent species are these of Se(IV), particularly selenite, as well as selenate (SeO_3^{2-}) and hydrogen selenate ion ($HSeO_3^-$) present in dietary supplements and water. Symptoms of Se deficiency may occur on very Se-poor soil. In some regions, Se is lacking in soils, where this selenium deficiency causes diseases like Keshan cardiomyopathy disease and Kashin-Beck osteochondropathy disease. Keshan disease (Keshan syndrome) was the first illness associated with selenium deficiency. The deficiency of Se contributes synergistically with the lack of iodine to progressive development of hypothyroidism, goiter and additionally liver necrosis, epilepsy, cardiovascular disease, and an elevated predisposition for liver cancer. It has been observed that the lesser the Se amount in blood, the higher the danger of developing different cancers. Categorically, it is supposed that selenium and its compounds could be powerful cancer-preventing substances. Its protective effect has been observed against colon, prostate, and breast cancer [165].

Toxicity: Selenium is a vital trace element for both prokaryotic and eukaryotic biosystems. Although essential for life, Se can be toxic if present in high doses [161, 162]. Nutritional Se supplementation with different origins and chemical forms is commonly used for overcoming Se deficiency, alleviating the deleterious effects of various toxic metals and maintaining high productive and reproductive performance of farm animals. Extreme nutritional amount of selenium is found as pro-oxidant and causes Se poisoning in all animal classes and humans depending on the concentration and duration of consumption. The mechanism of Se-mediated toxicity has not been precisely elucidated but there are some suggestions as oxidative stress mechanism, established by *in vitro* and *in vivo* investigations.

Excessive dietary intake and overexposure of Se fumes produce accumulation of fluids in the lung, pneumonia, asthma, bronchitis, fever, nausea, chills, headache, sore throat, conjunctivitis, diarrhea, vomiting, abdominal pain, *etc.* Typical symptoms of Se excess are loss of hair, red stain of nails and teeth, as well as CNS disorders. Selenosis is a poisonousness caused by extreme Se intake. The typical symptoms of selenosis include neurologic and dermatologic problems. High Se intake has been associated with an intensely lower prevalence of heart diseases. The mechanism of Se toxicity has not been completely clarified. It is identified that some compounds like selenite, selenocysteine, methylselenic acid are redox-reactive substances generating ROS and inducing OS.

Selenium compounds are very poisonous [161, 162]. SeO_2 interacts with moisture to form H_2SeO_3, which severely irritates and burns the eyes and skin. The toxic effect of selenite and selenate on farm animals has long been known. Selenium oxides (SeO_2 and SeO_3) and their derivatives cause skin burns and respiratory mucosa. The symptoms of intoxication with selenium and its compounds are almost identical. Acute Se intoxication is similar to As poisoning. A typical signal of toxic condition is the garlic breath due to volatile organic Se-containing compounds like dimethyl selenide (CH_3-Se-CH_3). Plants grown in soils containing large amount of Se may concentrate selenium.

However, micro doses of selenium preparations have recently found increasing use in medicine, for example, to prevent diseases of a necrotic nature, for the treatment of certain diseases of the eyes, liver, pancreas, dystrophic processes in various tissues, as well as for electrophoresis, especially in dental practice. Application of Se nanoparticles have potential therapeutic benefits in various OS and inflammation mediated disorders [166]. Nano-selenium forms have shown advanced bioavailability and lesser toxicity.

Tellurium

Tellurium, having the properties both of the metals and the non-metals, is constantly found in the body. Its biological functions are not clear. It has been observed as a noxious element, but some recent studies of the biological properties of tellurium inorganic and metalorganic compounds have exposed some possible capacity for their medical application [167].

Toxicity: As a member of the chalcogen group Te is a metalloid with no apparent biological functions and extremely low abundance in the planet. Due to its exceptional physicochemical properties, Te is broadly used in industry as alloys for photovoltaic modules, solar panels, for the production of optical magnetic disks, pigments, semiconductors, catalysis, quantum dots, *etc.* [167]. Along with the metallic tellurium, its volatile compounds are very toxic even at micromolar levels. Elemental Te^0 is classified as low toxic to living organisms compared to the soluble Te oxyanions tellurite (TeO_3^{2-}) and tellurate (TeO_4^{2-}). Tellurium compounds, particularly the oxyanions, possess numerous damaging effects on organisms and there is an existence of serious risk of exposure to Te in everyday life. Recent data indicate that growing environment al pollution with tellurium has a causal relation to autoimmune, neurodegenerative and oncological diseases [167].

When Te compounds penetrate into cells, they may change the cell membrane structure and glutathione metabolism, substitute vital metal ions in enzymes, and cause OS. It has been found that tellurium compounds are less poisonous than selenium compounds, however, the correspondence between their pathways is apparent.

Inorganic Te salts and organotellurium compounds have shown potential in pharmacology, therapy and diagnostics. They are active protein and enzyme inhibitors, killing a wide variety of microbes and can induce cancer cells apoptosis. Tellurium-based nanomaterials possess intrinsic biological potential for phototherapy and ROS-related applications [168].

Polonium

Polonium is a tremendously rare radioactive element which commonly exists in uranium-containing minerals [3 - 5]. It has primarily scientific application as an α-emitter.

p-Elements of Group VIIA

Fluorine

Fluorine is a very abundant halogen element mainly in combined form [5 - 10]. The halogen elements display extreme resemblance to each other in terms of their chemical properties. The most pronounced is the difference in the properties of fluorine and its analogs chlorine, bromine, and iodine [3, 4]. Although its abundance in nature, fluorine is almost absent from the biosphere. The reason is its high oxidation potential and hydration energy of F^- anion, making it inappropriate in forming carbon-fluorine bonds and a characteristic xenobiotic. Fluorine is the most active of the halogen elements and, in fact, of all chemical elements. It is one of the vital trace elements. There is lots of fluorine in the human body (around 3 g in skeleton and teeth) and as F^- anion it is crucial, although little is known about the mechanisms of its biological action. There are specific HF transporting proteins and F^-/H^+ co-transporter or F^-/OH^- antiporter proteins in acidic conditions.

In the living organism, fluorine participates in many bio reactions. It stimulates the activation adenylate cyclase, inhibits lipases, esterases and lactate de hydrogenases. Fluorine occurs in organisms in the form of a negatively charged ion, fluoride anion F^-. Fluoride anion contributes in mineral metabolism of teeth and skeletal tissues [169]. In the human body, fluorine in the form of fluorapatite $(Ca_5(PO_4)_3F)$ is concentrated most of all in the enamel of the teeth and bone. F^- anion possesses a strong affinity for hard metal cations like Ca^{2+}. Its small ionic radius lets it to shift the bigger OH^- anion in hydroxyapatite $Ca_5(PO_4)_3OH$, the predominant component of teeth and skeleton, forming the stronger and harder fluorapatite $Ca_5(PO_4)_3F$. This way, fluoride anion rises the crystal density. The formation of hydroxyapatite can be expressed by the equation:

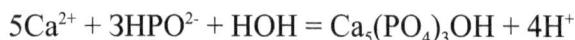

$$5Ca^{2+} + 3HPO^{2-} + HOH = Ca_5(PO_4)_3OH + 4H^+$$

Fluoride anion replaces OH^- ions of hydroxyapatite easily and forms a protective film on the enamel composed of solid $Ca_5(PO_4)_3F$:

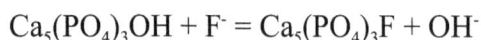

$$Ca_5(PO_4)_3OH + F^- = Ca_5(PO_4)_3F + OH^-$$

Additionally, F^- ions help in depositing $Ca_3(PO_4)_2$, accelerating the remineralization process or the crystal formation:

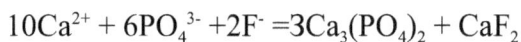

$$10Ca^{2+} + 6PO_4^{3-} + 2F^- = 3Ca_3(PO_4)_2 + CaF_2$$

Caries initiates with the formation of a destroyed enamel zone in the form of spots on the surface [169]. Under the action of acids produced by bacteria, the hydroxyapatite constituent of enamel dissolves:

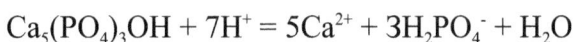

$$Ca_5(PO_4)_3OH + 7H^+ = 5Ca^{2+} + 3H_2PO_4^- + H_2O$$

Fluorine is the most electronegative halogen element and the least stable. Fluoride anion is the most basic of the halide anions. Small concentrations of 25-35 μM of fluoride are recommended to strengthen enamel. Thus, the main source of fluoride received by a person is drinking water, which should contain about 1 mg/L of fluoride [169]. It has been observed that in areas with high fluorine contents in drinking water, the risk of dental caries is small. Toothpastes should be supplemented with fluorine.

Chronic toxicity of fluoride is caused as a result of lasting ingestion of small quantities of fluoride. With a fluoride content of < 0.5 mg/L in drinking water, caries and destruction of enamel are developed, and if its content is over 1.2 mg/L, enamel spotting is observed. That is, in both cases, the teeth are quickly destroyed. The most important means of preventing caries is water fluoridation [169]. Fluoridation of drinking water in order to bring the fluoride content in it to the norm is carried out by adding a certain amount of sodium fluoride.

With an excessive content of fluoride in drinking water, an endemic disease develops, the so-called fluorosis [169, 170]. It is manifested by darkening of the enamel of the teeth in the spotting of tooth enamel, renal failure, deformation of bones, and muscle weakness. Extreme exposure to fluorides affects bones homeostasis and enamel growth. Fluorosis depends on the fluoride amount and the period of exposure. In many regions, the quantity of fluorides in groundwater exceeds the optional levels causing skeletal fluorosis.

Fluorine in the body forms complex compounds with calcium, magnesium, and other activators of enzyme systems. In various bioprocesses, F^- ion acts as an inhibitor, which blocks the active centers of several enzymes containing Ca^{2+}, Mg^{2+}, and other vital metal ions by binding of fluoride ions to the metal centers or because of the formation of low soluble CaF_2 thus removing physiologically important Ca^{2+} cations, for instance. In large quantities, fluoride ions replace the iodide ions in tyrosine and inhibit the activity of the thyroid gland, block the active centers of many enzymes, and affect the exchange of vitamins [169, 170].

Acute toxicity of F⁻ is rare and usually occurs as a result of ingestion of high concentrations. Acute toxicity symptoms occur quickly as diarrhea, vomiting, diffuse abdominal pain, excess salivation, thirst.

F⁻ ions can be absorbed mainly in the gastrointestinal tract. When entering the blood, F⁻ anions quickly pass in bones and teeth. At normal consumption level, F⁻ ions are not accumulated in soft tissues. The metabolism of fluoride in the body depends on pH as the coefficient of permeability of lipid layer membrane to HF is million times that of F⁻ anion [170]. Thus, fluoride becomes able to easily cross the membrane as hydrogen fluoride in interaction with the pH gradient between body fluids. That is why at the next ingestion, fluoride levels in the blood quickly rise due to the fast absorption in the intestinal tract. The release of fluorides is a slow process.

It has to be mentioned that fluorides (aluminum fluoride and beryllium fluoride) are known to inhibit microbial enzymes, leading to decreased acid production by cariogenic microorganisms. These fluorides prevent bacterial infections on the teeth. The enzyme inhibitors aluminum fluoride and beryllium fluoride act as mimics of phosphates [171].

In the free state, fluorine gas is a very strong poison. F_2 gas is released by the industrial processes. F_2 is dangerous, its inhalation produces instant respiratory damage and death at very high doses [172]. In skin contact, fluorine vapors at low concentrations, cause itching, eye, and nose irritation, up to the appearance of blisters. Hydrofluorocarbons are the most common type of organofluorine compounds. Organic fluorides are commonly used in air conditioning and as refrigerants and lubricants instead of older chlorofluorocarbons with detrimental effects on the ozone layer.

Currently, F-containing substances constitute about 30% of newly introduced medications. Synthesis of ¹⁸F-based radiopharmaceutical compounds is an emerging area in nuclear medicine [172].

Chlorine

Chlorine belongs to very essential biogenic macroelements being predominant and widely distributed in large concentrations in the body (around 96 g) as NaCl in the body [5]. Chloride ions are found mainly in extracellular fluids (100 mM in blood, ≈25 mM in cytoplasm, and ≈4 mM in nucleus). Anions of chlorine Cl⁻ are actively involved in biochemical transformations. They maintain the proper pH levels in the body, stimulate stomach acid needed for digestion, control the electroconductivity of cell membranes, stimulate the action of nerve and muscle cells, and facilitate the flow of oxygen and carbon dioxide within cells, activate some enzymes, *etc.*

Although Cl⁻ ions do not participate directly in bioreactions, they are essential for ionic balance, because they provide negative charges for neutralizing the metal cations [3 - 5]. Chloride anions Cl⁻ along with Na^+ ions are the main osmotic constituents of biofluids (blood, cerebrospinal fluid, lymph, *etc.*). Along with sodium and potassium cations, chloride ions carry electrical charges when dissolved in biofluids, the so-called electrolytes. This electric charge allows nerve cells to work properly. Chloride ion works with Na^+ and K^+ to regulate the amounts of fluids and to control pH. This element also helps muscles flex and relax normally. Chloride anion together with hydrogen carbonate HCO_3^- anion are the most vital free anions. It is important for the regulation of acid-base balance and osmotic pressure. Together with H^+ cations it participates in the maintenance of gastric juice pH.

Unlike F_2, but in common with Br_2 and I_2, Cl_2 can exist in its oxidized forms in the organism. It is a powerful oxidizing, bleaching, and sterilizing agent. It is very efficient for the inactivation of pathogenic microbes and is one of the most frequently used decontaminators for H_2O disinfection. The higher oxidation states of chlorine are an important factor in the body. Among its oxoacids, hypochlorous acid HClO is the strongest oxidizing agent produced by neutrophils (white blood cells) [173]. HClO eradicates all types of microorganisms. Bactericidal and bleaching properties of chlorinated H_2O are associated with its content. Atomic O, produced by HClO decomposition, bleaches paints and kills microorganisms. Hypochlorous acid interacts with organic and bioorganic compounds RH:

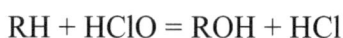

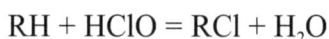

RH + HClO = ROH + HCl

RH + HClO = RCl + H_2O

Although HClO is used by the human immune system, it breaks down proteins and can be poisonous to human cells depending on the concentration. Myeloperoxidase in the white blood cells (neutrophils) uses hydrogen peroxide and chloride ions for producing HClO and eradicating bacteria, thus protecting the body [173].

Chlorine is essential in digesting the food suitably and in absorbing the other elements which the organism needs to survive because the stomach acid is a compound of chlorine [3, 4].

Hydrochloric acid HCl is an important constituent of the gastric juice. Its mass portion is around 0.3%. To obtain HCl in the stomach, table salt NaCl must be present. HCl is formed as follows:

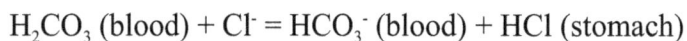

H_2CO_3 (blood) + Cl^- = HCO_3^- (blood) + HCl (stomach)

Hydrochloric acid of the gastric juice provides the breakdown of peptide R-CO - NH-R_1 under the action of pepsin into the respective carboxylic acid RCOOH and amine NH_2R_1. Pepsin affords the assimilation of proteins by hydrolytic cleavage of the peptide bonds. The Cl^- ion is also part of other enzyme systems, for example, it activates the enzyme amylase secreted by the salivary glands.

The concentration of Cl^- anions is relatively high in body biofluids. In the organism, the concentration of Cl^- is closely regulated by cystic fibrosis transmembrane conductance regulator (CFTR) membrane protein. Any substantial decrease or increase of this concentration may have damaging or fatal consequences. Excessive vomiting can cause a serious loss of Cl^- anions in the body [3, 4]. Hypochloremia, extreme reduction of Cl^- anions through loss of some digestive fluids by vomiting, by substantial sweating or by kidney conditions, may cause alkalosis as a result of HCO_3^- excess, as the insufficient concentration of Cl^- ions is partly compensated or substituted by hydrogen carbonate anions. All this leads to a hazardous disbalance of pH, which can cause loss of appetite, dehydration, muscle weakness, and finally coma. It is easy to take up sufficient chlorine from natural, untreated food, therefore deficiency of chlorine is quite rare. On the contrary, extreme Cl^- anions levels in blood or so-called hyperchloremia results in acidosis.

Elemental Cl_2 gas is poisonous and dangerous [3 - 5]. Breathing low quantities of Cl_2 for a short period affects the respiratory tract. This may vary from chest pain and coughing to H_2O retention in lungs. Cl_2 irritates mainly the eyes, skin and respiratory tract. Such effects are not expected to happen at Cl_2 levels which are usually found in the atmosphere. Health impact related to breathing or consuming small quantities of Cl_2 over long terms have not been identified.

Chlorine Compounds

Although Cl^- anion has an essential role, the covalently bonded chlorine is far less benign. Chlorine has found dangerous applications in the form of chlorinated hydrocarbons, used as work solvents for degreasing, paint removal, and dry cleaning (C_2HCl_3, CH_2Cl_2, CCl_2CCl_2) [3 - 5]. These types of hazardous agents injure the brain, irritate mucous, eyes, and skin membranes, and have possibly oncogenic effects. In many regions, such chlorohydrocarbons are banned. The use of chlorofluorocarbons (freons) was abandoned because of their influence on the ozone layer. The complete prohibition of the manufacture of chlorine-based covalent organic compounds may lead to the exclusion of numerous beneficial materials for instance polyvinylchloride.

The insecticide DDT (dichlorodiphenyltrichloroethane) was found to limit the spread of the insect-borne diseases malaria and typhus. The effectiveness of DDT against lice, mosquitoes, typhus, and malaria distribution, and its capability to defend crops, made this insecticide valued in the last century. However, DDT has fatal characteristics, common to other chlorohydrocarbons, connected with its fat solubility. DDT is a stable compound, which metabolizes very slowly, and is usually deposited in the fatty tissues. Nowadays, DDT is considered an endocrine-disrupting compound which alters and disrupts important hormones, including reproductive health, as well as neurological and immune systems and functions [3 - 5, 6 - 10].

Polychlorinated biphenyl (PCB) belongs to the group of chlorinated hydrocarbons. It was utilized as an additive in paints, polyvinylchloride plastics, electrical condensers and transformers, copying papers, and glues, rather than as an insecticide because it was classified as carcinogenic to humans [174]. Polychlorinated biphenyls and organochlorine pesticides are persistent organic pollutants that have been linked to many health concerns involving the skin, liver, endocrine, reproductive, neurological and immune systems. The burning of products containing chlorine at low temperature is the major source of toxic dioxins.

Disinfection of Water

Chlorine makes a major contribution to epidemics of cholera and typhoid. It is an effective water disinfectant against parasites, bacteria, and viruses. It provides a durable protection, easy and inexpensive usage. It can be used as Cl_2, NaClO, $Ca(ClO)_2$. In water all of them yield the strong oxidizer - hypochlorite anion ClO^-:

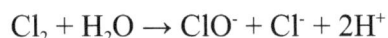

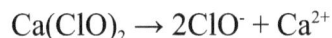

$$Cl_2 + H_2O \rightarrow ClO^- + Cl^- + 2H^+$$

$$NaClO \rightarrow ClO^- + Na^+$$

$$Ca(ClO)_2 \rightarrow 2ClO^- + Ca^{2+}$$

The chlorine bactericidal effects are due to its reaction with organic compounds and NH_3 to form chlorinated organic compounds and chloramines [3, 4, 6 - 10]. A group of compounds of specific concern are trihalomethanes THMs, produced by chlorination and disinfection of water, rich in organic matter. This process of chlorination leads to the decomposition of the organic compounds to give small

Cl-containing substances like trichloromethane ($CHCl_3$). That is why, there are suggestions to decrease the permitted THM concentrations to use ozone or chlorine dioxide as water disinfectants in order to reduce the generation of THMs.

Bromine

Bromine belongs to biogenic elements. It is supposed to be a vital trace nonmetal in red algae and perhaps in animals and humans. In the human body, the mass of bromine is about 7 mg (around 10^{-5}%) which is a significant amount. Unlike other halogens, for bromine, endogenous compounds are atypical [3 - 5,6-10]. It is localized mainly in the pituitary gland. Although no definite role for bromine in health was identified, there is increasing evidence that bromine is essential. Eosinophil peroxidase, found in human and mammalian immune cells, catalyzes the formation of hypohalous acids, particularly HBrO, which plays an essential role in posttranslational modification of proteins for tissue development. Recent investigations have established that bromine is essential for all animal species, since bromide anions on translation to HBrO are vital cofactors for peroxidase-catalyzed formation of sulfonimine cross-links. Some peroxidases are haloperoxide enzymes and can produce both HBrO and HClO [175]. Although peroxidase can produce HClO, it favorably chooses Br⁻ over Cl⁻ anions to produce bromine-based compounds at physiological conditions, when Cl⁻ anions are much more abundant.

Actually, there are some doubts about the role of bromine as a trace element, although its sedative effect is reliably known. CNS is most sensitive to the influence of bromide anions. It takes part in the biosynthesis of sex hormones and the regulation of the function of the sex glands. Bromine has a healing effect on CNS, enhancing the processes of inhibition, thus many salts and organic compounds of bromine (carbromal, bromizoval, bromural, bromital, bromocamphor) are used in medicine, which have a calming and hypnotic effect. More investigations are required to approve the nutritious benefits of Br_2 [3,4,175]. No bromine deficiency has been documented. Br_2 has similar properties to Cl_2 as a water disinfectant.

Bromine vapors are highly poisonous [3 - 5,6-10]. Bromine burns are very painful and do not heal for a long time. Organic compounds of bromine (bromoacetone, bromobenzyl cyanide), causing severe tearing (lacrimators), are used as toxic substances with irritating action. The toxicity of bromide ions is small. The accumulation of bromide ions due to their slow removal from the organism (1-2 months), leads to chronic toxic condition "bromism".

The most controversial Br-based organic compound is bromomethane CH_3Br, referred to as methylbromide. Bromomethane is a wide-ranging fumigant used against insects, pathogens and rodents. It is highly volatile and hence leaves little residue. CH_3Br is significant to the agricultural community. Various marine organisms synthesize organo-bromine compounds and some of the metabolic pathways lead to the formation of CH_3Br. The problem is that CH_3Br is an efficient ozone-depleting substance, because bromine destroys ozone much more efficiently than chlorine [3 - 5, 175]. Another problem is that bromomethane is fatal to nontargeted organisms being extremely poisonous. It can cause CNS and respiratory system failures. At low amounts it causes headaches and sickness. At higher concentrations it causes muscle spasms, convulsions, coma and death. Br_2 is used essentially for preparing the gasoline additive, ethylene dibromide, that prevents Pb deposits in engines.

Iodine

Although there is a small amount of this element in the body, iodine is a vital trace nonmetal and an important micronutrient for animals and humans essential at all stages of life [3 - 5]. The heaviest stable halogen is mostly vital for the thyroid gland. Embryonic life and early childhood are the most critical stages of its necessity. Essential nonmetals, like iodine with their roles in enzymes, hormones *etc.,* spread to different body parts.

In 19th century, iodine was firstly documented as a crucial element for organisms. Iodide ions are localized in the body, mainly in the thyroid as polyiodinated bioorganic compounds [176]. The thyroid captures iodine from the bloodstream and includes it in thyroid hormones which are deposited and put into circulation if required. Iodine is a main constituent of the thyroid hormones thyroxine (T4) and 3,3′,5-triiodothyronine (T3), critical for kidney, liver, muscles, brain, and CNS functions. Thyroid hormones are produced from iodide and tyrosine from thyroglobulin protein through the enzyme thyroid peroxidase. Particularly, the most active of the tyrosine derivatives is triiodotyrosine $(HO)(I)-C_6H_3-O-C_6H_3(I_2)-CH_2\ CH(NH_3^+)\ COO^-$. The above-mentioned hormones play a key role in controlling numerous biological functions, involving growth, production, and control of energy as well as all accompanying processes. These hormones influence cardiovascular, CNS, and reproductive systems as well. Of the entire quantity of iodine in the body (25 mg), more than half is accumulated in thyroid glands, as a part of the hormone thyroxine, which determines the overall intensity of body metabolism.

The importance of carbon-iodine bonds can be contrasted with the behavior of the lighter halogens in the body. The Na^+/I^- symporter (NIS) plays a vital role in iodine metabolism and thyroid control [177]. NIS is a fundamental plasma membrane glycoprotein and thyroidal iodide ion transport from the blood is made likely by selective targeting of Na^+/I^- symporter to the basolateral membrane. It also controls the transport of iodide ions in other tissues, including the gastric mucosa, salivary glands, and lactating mammary gland, where iodide ion is transferred into the milk for thyroid hormone synthesis to the nursing newborns.

Owing to the iodine metabolic role, symptoms of its deficiency could be far reaching. With an absence of iodine in the body, the formation of thyroxine in the thyroid gland is delayed which causes the disease hypothyroidism, in which endemic goiter excessively grows. In this way, the thyroid gland, by increasing its size, tries to increase the amount of hormone produced. Low thyroid activity due to iodine deficiency leads also to the increased tendency for tumor formation. Goiter must be treated by additional KI or iodine casein [178]. Symptoms of decreased thyroid activity (hypothyroidism) consist of weight gain, fatigue, and cold intolerance. In technologically advanced countries, iodine deficiency is nowadays rare since iodine is constantly supplemented to the table salt. In a number of areas, the iodine content in water and soil is negligible, which also leads to its extremely low content in food products. In these cases, drinking water and ordinary food do not cover the body requirement for iodine, forcing to resort to iodination of food (usually by the addition of 15-20 mg of soluble iodides per kg of the salt). For iodization of the table salt, KIO_3 is also applied, which under physiological conditions turns into I_2. One of the most disturbing effects of maternal iodine deficiency has a particularly strong effect on the health of children. This is so-called congenital hypothyroidism, which leads to irreversible mental retardation and child lag behind in physical and mental development. An iodine deficiency diet during pregnancy leads to the birth of hypothyroid babies (cretins).

Excess iodine leads to active functioning of the thyroid gland (hyperthyroidism), which is expressed in increased metabolic processes, excitability, tachycardia [3, 4]. Iodine overload is not as much common compared with its deficiency although it is unfavorable. Excessive amount of thyroid hormones causes tachycardia, nervousness, weight loss, and heat intolerance. In exceeded iodine intake, it is rapidly excreted in urine.

Iodine possesses antimicrobial activity. Correspondingly to chlorine, it replaces hydrogen atoms bonded to N atoms in protein molecules of microbes, which causes their eradication:

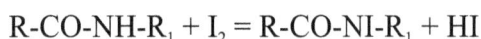

$$R\text{-}CO\text{-}NH\text{-}R_1 + I_2 = R\text{-}CO\text{-}NI\text{-}R_1 + HI$$

Povidone-iodine has the broadest spectrum of activity versus other antiseptics [179]. It has acceptable tolerability and promotes effective wound healing acting against bacterial biofilms.

Elemental I_2 is poisonous, and its vapor causes severe mucous inflammations. The maximal tolerable concentration of iodine in the air at working places is only 1 mg/m^3. All iodide compounds are poisonous if taken in an overdose.

Organically bound iodine, as the intake of iodine from seaweed, is innocuous, even in continued use at high amounts. Bound to C, iodine cannot participate in redox functions, and is not chemically accessible for covalent attachment to other biomolecules [3 - 5]. Because iodine electronegativity is near to that of C, it is not likely that I atoms make any substantial changes to the total electronic structures of the organic biomolecules, except the volume as the covalent radius of I atoms is twice the radii of C, N, and O atoms. The I atoms of the iodoorganic molecules appear to fit into some large cavities in enzymes, holding unique enzyme conformations. For example, replacing the large isopropyl component $(CH_3)_2CH-$ for iodine could result in a molecule with analogous activity.

Radioactive iodine isotopes are spreading in nature [180]. Particularly important is the isotope ^{131}I (β- and γ-ray emitting radioisotope with a low cost and long half-life of 8 days). This long-lived theranostic radionuclide, taken up by the thyroid, for many years produced and continues to produce an increased risk of thyroid cancer and diseases caused by thyroid hormonal deficiency [181]. ^{131}I is used in radioactive iodine therapy, but is nevertheless very harmful for persons living near or working in nuclear power plants. Iodine tablets are recommended to block the acceptance of the radioactive isotope.

Astatine

Astatine is a solid substance of the metallic type, the heaviest halogen. It is not found in nature since it contains only short-lived radioactive isotopes. Astatine is somewhat less volatile than iodine and exhibits typical metallic properties. Its physiological role is unclear. It is only known that it selectively concentrates in the thyroid, spleen, and lungs and has an effect similar to iodine [3, 4]. Nevertheless, the chemistry of At differs considerably from that of iodine because of the greater metallic character of this element. Another factor explaining its performance in biochemical systems is that all At isotopes except three (^{221}At, ^{222}At, ^{223}At), are α-emitters. α-Induced radiolysis plays an important role in the At behavior in many systems in comparison to that of the stable β-isotopes of iodine. ^{211}At ($T_{1/2} = 7.2$ h) is of particular interest for usage in cancer targeted α-therapy. Only a small number of α-radionuclides, such as astatine-211, radium-223, thorium-227, bismuth-213, actinium-225, lead-212, and bismuth-212, meet the requirements for nuclear medical applications. Among them ^{211}At is one of the most promising candidates [182, 183].

Concluding Remarks

Examination of the biological and chemical properties of halogen elements demonstrats that chlorine and bromine in the body are typically found as hydrated ions Br^-, Cl^-. F_2 and I_2 have different behavior in the same conditions. I_2 characteristically forms carbon-iodine bonds. Fluorine usually binds to metals, like Ca, Mg, Fe. Regarding physicochemical characteristics and the tendency to coordinate with biogenic metal cations, F^- ion differs substantially from the other halogen analogues. It is practically not involved in the replacement of Cl^-, Br^- and I^- ions. These anions are similar in their chemical properties and can easily replace each other *in vivo*, while showing synergy and antagonism.

Most of the p-elements are nonmetals. These nonmetals are parts of bioorganic molecules participating in the formation of living tissues. Six nonmetallic elements (C, N, O, P, S, Cl) occur in the body in large amounts and five (B, Si, As, Se, I) are essential for humans. Some other elements are vital in one form and toxic in another. The value of bromine for organisms is not fully understood. As blocks -SH groups and is a lethal toxin. Conversely, for some animals, arsenic is essential supporting their growth. Some bismuth substances are useful in medical practice. Nevertheless, most of the p-metals are highly toxic. The most hazardous for humans are lead compounds commonly used in manufacturing. Lead compounds disturb the normal porphyrin synthesis, participate in the synthesis of hemoglobin and other vital hemo-proteins.

Most p-elements, even essential ones, are harmful to living organisms if their intake is higher. Se is a typical example. It is noxious to the human body even in concentrations that slightly exceed the optional intake standards. Conversely, it is certainly not healthy if the intake is very low. Chlorine in the form of Cl^- anions is very significant for the life but as a Cl_2 gas it is very poisonous. Chlorine gas converts hydrocarbons to the insecticide DDT and to the polychlorinated biphenyls (PCBs), that are very damaging to the biosystems.

p-Elements of the VIIIA Group

At normal conditions, noble gases (He, Ne, Ar, Kr, Xe, and Rn) are colorless, odorless monatomic elements with a filled outer shell of electrons, making them less capable of chemical interactions. Noble gases are known as chemically inert. Remarkably, some of them possess biofunctions, and in recent years, a lot of reports have revealed their neuroprotective and organ protective effects [184, 185]. It has been reported that most of these elements have essential bioeffects, including cell death modulation, immunomodulation, anti-inflammatory effects, gases interaction, and oxidative stress [186]. Having strong cytoprotective effects,

He, Ne, Ar, Kr, and Xe are also good protective and therapeutic agents for cardio- and cerebrovascular diseases.

Helium

The lightest noble gas (He) is the second (after H_2) most prevalent element in the universe. Helium and xenon, have been reported to display neuroprotective functions following many disease states, including cardiopulmonary bypass-induced dysfunction, acute ischemic stroke, perinatal hypoxia, ischemia, cerebral hemorrhages, and traumatic brain injury. Helium and xenon are used in balneotherapy or medical rehabilitation [187].

Argon

Approximately 1% of the air is argon, frequently growing from the radioactive decay of the radioisotope ^{40}K in the Earth. Ar isotopes have found important applications in hydrology [188].

Krypton

The bioeffects of neon and krypton have been comparatively little examined which merit further study. The long-lived radioisotopes of krypton and argon are predominantly suitable tracers in the earth sciences [189]. Radioisotopes of xenon and krypton are recognized for diagnostic applications in nuclear medicine. Among them ^{133}Xe is the best known as a γ-tracer for the diagnostic of lung diseases.

Xenon

Xenon has neuroprotective activity. Xenon therapy has shown protection of cell viability. Xenon has been firstly revealed to possess anesthetic activity in 1951, while none of the other analogues have anesthetic action at normal conditions. It shows a high affinity for the glycine site on the receptor N-methyl-D-aspartate (NMDA). In comparison with other clinically used NMDA antagonists, it does not show neurotoxic effects [190]. Results for Xe are more coordinated than those for Ar. The mechanisms of action of Xe (noncompetitive NMDA-receptor inhibition) have been better studied compared with those for argon. Particular attention should be paid to the use of Xe as an additive to the ventilation mixture for newborns in the prevention of traumatic brain injury.

Radon

Radon is a dense and toxic radioactive gas formed as a result of the decay of long-lived radioactive uranium and thorium through ^{226}Rn in soil, rocks and water. The decay of Rn leads to the formation of radioactive solids (α-emitters) which attached to dust particles can be breathe in. This inhalation is associated with human lung cancers [191]. Exposure to radon can also lead to the formation of toxic ROS. Radon build-up in nature is a potential problem because exposure to radon accounts for around 50% of natural radioactivity, which is the major single fraction of natural radiation. Predominant isotopes are ^{222}Rn (α-emitter, $T_{1/2}$ = 3.8 days), produced by the decay of ^{238}U, as well as ^{220}Rn (α-emitter, $T_{1/2}$ = 56 s) obtained from the α-decay of ^{224}Rn. These processes happen continuously in rocks and soil, and the produced Rn usually escapes into the air. It is not really Rn that is the problem but the solid radioisotopes produced by its decay, such as polonium-218. These radioisotopes attached to lung tissue, irradiate it with α- and β-particles (electrons).

The biological functions of the elements have been discussed in the respective elements' chapters. Some overall information and brief conclusions on the reviewed main groups' elements of the periodic table are listed in Table **8**.

Table 8. Examples of the biological role of the elements from IA to VIIIA groups.

Atomic number	Element	Biological role	Deficiency	Excess
1	H	Uptake and transport of H-based molecules with C–H, N–H, *etc.* bonds, bicarbonate/CO_2 for pH control.	-	-
6	C	C–H, C=O, *etc.* bonds in the building blocks (amino acids, fatty acids), regulation of CO_2, carbonates, CO.	-	-
7	N	N–H, N–C bonds in amino acids and nucleotides NOSs; conversion of NH_3 to urea (enzymes and transporters)	-	-
8	O	O_2 uptake and transport (hemoglobin), O_2 storage (myoglobin), conversion of O_2 to H_2O_2 and H_2O by mitochondria proteins, enzymes (superoxide dismutase, catalase) O_2-sensor proteins (HIF).	Hypoxia - a chief factor in the progress of serious pathologies including myocardial and cerebral ischemia and cancer [129]	Hyperoxia, ROS production, oxidative stress disrupting the balance between oxidants and antioxidants [128].
9	F	Fluorine favors structural resistance of teeth; F^-/H^- cotransporter or a F^-/OH^- antiporter; its biochemistry is poorly understood.	Increased incidences of dental caries [169].	Fluorosis. Spots on the teeth [170].

(Table 8) cont.....

Atomic number	Element	Biological role	Deficiency	Excess
11	Na	Membrane pumps Na^+/K^+ ATPase	Hyponatremia [31]	Hypernatremia [30]
12	Mg	MAGT1 - protein coding gene	Hypomagnesemia, cardiac arrest [51]	Hypermagnesemia, hypotension [52]
15	P	Kinases, phosphatases, nucleotides	Hypophosphatemia [109], respiratory failure, hemolysis and cardiac failure	Hyperphosphatemia [110], chronic kidney disease
16	S	Thiol and Met in proteins; sulfide in ferredoxins	Acne, rashes, depression, memory loss, arthritis [154, 155].	Asthma-like allergy, breath shortness, coughing, wheezing [154, 155].
17	Cl	Chloride channel: CFTR gene; balance of salts and water	Hypochloremia, alkalosis due to an excess of HCO_3^- [3, 4].	Hyperchloremia - results in acidosis [3, 4].
19	K	Na^+/K^+ ATPase membrane pumps	Hypokalemia [33]	Hyperkalemia [32]
20	Ca	Ca^{2+}-sensor protein troponin; Ca^{2+}-ATPase membrane pump; calmodulin transduces Ca^{2+} signals.	Hypocalcemia [56], demineralization of bone.	Hypercalcemia [57], hyperparathyroidism or malignancy.
34	Se	Component of glutathione peroxidase; Contributes to neutralizing ROS; $\approx$25 selenoproteins with redox and signaling functions.	Kesham disease of heart muscle [160] Osteoarthropathy or Kashin-Beck disease (thickening of the fingers tips).	Selenosis; blind staggers and chronic alkali disease (grazing cattle) [164]
53	I	Component of thyroid hormones thyroxine (T4) and triiodothyronine (T3) synthesized from tyrosine residues in protein thyroglobulin.	Goiter and cretinism [176, 178]	Goiter and thyrotoxicosis [176]
Potentially essential elements				
5	B	Essential for healthy bones and joints.	Arthritis, decreased brain activity [61, 62].	Inhibits amylase, proteinase, and adrenaline [64].
14	Si	Role in bone mineralization, synthesis of collagen.	Deficiency is extremely rare [82].	Silicon compounds - respiratory effects, silicosis, and asbestosis [83]

(Table 8) cont.....

Atomic number	Element	Biological role	Deficiency	Excess
33	As	Blocks -SH groups of enzymes.	Damage of growth and reproduction (in animals) [111]	Poisonous, arsenolysis. [112 - 115]
35	Br	Essential (as HBrO) for killing invading microbes; essential for assemblage of collagen IV scaffolds in tissue development, sedative effect	No deficiency has ever been recognized [175]	Chronic poisoning, called "bromism" [175]
50	Sn	Supposed to be essential for animal growth	Baldness in humans [88]	Non-toxic, safely used in the body; organic tin compounds - toxic [89, 90]
83	Bi	Inhibits enzymes of amino- and carboxypolipeptidaze	Deficiency is extremely rare [123]	There is no serious health risk [122]

CHAPTER 3

Biological Functions of d- and f- Block Elements General Characteristics of d-Elements and Their Compounds

In the periodic table of elements, there are currently 40 d-elements: each of the fourth, fifth, sixth, and seventh periods contains 10 d-elements. They are located between s- and p-elements.

d-Elements are in the group the trace microelements [11 - 13]. Transition metals have some common features:

1. d-elements are rather common in nature and thus available for absorption from the soil;
2. d-elements have high affinity to various donor atoms;
3. d-elements have various stable oxidation states and easily change their oxidation states.

These microelements take part in the most important life processes:

1. Enzymatic catalysis of synthetic reactions and cellular energy processes;
2. Electron transfer, transfer of ions, biomolecules, and molecular enzymes;
3. Regulating the activity of cellular mechanisms and biosystems.

Free ions of transition metals cannot exist in the organism. In biochemical interactions, most often d-elements participate in the form of metal-based bioinorganic complexes [3,11-13].

A characteristic feature of d-elements is that in their atoms, the orbitals are filled not with the outer shell (as in s- and p-elements), but with the pre-external shell. In d-elements, the valence orbitals are the energetically close nine orbitals: one ns-orbital, three np-orbitals, and five (n - 1)d-orbitals.

At the external level, the atoms of d-elements usually have two s^2 electrons. However, nine d-elements (Nb, Rh, Cr, Mo, Ru, Pt, Cu, Ag and Au) have a half-filled 4s subshell. In the palladium atom, there is a "double dip", and its outer level does not contain electrons. This structure of the electron configuration of the atoms of d-elements determines a number of their common properties [3,4,11-13]. All d-elements are metals, but their metallic properties are less pronounced than those of s-elements. In each large period, d-elements form families of 10 d-elements consisting of two subfamilies (s^2d^1 - s^2d^5 and s^2d^6 - s^2d^{10}).

d-Elements are characterized by a large set of oxidation states and, as a consequence, changes in acid-base and redox properties within wide limits. Since part of the valence electrons reside in s-orbitals, the lower oxidation state exhibited by them is usually +2. The exceptions are elements whose ions E^{+3} and E^+ have stable electron configurations d^0, d^5 and d^{10}, such as Sc^{+3}, Fe^{+3}, Cr^+, Cu^+, Ag^+, Au^+. Compounds in which d-elements are in their lowest oxidation state form ionic crystals, exhibit basic properties in chemical interactions and are, in general, strong reducers [4,9-13]. All d-elements, except for Zn, Cd, Sc, Y, and Ag, exhibit variable oxidation states. For almost all d-elements, the oxidation states of +2 and +3 are possible.

d-Elements from IIIB to VIIB groups in the higher oxidation states are comparable in properties to the corresponding p-elements. Thus, in the higher oxidation states, Mn(VII) and Cl(VII) are electron analogues. The resemblance of their electronic configurations (s^2p^5) leads to similar properties of Mn(VII) and Cl(VII) compounds. Mn_2O_7 and Cl_2O_7 under standard conditions are unstable liquids, anhydrides of strong acids with the general formula HEO_4. In the lower oxidation states, Mn and Cl have different electronic structures, which causes a difference in the chemical properties of their compounds [3,4,9-13]. Cl_2O is a gaseous compound, an anhydride of HClO, while MnO is a solid crystalline substance of a basic nature. The similar properties of d-elements with those of the main groups elements is fully demonstrated in the elements of the III groups ns^2np^1 and $(n-1)d^1ns^2$. With increasing the number of the group, this similarity decreases. Elements of the VIIIA group are gases, these of VIIIB are metals. The similarity is also typical for the first and second groups.

From a chemical point of view, d-elements are characterized by three main features: a tendency to exhibit oxidation-reduction properties; acid-base and amphoteric properties; high ability to complexation reactions.

TENDENCY TO EXHIBIT OXIDATION-REDUCTION PROPERTIES

All d-elements, like all metals, are reducing agents. Their reducing capacity is determined both by the structure of the electronic configurations and the size of ions. In the period with the increasing of Z, the reducing properties of metals decrease, reaching a minimum in the elements of group IB. Heavy metals of VIIIB and IB groups are termed noble for their inertness. Due to the negative values of the standard electrode potential, all d-elements, except copper, must dissolve in diluted solutions of acid with the release of hydrogen [3,4,11-13].

Metals with negative potentials are oxidized in the air; metals with positive potentials are oxidized much more slowly or practically not oxidized at all (Pt, Au).

Compounds of d-elements in their highest oxidation state have strong oxidative properties [11 - 13]. For example, chromium(VI) compounds are strong oxidizing agents and in oxidation-reduction processes pass into chromium(III) derivatives in acidic and alkaline environments:

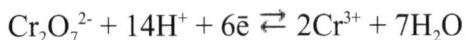

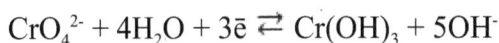

$$Cr_2O_7^{2-} + 14H^+ + 6\bar{e} \rightleftarrows 2Cr^{3+} + 7H_2O$$

$$CrO_4^{2-} + 4H_2O + 3\bar{e} \rightleftarrows Cr(OH)_3 + 5OH^-$$

The greatest oxidative activity of chromium(VI) compounds is observed in acidic solutions.

Chromate ions CrO_4^{2-} are able to pass into dichromate ions $Cr_2O_7^{2-}$ and vice versa:

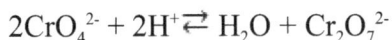

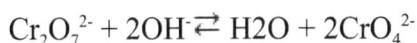

$$2CrO_4^{2-} + 2H^+ \rightleftarrows H_2O + Cr_2O_7^{2-}$$

$$Cr_2O_7^{2-} + 2OH^- \rightleftarrows H2O + 2CrO_4^{2-}$$

Chromates and dichromates have the same oxidation state of chromium equal to +6, but dichromate ions $Cr_2O_7^{2-}$ exist in an acidic environment, and chromate ions CrO_4^{2-} in an alkaline.

Strong oxidizing properties are also possessed by the salts of $HMnO_4$, permanganate salts. The most widely used is $KMnO_4$. Depending on pH, the reduction of permanganates can occur with the formation of various final products [4,11-13]. In an acidic medium, the reduction reaches manganese ions Mn^{2+}, in a neutral environment, the final product is usually the hydrated manganese oxide MnO_2, and in a highly alkaline medium, a fragile manganate MnO_4^{2-} is formed:

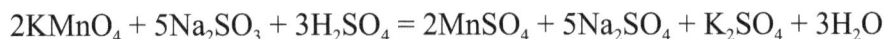

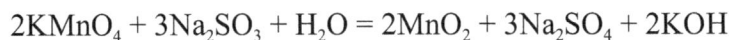

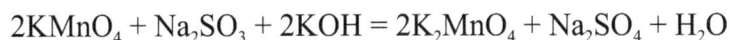

$$2KMnO_4 + 5Na_2SO_3 + 3H_2SO_4 = 2MnSO_4 + 5Na_2SO_4 + K_2SO_4 + 3H_2O$$

$$2KMnO_4 + 3Na_2SO_3 + H_2O = 2MnO_2 + 3Na_2SO_4 + 2KOH$$

$$2KMnO_4 + Na_2SO_3 + 2KOH = 2K_2MnO_4 + Na_2SO_4 + H_2O$$

The oxidizing properties of $KMnO_4$ solutions are used for the quantitative analytical determination of reducing agents for instance Fe(II) salts, hydrogen peroxide, sulfites, nitrites, oxalic acid, chlorides, iodides, *etc.*

FEATURES OF THE ACID-BASIC PROPERTIES

In chemical reactions involving d-elements, the formation of a bond is caused by both s-electrons and all or part of the d-electrons. Compounds with different valence states of d-elements exist [9 - 13]. For example, $TiCl_2$, $TiCl_3$, and $TiCl_4$. The same applies to metal hydroxides, depending on the oxidation state. The oxidation state dramatically affects the acid-base properties of hydroxides. Hydroxides in which the d-element is in a low oxidation state usually exhibit basic properties, and if the d-element is in the highest oxidation state, the hydroxides have acidic properties. The boundary between the two most often corresponds to oxidation states of +3 and +4 and shifts to lower oxidation states with an increase in atomic number. Hydroxides corresponding to these oxidation states are often amphoteric hydroxides. The alteration in the acid-base properties of hydroxides with the variation in the oxidation states is specifically pronounced in Mn compounds. In the sequence $Mn(OH)_2$ - $Mn(OH)_3$ - $Mn(OH)_4$ - H_2MnO_4 - $HMnO_4$, the properties of hydroxides change from a weak base $Mn(OH)_2$ *via* amphoteric $Mn(OH)_3$ and $Mn(OH)_4$ to strong acids H_2MnO_4 and $HMnO_4$.

Dissolution of amphoteric hydroxides in alkali solutions occurs with the formation of complex compounds:

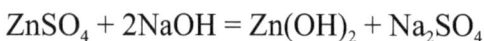

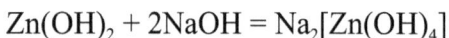

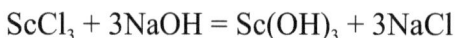

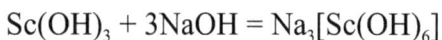

$ZnSO_4 + 2NaOH = Zn(OH)_2 + Na_2SO_4$

$Zn(OH)_2 + 2NaOH = Na_2[Zn(OH)_4]$

$ScCl_3 + 3NaOH = Sc(OH)_3 + 3NaCl$

$Sc(OH)_3 + 3NaOH = Na_3[Sc(OH)_6]$

The reactions of the formation of complex compounds of the above equations can be expressed by one general equation:

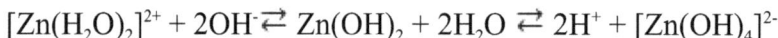

$[Zn(H_2O)_2]^{2+} + 2OH^- \rightleftarrows Zn(OH)_2 + 2H_2O \rightleftarrows 2H^+ + [Zn(OH)_4]^{2-}$

ABILITY TO COMPLEXATION REACTIONS

Due to the incompleteness of the d-shells and the presence of energetically similar unfilled ns- and np-level, d-elements are predisposed to complexation; their complex compounds are usually colored and paramagnetic. All d-elements are active complexing agents [3,4,11-13]. The maximum capacity for complexation falls on those d elements that are located in the VIIIB group (Fe, Co, Ni, Pt, *etc.*). They are adjacent to the elements of the VIB and VIIB groups. These are elements with unfilled d-subshells. When moving along a large period, an increase in the ability to chelate in both directions toward the center of the period is clearly observed. Although the elements of small periods (s- and p-elements) are much worse complexing agents, but they also have the greatest tendency to complexation approximately in the middle of the period.

When moving down group B, the ability to form complexes changes in a complex manner [9 - 13]. It is related to the charge of the ion and its radius. Low charges of ions and their large radii lead to a decrease in the strength of complex ions, but a greater variety of complex compounds is often observed. On the contrary, high-charge ions and their small radii contribute to an increase in the strength of the complexes, but at the same time, the number of possible complex compounds decreases.

Stable compounds are the complexes of Hg(II), Fe(II), Fe(III), Co(III), and Ni(II):

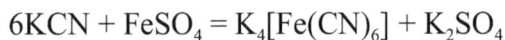

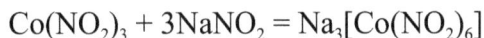

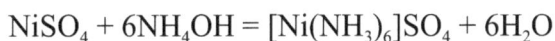

$$2KI + HgI_2 = K_2[HgI_4]$$

$$6KCN + FeSO_4 = K_4[Fe(CN)_6] + K_2SO_4$$

$$Co(NO_2)_3 + 3NaNO_2 = Na_3[Co(NO_2)_6]$$

$$NiSO_4 + 6NH_4OH = [Ni(NH_3)_6]SO_4 + 6H_2O$$

d-Elements can form neutral, cationic, and anionic complexes [3,11-13]. For some d-elements, complexation is manifested even in the behavior of their ions in relation to water. It is known that the anhydrous ion Cu^{2+} is colorless, but the dissolution of dehydrated copper(II) salts in water is accompanied by the formation of blue aqua-complexes $[Cu(H_2O)_6]^{2+}$. The most stable cationic complexes are amino complexes of the type $[E(NH_3)_4]^{2+}$ and $[E(NH_3)_6]^{2+}$, which are easily formed by ammonia in salt solutions:

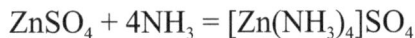

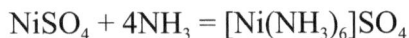

$$ZnSO_4 + 4NH_3 = [Zn(NH_3)_4]SO_4$$

$$NiSO_4 + 4NH_3 = [Ni(NH_3)_6]SO_4$$

THE SIGNIFICANCE OF COMPLEX COMPOUNDS OF D-ELEMENTS IN BIOLOGICAL SYSTEMS

Of the d-elements, some of the transition metals are significant to the chemistry of living systems, the most pronounced examples being eight of them (Fe, Cu, Zn, Mn, Co, Mo, Ni, Cr), which are broadly studied with regard to their biological functions [9 - 13]. The ions of these biogenic metals are the best-known components of a large number of enzymes, bioproteins, and some vitamins. These elements exist mostly as coordination complexes in the body. The biogenic d-elements are often termed metals of life. The typical chemical properties of vital d-elements and their compounds are oxidation-reduction reactions and complex formation reactions. The transition metals have unfilled d-orbitals, therefore their oxidation states in the compounds are variable, which explains their affinity to participate in a great range of oxidation-reduction bioreactions. All these elements have a high capability to form coordination complexes because of the free s- and p-orbitals and partially vacant d-orbitals, which enables them to form additional donor-acceptor bonds in the coordination complexes acting as good complexing agents in a variety of bioreactions.

The biofunctions of d-elements have dual roles [11 - 13]. At standard levels, they can be vital for the stabilization of cell structures, in deficiency conditions, may activate alternative pathways, and cause diseases, and in high levels they are poisonous.

Elements whose content does not exceed $10^{-3}\%$, are part of enzymes, hormones, vitamins, and other vital compounds [11]. For protein, carbohydrate, and fat metabolism, necessary are the next metals: Fe, Co, Mn, Zn, Mo, V, B, W; in the synthesis of proteins the main participants are: Mg, Mn, Fe, Co, Si, Ni, Cr, in hematopoiesis - Co, Ti, Si, Mn, Ni, Zn; in respiration - Mg, Fe, Cu, Zn, Mn and Co. Therefore, trace elements are widely used not only in human medicine but also as micro fertilizers for crops in animal and fish farming. There is a remarkable number of trace microelements, especially among the transition metals, that have been revealed to assist as essential growth factors at extremely low amounts. Trace elements are part of a large number of bioregulators of living systems, which are based on biologically active complexes.

Most of the existing information about the biofunctions of transition metals is focused on their role as metalloenzymes [11]. Many transition metals form coordination complexes with bioproteins in metalloenzymes. These metals are vital since they serve as required prosthetic groups in active sites as coenzymes for many metalloenzymes.

Biological complexes vary in their stability. Some of them are so strong that they are constantly in the body and perform *specific functions*. In cases where the bond between the cofactor and the enzyme protein is strong and difficult to be separated, it is called the "prosthetic group". The role of metals of such complexes is very specific: replacing them even with an element similar in properties leads to a significant or complete loss of physiological activity. In metalloenzymes, Fe,

Zn, Cu, Mn, Mo, Co, Ni, and other trace elements are definitely associated with specific proteins, thus producing unique catalytic functions [9 - 13]. Examples of specific enzymes are chlorophyll, polyphenyl oxidase, vitamin B_{12}, hemoglobin, *etc.* Few enzymes are involved in only one specific or single reaction.

The catalytic properties of most enzymes are determined by the active site formed by different trace elements [11 - 13]. Enzymes are synthesized for the period of performance of the function. The metal ion acts as an activator and can be replaced by an ion of another metal without losing the physiological activity of the enzyme (*non-specific enzymes*). One trace element can activate the work of various enzymes, and one enzyme can be activated by various trace elements. Some enzymes in which ions of different metals perform similar functions are listed in Table **9**.

Table 9. Enzymes in which ions of different metals perform similar functions.

Enzyme	Trace elements that activate the enzyme
Carboxylase	Mn^{2+}, Co^{2+}, Cu^{2+}, Fe^{2+}, Ca^{2+}, Zn^{2+}
Polypeptidase	Zn^{2+}, Co^{2+}
Lecithinase	Zn^{2+}, Mg^{2+}, Co^{2+}, Zn^{2+}, Mn^{2+}
Arginase	Co^{2+}, Mn^{2+}, Ni^{2+}, Fe^{2+}

The greatest proximity in biological action is exerted by enzymes with trace elements in the same oxidation state, for instance, +2. As can be seen for the transition trace elements in their biological action, a horizontal similarity is more characteristic than the vertical one (in the Ti-Zn series) [11].

The intermediate position between specific and non-specific enzymes is occupied by some metalloenzymes [11 - 13]. Metal ions perform the function of a cofactor. Increasing the strength of the enzyme, and the bio-complex increases the specificity of its bioaction. The effectiveness of the enzymatic action of the metal ion of the enzyme is influenced by its oxidation state. According to the intensity of the effect, the trace elements are arranged in the following row: $Ti^{4+} \rightarrow Fe^{3+} \rightarrow Cu^{2+} \rightarrow Fe^{2+} \rightarrow Mg^{2+} \rightarrow Mn^{2+}$. Ion Mn^{3+} in contrast to the ion Mn^{2+}, is very strongly bound to proteins, and mainly with oxygen-containing groups together with Fe^{3+} is part of the metalloproteins.

Trace elements in the complex form act in the body as a factor that apparently determines the high sensitivity of cells to trace elements by their participation in the creation of a high concentration gradient [11]. The values of the atomic and ionic radii, ionization energy, coordination number, and the predisposition to form bonds with the same donors in biomolecules determine the effects detected in the mutual ionic substitution occurring with an intensification (*synergy*), and with an inhibition of their bioactivity (*antagonism*) of the replaced elements.

Ions of d-elements in the oxidation state +2 (Mn, Fe, Co, Ni, Zn) have similar physicochemical characteristics of atoms (electronic structure of the external level, a close radius of ions, type of hybridization of orbitals, close values of stability constants of bioligands. The similarity of the physicochemical characteristics of the complexing agents determines the closeness of their biological functions and interchangeability. Such transitional elements stimulate the processes of hematopoiesis, which enhance metabolic processes [11 - 13]. The role of copper as a plasma Cu protein, ceruloplasmin, is typically positive in promoting Fe mobilization and hemoglobin synthesis. The synergy of elements in the processes of hematopoiesis is possibly associated with the participation of ions of these elements in various stages of the process of synthesis of human blood cells. Numerous antagonistic and synergistic effects have been detected. Zinc absorption is diminished by Fe(II). Zinc also induces Cu deficiency, perhaps by interfering with Cu absorption. Mo and S antagonize Cu as well, probably by the formation of Cu thiomolybdate, causing a reduced Cu uptake. W has an antagonistic effect on Mo in some Mo-dependent enzymes such as xanthine oxidase.

The same is true not only for d elements. The highest similarity of lithium with sodium (s-elements of the IA group) determines the interchangeability and synergy of their activity. Destructive properties of aqueous solutions of potassium, rubidium, and cesium ions, provide their better membrane permeability, interchangeability, and synergy of their bioactivity [29]. s-Elements of the IIA group *in vivo* are in the form of compounds formed by phosphoric, carbonic, and carboxylic acids. Ca, contained mainly in bone tissue, is close in its properties to strontium and barium, which can replace it in bone tissues. The concentration of K^+ inside the cells is 35 times higher than outside it, and the concentration of Na^+ in the extracellular fluid is 15 times greater than inside the cell. These ions in biosystems are antagonists. Ca^{2+} ions are also antagonists of sodium, potassium, and magnesium ions [37]. The similarity of physical and chemical characteristics of Be^{2+} and Mg^{2+} cations cause their interchangeability in bio-compounds containing Mg-N and Mg-O bonds. This may explain the inhibition of magnesium-containing enzymes when beryllium enters the body. Beryllium is a magnesium antagonist.

In humans, many d-elements form complex compounds with various endogenous (initially present in the organism) and exogenous (entering the body from the external environment) with significant biological functions [3,4,11-13,192]. The exogenous ligands include vitamins, drugs, toxic compounds, *etc.* Some examples of biologically active natural and synthetic complex bio-compounds are shown in Table **10**.

Table 10. Biologically active complexes.

Metal	Biological system
Fe	Hemoglobin, cytochromes, catalases; peroxidases, NO-synthase, hydroxylases
Zn	carbonic anhydrase; $Zn(gluconate)_2$, $Zn(His)_2$ in carbonic anhydrase
Cu	cytochrome; NO-synthase, hydroxylases, $Cu(His)_2$ in carbonic anhydrase
Mn	carboxylase, galactose oxidase, ribonucleotide reductase
Mo	xanthine oxidoreductase, nitrate reductase, CO-dehydrogenase, sulphite oxidase
Mg	chlorophyll, Mg complex with ATP in the enzyme kinase
Hg	$K_2[HgI_4]$ — Lugol's solution
Co	Vitamin B_{12} (cobalamine), cyanocobalamine

Natural coordination compounds are significant in many characteristics. Most of the chemical elements contained in the organs and tissues form complex compounds with proteins and other biopolymers, including amino acids, peptides, nucleic acids, fatty acids, carbohydrates, enzymes, vitamins, and hormones. The complexing capability of biological ligands can be elucidated by the presence in their molecules of some essential functional groups -COOH, $-NH_2$, primary, secondary, and tertiary amines, which can coordinate with the metal cations. The porfinic system is composed of tetradentate macromolecules [3,4,11,192]. Nitrogen donor atoms are located on square corners, tightly coordinated in space. The metal complexes of porphyrins (Fig. **5**) are among the most significant in the living systems (chlorophyll, hemoglobin, myoglobin, *etc.*). Porphinic structure forms stable complexes with metal cations like Mg^{2+}, Fe^{2+}, which act as the central atoms in important biological molecules. Heme, the constituent of hemoglobin which transports O_2 in blood, is a complex (chelate) of porphyrins and ferrous cations. Chlorophyll is a complex of porphyrin and magnesium(II) ions. Cobalt(III) complex with corrin (similar to the porphyrin ring) is a part of cobalamin (vitamin B_{12}), (Fig. **6**), which plays a significant role in the formation of red blood cells and its deficiency causes pernicious anemia. Flavin (Fig. **5**) is a constituent of dehydrogenases.

Together with the widely studied bimetallic complex compounds of porphyrin, corrin, and flavin, there are additional systems in which transition metal ions and redox-active cofactors cooperate in electron transfer and substrate activation. The typical representatives are pterin (in molybdopterin), alloxazine, isoalloxazine (in NO-synthase and aromatic amino acid hydroxylases), histidine (Cu(II) and Zn(II) complexes in carbonic anhydrase), quinone, topaquinone (Cu-dependent quinoproteins as amine oxidases), phenoxyl radical, tyrosyl radical (copper(II), iron(II) and manganese(II) complexes in galactose oxidase and ribonucleotide reductase), *etc.* [192], (Fig. **7**).

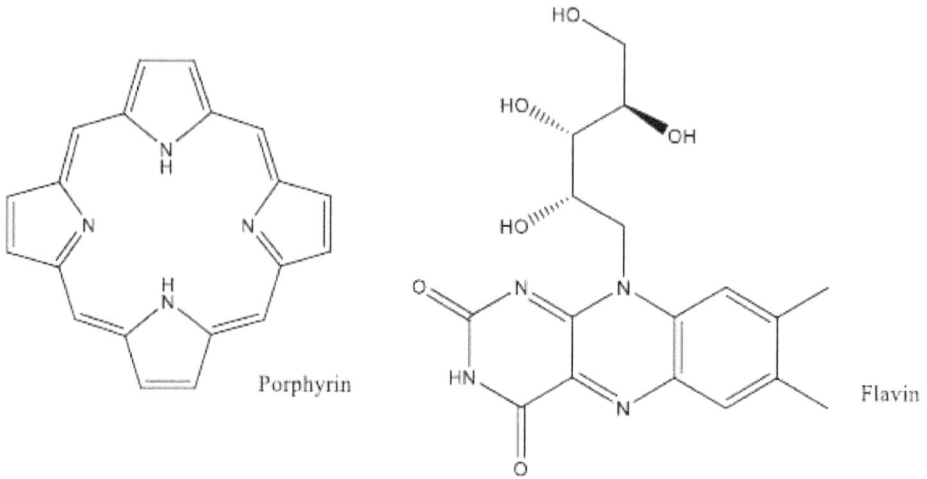

Fig. (5). Structures of porphyrin and flavin.

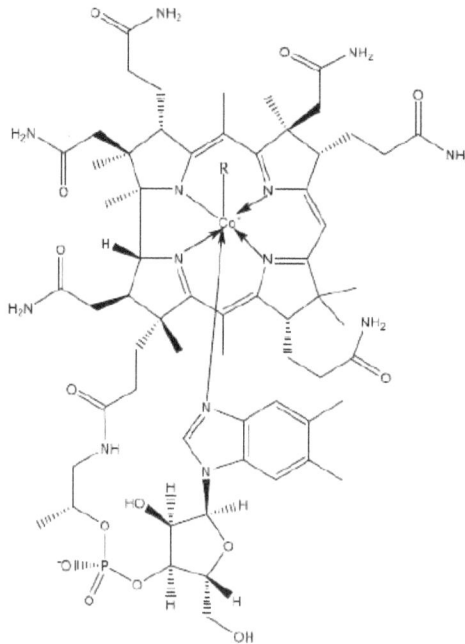

Fig. (6). Structure of Vitamin B$_{12}$.

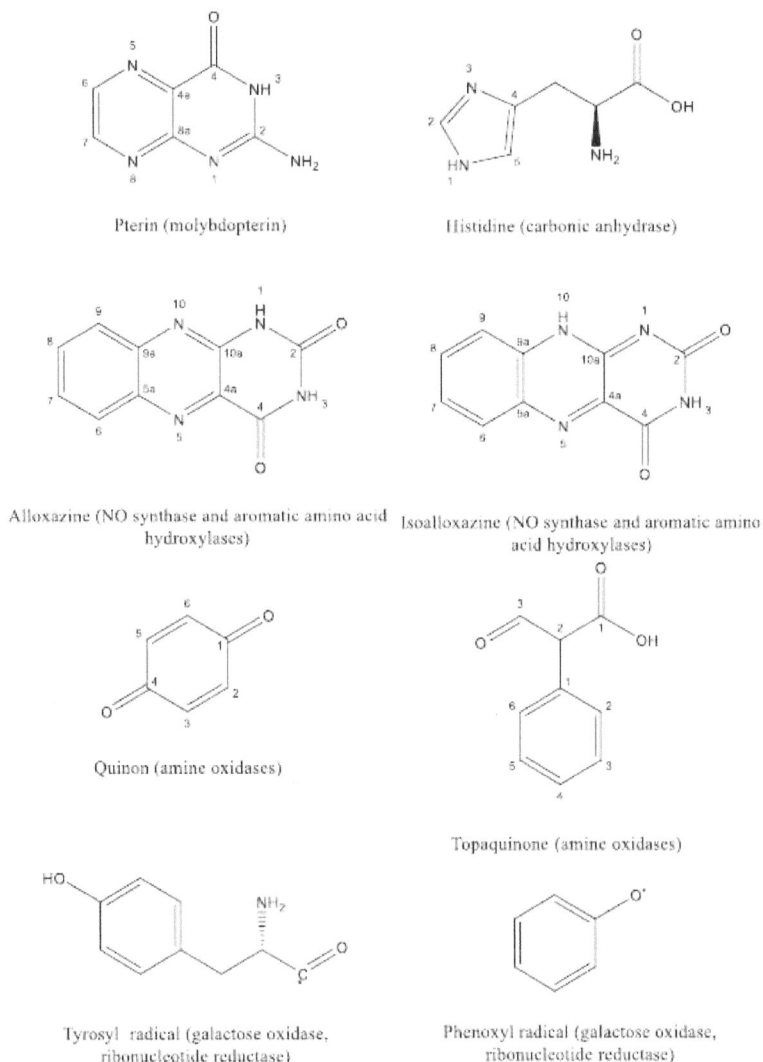

Pterin (molybdopterin)

Histidine (carbonic anhydrase)

Alloxazine (NO synthase and aromatic amino acid hydroxylases)

Isoalloxazine (NO synthase and aromatic amino acid hydroxylases)

Quinon (amine oxidases)

Topaquinone (amine oxidases)

Tyrosyl radical (galactose oxidase, ribonucleotide reductase)

Phenoxyl radical (galactose oxidase, ribonucleotide reductase)

Fig. (7). Redox-active bioorganic compounds in biological systems.

Many coordination compounds are used as therapeutics, which are widely discussed in the next sections [9 - 13, 192]. Iron compounds are used for the treatment of iron deficiency anemia, zinc preparations - in dermatology, platinum complexes - as antineoplastic agents. Chelation agents are applied as antioxidants and for detoxification of heavy metals at intoxication (Pb, Hg, Cd *etc.*). In body fluids, some metal ions *(e.g.,* Fe^{3+}, Ca^{2+}, Cu^{2+}) are chelated by low molecular chelating agents like citrate, polyphenols, *etc.* The metal cations coordinated with various synthetic low-molecular ligands also exhibit some important bioeffects, like the anti-inflammatory effect of Cu^{2+} complexes with indomethacin, D-penicillamine and some salicylates. Human body metabolism supports the complexation processes, *viz.,* metal-ligand homeostasis, the destruction of which leads to numerous diseases, for example, different types of deficiency anemia.

The toxic effects of many transition metals are also connected with their ability to form coordination complexes [11 - 13]. Consequently, poisoning with the compounds of d-elements is because of the formation of stable complexes with proteins or enzymes, resulting in the disruption of significant metabolic processes. Raw materials and foods are polluted with toxic metals through gas, liquid, and solid emissions and contaminated waste from industrial, communal, agro-industrial and energy enterprises, vehicles, through technological equipment, *etc.* These metals get into plants, animals, and fish in air, water, and soil, and as a result they get into the human bodies with food products. Metal chelation activity depends on the occurrence of toxic compounds, for instance, CO, HCN, cyanides, and salts, which are hazardous when inhaled. Typical metal complex compound is carbonyl hemoglobin HbCO, the stability of which constants are 200 times more than that of HbO_2. So even a small amount of CO is dangerous. As a result, the access of O_2 to tissues decreases, displaying signs of hypoxia. Similar is the mechanism of action of cyanides, but their toxic effects are higher. The higher toxicity is attributed to the higher resistance of the $Fe=CN^-$ bond in cyanide hemoglobin. The toxic effects of Cu compounds are associated with the affinity of copper ions to -SH and $-NH_2$ groups, which block proteins. This is a typical chelating interaction, as a consequence of which proteins become insoluble, losing enzyme activity, and disrupting vital body functions. The toxic effects of Ag compounds are connected with the fact that silver ions react with toxic sulphur- and nitrogen-based proteins and nucleic acids. There are similar compounds of Au and many other metals. Toxicity rises with the atomic number of the metals.

One of the most broadly used, inexpensive, and simple chemical methods of decontamination are chelation therapy [193, 194]. Compounds used as antidotes allow to change the composition, charge, size, properties, and solubilities of toxic particles, turn them into low-toxic ones, stop their toxic effects, and remove them from the body. Chelating agents can be organic or inorganic compounds which are able to bind metal ions forming complex structures. In most cases of metal intoxication, S, N, and O donor atoms function as effective ligands. These donors are in the form of chemical functional groups of biomolecules, such as $-NH_2$, $=NH$, -SH, -S-S, -OH, $-OPO_3H$, $>C=O$. The chelating agents are mainly bidentate or multidentate ligands which form stable structures with toxic metals. The most widely used detoxifiers (antidotes) in clinical practice are presented in Fig. (**8**).

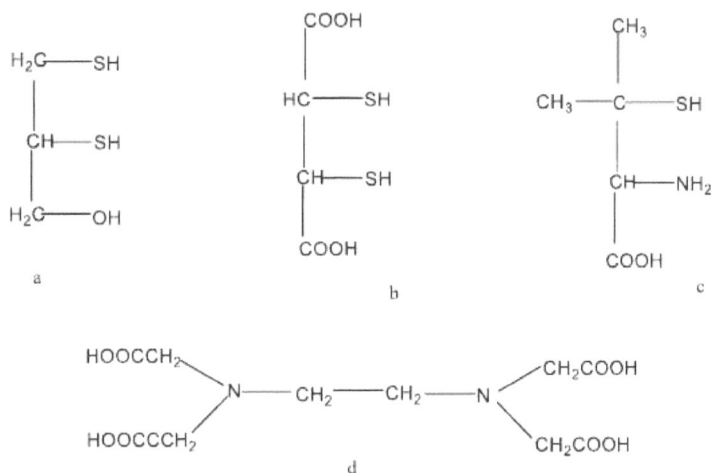

Fig. (8). Antidotes for heavy metal intoxication: (**a**) Dimercaprol; (**b**) Dimercapto-succinic acid; (**c**) Penicillamine; (**d**) EDTA.

Dimercaprol is used for the detoxification of As, Hg, Te, Au. Meso-2,3-di mercaptosuccinic acid (DMSA) is very effective against Hg intoxication with no substantial damage to essential metals like Zn, Ca, Fe and Mg. The α-amino acid metabolite of penicillin, penicillamine, detoxifies Pb, Cu, and Hg. The medicinal form is D-penicillamine, because L-penicillamine inhibits the action of pyridoxine and has toxic effects. D-penicillamine is mainly recommended for the removal of excess Cu in patients with Wilson's disease. Ethylenediamine-tetraacetic acid (EDTA) and its soluble salts are the most extensively used antidotes in cases of various heavy metal intoxications and radioactive isotopes. CaNa$_2$EDTA is frequently used for the treatment of Pb poisoning (Pb^{2+} displaces Ca^{2+} in the chelate), [193, 194].

BIOLOGICAL ROLE OF D-ELEMENTS

d-Elements of the IB Group

Copper

Copper is the third most abundant essential transition element (10^{-4}%). The human body contains around 100-150 mg of copper. Approximately 30% of the total amount of copper is contained in the muscles. Copper is found in cells of all organs, but accumulates mostly in the liver, kidney, and brain. Copper enters the body mainly with food. A person's need for copper is 2-3 mg per day [195].

Copper ions, in comparison with ions of other metals, interact more actively with amino acids, proteins and other biomolecules, so Cu forms the most stable chelates with biologically active substances. It is assumed that during evolution when nature created an oxygen transport system, it had a choice between iron and copper [3 - 5]. Apparently, initially, in most animals, the copper-containing protein hemocyanin served as a blood pigment, but later hemoglobin received an advantage. Hemocyanins are found only in plasma, while hemoglobin is located inside red blood cells (erythrocytes) so that the blood can carry much larger amounts of oxygen. It is clear that higher animals with their increased need for oxygen had to switch to hemoglobin, while mollusks and arthropods retained hemocyanin, which fully meets their needs.

Copper is necessary for growth and bone formation, for the formation of myelin sheaths in the nervous system. Copper with iron participates in blood formation. It helps in the incorporation of iron in the hemoglobin of red blood cells, in the absorption of iron, and in the transfer of Fe from tissues to blood plasma. With Cu deficiency, Fe exchange between blood plasma and erythrocytes is disturbed which leads to the destruction of the red blood cells in the body. Copper also enhances the action of insulin and pituitary hormones. It additionally has a hypoglycemic effect as well as some impact on water and mineral metabolism [195].

Copper is part of proteins and enzymes that regulate such vital processes as hematopoiesis, tissue respiration, growth of the body, and particularly oxidation-reduction processes. In the form of the couple, Cu^+/Cu^{2+} copper has redox properties, which are similar to that of Fe^{2+}/Fe^{3+}. Copper acts as both an antioxidant and a prooxidant. Being an antioxidant, Cu scavenges and neutralizes reactive oxygen species and reduces or helps prevent some damage. When it acts as a prooxidant, Cu promotes ROS damage and may contribute to the development of some diseases. In non-complexed free form, copper has to be tightly controlled to prevent damaging cells because of its potential to accelerate the generation of toxic free radicals [196]. High Cu intake for a prolonged period of time causes increased Cu concentration in serum and tissues, which in sequence, causes OS and affects some immune functions. Irregularities in copper homeostasis are supposed to play roles in Alzheimer's and Parkinson's diseases and amyotrophic lateral sclerosis [197].

Copper participates in many vital bioprocesses including angiogenesis, neuromodulation, and respiration processes, although the complete role of Cu has yet to be clarified. The main function of copper in higher organisms is catalytic [195]. It has a very imperative role in human metabolism mainly because it allows numerous important enzymes to work properly. Various metalloproteins and metalloenzymes (around 1% of the total proteome found in eukaryotes and prokaryotes) contain copper as an important constituent in their active sites (cytochrome oxidase, ceruloplasmin, catalase, tyrosinase, peroxidase, cytosolic superoxide dismutase, ascorbic acid oxidase, uricase, *etc.*). The structure and activity of Cu enzymes and chaperones became well clarified. Examples of enzymes, in which copper is the component, are given in Table **11**.

Table 11. Copper enzymes and their functions.

Cu enzymes	Biological function
Hemocyanin	Dioxygen transport in mollusks and arthropods $Hc + O_2 \leftrightarrow Hc{\cdot}O_2$
Cytochrome-c-oxidase	Electron transfer from cytochrome c to O_2 in tissues respiration $O_2 \rightarrow 2O^{2-}$ in mitochondria
Monoamine oxidases	Oxidative deamination of biogenic amines primary amine $\rightarrow$ aldehyde
Methane monooxygenase (MMO)	Methane $\rightarrow$ methanol in methanogenic bacteria
Dopamine β-hydroxylase	Noradrenaline synthesis in the adrenal gland and brain Dopamine $\rightarrow$ norepinephrine dopamine $\rightarrow$ noradrenaline
Tyrosinase	Tyrosine oxidation in fungal and mammal Melanin biosynthesis DOPA $\rightarrow$ melanin
Lysyl oxidase	lysine $\rightarrow$ allysine, maturation of collagen and elastin
Ceruloplasmin	Dismutation of superoxide anion radical to H_2O_2; Fe metabolism; ferroxidase, $Fe^{2+} \rightarrow Fe^{3+}$, acts in blood plasma
Ascorbate oxidase	Oxidation of L-ascorbate in plants L-Ascorbate + O_2 $\rightarrow$ dehydroascorbate + H_2O
Laccase	Phenol and diamine oxidation in a tree, fungal p-diphenols + O_2 $\rightarrow$ p-quinones + H_2O
Cu,Zn-superoxidedismutase	Dismutation of O_2^- anion radical to hydrogen peroxide $2O_2^- + 2H^+ \rightarrow H_2O_2 + O_2$ (in red blood cells)
Aminooxidases	Oxidative deamination of amines; Elastin, collagen formation in animals
Glycosylphosphatidylinositol (GLI)-ceruloplasmin	Iron elimination from macrophages
Peptidylglycine-α-amidating monooxygenase (PAM)	Oxidative N-dealkylation in the pituitary and heart Neuropeptide transformation
Hephestin	Iron elimination from enterocytes

A variety of Cu-based metalloenzymes, found in flora and fauna, are utilized for electron transfer reactions (azurin, plastocyanin, laccase), oxygenation processes (tyrosinase, ascorbate oxidase), and O_2 transport (hemocyanin). Cu^{2+} ions are normally coordinated with N-donor atoms or with a combination of N- and S-donors [195]. Cu-containing metalloproteins and metalloenzymes can contain Cu(I), Cu(II) and Cu(III) ions in d^{10}, d^9, and d^8 configurations with linear, tetragonally distorted octahedral and square-planar geometries, respectively. The soft Cu(+1) ion prefers S-based bioligands or unsaturated bioligands with large polarizable electron shells. The comparatively hard Cu(+2) ion prefers the hard N-based ligands. Normally, the Cu metalloenzymes, involved in redox reactions, include both kinds of ligands, so that the metal center can easily exist in both oxidation states.

The Cu-containing metalloproteins and metalloenzymes are classified into three categories; type 1, type 2, and type 3, which have characteristic geometries and ligand environments surrounding the metal centers as well as recognizable properties [3,4,195]. Type 1 copper(II) proteins (blue copper proteins), with a distorted tetrahedral structure, act in single electron transfer processes. Biologically, type 1 Cu ions prefer the combination of N-donor (histidine) and S-donor (cysteine) bioligands. In type 2 copper sites, Cu functions as a catalytic center and can bind directly to substrates, for instance, laccase and ascorbate oxidase. The type 3 copper(II) proteins include a binuclear Cu(II) center and occur in oxygen transporting proteins (hemocyanin) as well as in many oxidases (tyrosinase, cytochrome *c* oxidase).

Copper transport in the liver involves the protein ceruloplasmin, which carries the majority of Cu in human blood plasma and possesses enzymatic properties [195, 196]. The major Cu-containing protein ceruloplasmin catalyzes the conversion of Fe(II) to Fe(III). That is why patients, deficient in ceruloplasmin, accumulate Fe in the liver (aceruloplasminemia). Ceruloplasmin contains Cu(I) and Cu(II) ions. It has a blue color and accounts for 3% of Cu contained in the organism. Ceruloplasmin participates in the transport of Cu, in keeping its level in tissues, especially in the liver. With a lack of copper in the body, the content of ceruloplasmin decreases, which can cause anemia.

Hemocyanin binds to O_2 reversibly for the transport and storage of oxygen [3,4,195]. In the deoxygenated form, copper in the form of Cu^+ cation changes its color upon O_2 binding due to the oxidation state transformation from +1 to +2:

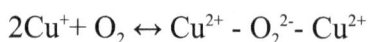

$$2Cu^+ + O_2 \leftrightarrow Cu^{2+} - O_2^{2-} - Cu^{2+}$$

Tyrosinases, the first enzymes in which Cu was shown to be essential to function, catalyze melanin biosynthesis [3,4,195,196]. The enzyme tyrosinase oxidizes catechol to quinone in the presence of O_2 (Fig. **9**).

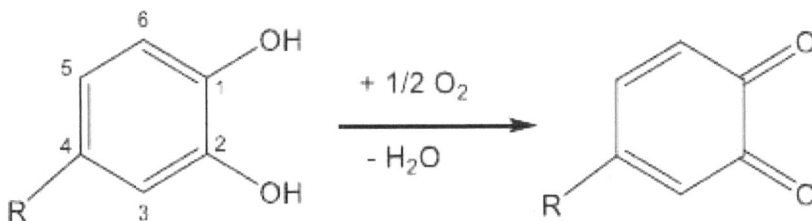

Fig. (9). Oxidation of catechol to quinone.

Metalloenzymes such as CuZn-superoxide dismutase (CuZnSOD), copper metallothionine (CuMT) modulate the ROS production and the level of OS in the body [195]. CuZn-SOD, which contains one Cu and one Zn ion per subunit, catalyzes the dismutation (disproportionation reaction) of the biologically harmful $\cdot O_2^-$ to molecular O_2 and H_2O_2. The overall mechanism of superoxide dismutation catalyzed by SOD can be illustrated by the chemical equations, given below. It is characterized by the copper redox cycle $Cu^{2+}/Cu^+/Cu^{2+}$ *etc.*

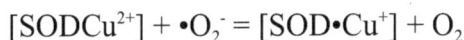

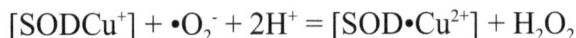

$$[SODCu^{2+}] + \cdot O_2^- = [SOD\cdot Cu^+] + O_2$$

$$[SODCu^+] + \cdot O_2^- + 2H^+ = [SOD\cdot Cu^{2+}] + H_2O_2$$

Consequently, superoxide dismutase converts $\cdot O_2^-$ into H_2O_2, which is a comparatively slight oxidant that decomposes quickly to H_2O and O_2 by the heme iron metalloenzyme catalase according to the following equation:

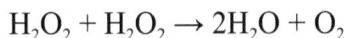

$$H_2O_2 + H_2O_2 \rightarrow 2H_2O + O_2$$

The common aerobic organisms, apart from some algae and bacteria, comprise catalase in the peroxisomes [195]. In prokaryotes, SODs have been found to contain some redox-active manganese and iron metal centers (MnSOD and FeSOD). The Cu-Zn superoxide dismutase enzyme (CuZnSOD), occurring in eukaryotic and some bacterial species, is mainly located in mammalian blood cells, liver and brain tissues. SODs act as antioxidants that can inhibit aging and carcinogenesis.

There are many other copper-containing proteins and enzymes. Other proteins (erythrocuprein, cerebrocuprein, hepatocuprein) occurring in the erythrocytes, mammalian brain and liver, respectively, contain around 60% of the total Cu amount in these tissues, although their biofunctions are still unidentified. Ascorbic acid oxidase, which contains eight Cu atoms per molecule, is widely distributed in vegetation and some microorganisms [3,4,195,196]. Cytochrome oxidase with a 1:1 ratio of heme to copper contains a binuclear complex where two copper atoms are bonded through bidentate cysteine residues, with each copper atom coordinating the heterocyclic N-atom of imidazole. The center of the enzyme is similar to N_2O-reductase.

Copper homeostasis is crucial in the human body because the genetic copper deficiency and excess lead to Menkes and Wilson's diseases, respectively, which cause liver failure, neuromodulation, respiration failure, and angiogenesis. In the absence of Cu in the body, copper-deficient anemia can progress [196, 198]. The symptoms of Cu deficiency are neutropenia, hypochromic anemia, hair and skin hypopigmentation, lowered immunity, vascular abnormalities, anomalous bone formation with skeletal brittleness and osteoporosis, joint pains, *etc.* Copper is necessary for the absorption of Fe, particularly in the biosynthesis of cytochrome oxidase. With a Cu deficiency, the normal growth of connective tissues and hematopoiesis are disturbed. The resulting symptoms of genetic Menke's disease in infants include neuropathy, impaired immune responses, and severe disorders in mental and physical growth. Effective therapy should rely on soluble Cu compounds, administered intravenously. The deficiency of copper is a very rare hematological and neurological disorder because the daily requirement for copper is relatively low.

In high amounts, copper is in a metallic state and its soluble compounds are poisonous. The toxic effects of copper in plants are very rare in comparison to the Cu deficiency, while in animals and humans, the intoxication is frequently induced by high concentrations in genetically anomalous levels. Similar to Fe, copper ions tend to participate in the formation of ROS. Cu concentrations in the atmosphere are generally rather low meaning that the exposures to Cu through breathing are negligible. Nevertheless, people living near the smelters of copper ore do experience this kind of occupational exposure to copper. In the working environment, Cu contamination leads to a flu-like disorder, the so-called metal fever. This condition is produced by hypersensitivity and can pass within 2-3 days. Genetic copper overload gives rise to Wilson's disease, which leads to excessive Cu accumulation in the brain and liver, leading to progressive neurological disorders, psychiatric illness, and liver failure [196, 199]. A treatment of this disease and of acute Cu intoxication, involves the application of Cu-specific chelating ligands like D-penicillamine (Fig. **8**). The ligand contains sulphur (thiolate) and nitrogen (amine) donor atoms that guarantee copper specificity, as well as a hydrophilic carboxylic functional group, which makes the obtained complex excretable.

Excesses of copper-soluble salts are toxic [199]. Copper(II) sulfate in high quantities around 2g produces severe intoxication and probably a fatal consequence because Cu easily forms insoluble chelates. Copper ions entering blood plasma bind strongly to albumin and go primarily to the liver and kidney. Cu cations bind to the functional groups of the fungi and algae proteins causing protein denaturation, cell damage, and leakage.

Silver

The physiological role of silver in a living organism has not been studied enough. Silver is an ultra-microelement of plants and animals [3,4,11]. The human body contains silver in a concentration of less than 10^{-12}%. Silver is concentrated in the liver, pituitary gland, erythrocytes, and the pigment membrane of the eye.

Silver has no known vital function in biology. Silver compounds have a low acute or chronic toxicity [11]. This element is not as significant, but entering the body in high concentrations exhibits toxic effects, like other heavy metals. Interacting with sulfur-containing proteins, silver deactivates enzymes, coagulates and deconstructs proteins, and produces low-soluble albuminates. These possessions to form albuminates are the reasons for the antibacterial activity of silver compounds. The silver concentration of 10^{-8} mmol/l in water demonstrates antibacterial action.

Silver is best-known for its well-established bactericidal properties [11 - 13]. Silver(I) complex compounds with protein-proteinates represent colloidal solutions. Silver colloidal medications do not precipitate tissue proteins and are applied in the treatment of infectious diseases of mucous membranes, conjunctivitis, venereal, and skin diseases. The best-known silver colloidal preparations are the silver protein complex (Protargolum) and the colloid silver (colloidal Argentum). Ag(II) compounds are of interest as antibacterial agents because they are soluble in water, contrasting silver(I) salts (excluding nitrate and fluoride).

Silver(I) complexes have received great attention as potential antineoplastic agents, with pronounced cytotoxicity against different tumor cell lines. Silver nanoparticles have become a prevalent method of treating bacteria and viruses [200]. They are the most predominant nanomaterials used in consumer cleaning products, incorporated in air filters, and medical devices. One of the common water purification systems involves Ag nanoparticles.

Gold

Gold is a trace microelement found in the human body. Its role is just beginning to be studied. Gold has unique pharmacological properties which have to be explored. As a soft metal, Au(I) has a tendency to produce stable coordination compounds with easily polarizable soft donors, such as sulphur- and phosphorus-based ligands [3, 4]. Au(I) ions bind to -SH groups of blood protein molecules and block them. They also inhibit free oxygen radicals.

The application of gold compounds to medicine is known as chrysotherapy (aurotherapy). The gold compounds are predominantly effective in the therapy of rheumatoid arthritis reducing inflammation; however, the mechanism is still discussed [201]. Several gold compounds are used the best known being auranofin $(C_{14}H_{19}O_9)$-S-Au=P$(C_2H_5)_3$. Many Ag(I) and Au(III) complexes with biologically active ligands are known to be useful for treating other medical conditions, especially cancer, but some of them have not been confirmed.

The most promising Ag(I) and Au(III) candidates for clinical application in the treatment of rheumatoid arthritis and cancer are discussed in the next sections.

d-Elements of the IIB Groups

Zinc

Zinc is known as an essential trace element for plant and animal organisms. Zn is the second most important metal, present in an amount of around 2.5 g in the human body. It is placed between Fe ($\approx$ 4 g) and Cu ($\approx$ 0.2 g). Zinc is found in all body systems, in all organs and tissues of humans and higher animals [3, 4]. The most zinc-rich organs are the liver, muscle tissue, pancreas and sex glands, pituitary gland, and adrenal glands. The recommended daily amount is 10-15 mg.

Although the average human body contains only 2-3 grams of zinc, this metal has some very vital functions. Zinc is involved in numerous bioreactions in the body [11 - 13]. This element is used in the formation of connective tissues like ligaments and tendons. Bones, teeth, nails, hair, and skin need zinc to grow. Zinc is vital for a healthy immune system. It participates in the formation, release, and usage of hormones. In addition, the human sense of vision, taste, and smell depends on zinc. Zinc takes part in the replication processes of the genetic code of DNA and RNA. In the pancreas, Zn contributes to the formation of insulin.

The metal zinc has an amphoteric character. Therefore, it ionizes either in an acidic or alkaline environment. Zinc, although redox inactive in its constant oxidation state (+II), displays flexible coordination numbers in biological systems, allowing Zn-based enzymes to catalyze different biochemical transformations. Although zinc cannot serve a redox function, Zn^{2+} is a valuable ion for the organism, because of several reasons. First of all, it is widely available in the environment. Zn^{2+} is a strong Lewis acid and acts as such in enzymes. The tetrahedral geometry, a key feature for zinc enzymes, is preferable in zinc complexes, unlike the geometries of many other metals [3,4,11]. Zn^{2+} is almost entirely resistant to oxidation-reduction changes at biopotentials, which means that its role cannot be influenced by changing redox biopotentials in the body. Moreover, Zn^{2+} undergoes very rapid ligand exchange, facilitating its function in enzymes.

The biological functions of Zn are due to its connection with enzyme- active proteins (carbo xypeptidase, carbonic anhydrase, amino peptidase, lactate dehydro genase, alcohol dehydro genase, Cu/Zn superoxide dismutase [202], DNA and RNA polymerase, retinene reductase), in which zinc is a crucial constituent [203]. Zinc activates enzymes peroxidase, enolase, and arginase and inhibits phosphoglucomutase, alkaline phosphatase, and ribonuclease. In the human body, around 3000 Zn-based proteins are recognized and they play a crucial role in enzyme catalysis. Moreover, they determine the structural stability of other various proteins. The constant oxidation state of Zn explains its role in the non-electron transport hydrolysis reactions. The main zinc enzymes and their biological functions are presented in Table **12**.

Table 12. Zinc enzymes and their functions.

Enzyme	Function
Carbonic anhydrase	Catalyzes reversible hydration of CO_2: $H_2CO_3 \rightleftarrows CO_2 + H_2O$ Regulates acidic-base balance in tissues
Carboxypeptidase	Hydrolytic cleavage of amino acids from the C-terminal of proteins and polypeptides
Cu,Zn-superoxide dismutase	Antioxidant defensive function superoxide $\rightarrow O_2 + H_2O_2$
Alcohol dehydrogenase	Oxidation of alcohols and reduction of aldehydes ethanol $\rightarrow$ acetaldehyde
Metallothioneins	Antioxidant defensive function
Alkaline phosphatase	Hydrolytic cleavage of phosphate residues from organic compounds
Alanine aminopeptidase	Hydrolytic cleavage of N-end amino acid from peptides, amides or acrylamide
Protein kinase C	Phosphorylation of proteins and subsequent induction of signal transduction
RNA/DNA polymerases	Synthesis of nucleic acids

Zn enzymes that perform practically all enzyme-type functions are identified, but the most common one is hydrolysis. The Zn-based hydrolases are enzymes that activate the hydrolysis of C-O-C, P-O-C, and P-O-P bonds.

The high Zn content in erythrocytes can be explained by the fact that most of it is part of carbonic anhydrase (CA), which participates in gas exchange and tissue respiration [3,4,203]. CA, which keeps acidic-base equilibrium in the bloodstream and tissues to transport CO_2, contains zinc in its active position. In the lungs, carbonic anhydrase converts HCO_3^- into CO_2, suitable for exhalation, by catalyzing the reactions:

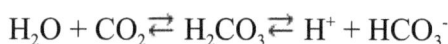

$$H_2O + CO_2 \rightleftarrows H_2CO_3 \rightleftarrows H^+ + HCO_3^-$$

$$OH^- + CO_2 \rightleftarrows HCO_3^-$$

In principle, the Zn complexes with proteins contain hard N- and O-donor atoms, and soft S-donors of histidine, aspartate, glutamate, *etc*. CA contains one Zn^{2+} ion per molecule, coordinated with three histidine imidazole ligands and one water molecule. Because Zn^{2+} is a Lewis acid, the pK_a of the Zn^{2+}-H_2O unit is around 8 versus 14 for pure H_2O. Therefore, at physiological pH 7-8, a significant fraction of the enzyme molecules contains Zn^{2+}-OH^- groups, which are more reactive than bulk H_2O [3,4,203]. When CO_2 binds to a nonpolar site next to the Zn^{2+}-OH^- unit, it can react quickly to give a coordinated HCO_3^- that dissociates from the enzyme:

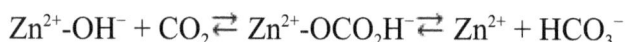

$$Zn^{2+}\text{-}OH^- + CO_2 \rightleftarrows Zn^{2+}\text{-}OCO_2H \rightleftarrows Zn^{2+} + HCO_3^-$$

Thus, the function of zinc in CA is to generate OH^- at neutral pH, far less than the pH required in the absence of the metal cation. In the enzyme, Zn activates the hydration of CO_2 in biofluids and transfers H^+ ions to CO_3^{2-}, which regulates one of the most significant buffers of the body.

The other Zn-based enzyme - carboxypeptidase (CPD) occurs in several forms, which differ in the number of amino acid residues and molar masses [203]. CPD participates in the reactions of peptide bond hydrolysis. Its mechanism of action is not clarified. There are Zn enzymes involved in the hydrolysis of dipeptides, called dispeptidases.

Oxidoreductases catalyze oxidation-reduction bioreactions, for instance, alcohol dehydrogenase catalyzes alcohol oxidation to aldehyde. It contains two independent Zn^{2+} centers. One of them is responsible for the detoxification and oxidation of alcohols to aldehydes by means of NAD^+ and the other one gives the structural stability of the enzyme. In CuZn-superoxide dismutase (CuZnSOD), accountable for the reduction of O_2^-, the Zn center is similarly supposed to give the enzyme's structural stability [202, 203].

Zinc-based enzymes form notable in their shapes Zn fingers [204]. Zinc fingers keep Zn^{2+} in a tetrahedral structure characteristically using a combination of Cys and His residues. The composition includes fragments of the type $(Cys)_3(His)$, $(Cys)_2(His)_2$, $(Cys)_4$ or thiolate cluster compounds with bridged cysteine residues to generate peptide domains, that react with DNA. The role of Zn^{2+} is not catalytic but structural. Zn^{2+} ions maintain the protein structures that bind specifically to DNA for the activation and deactivation of genes. Advances in zinc finger research are leading to an innovative understanding of zinc-finger-DNA reactions, together with the possibility of their use in gene therapeutic and medical applications.

Practically, many transition metals can substitute for Zn. Pb and Cd are toxic partially because they can replace zinc with their enzymes and make them inactive. Zn(II) ion shows differences from magnesium(II) and calcium(II) ions as it forms significantly more stable complexes with various bioligands. Zinc impacts the metabolism of calcium and phosphorus and activates the synthesis of vitamins C and B. Stimulating activity of zinc ions on the phagocytic action of leukocytes has been reported [202, 203].

With such a dependency on Zn enzymes, it is reasonable that Zn is one of the most vital metals in the human diet. It is estimated that many people suffer from Zn deficiency. Zinc deficiency, occurring because of insufficient dietary consumption, is manifested by impaired wound healing, and dermatitis, anemia, loss of appetite, loss of taste sensation, hair loss, damage to reproductive system, and mental apathy [205]. Additionally, zinc deficiency in children may cause delayed mental progress, retarded growth, or postponed puberty. The role of Zn in protein synthesis makes the necessity for this metal particularly pronounced for fetuses and newborns.

The excess of zinc is poisonous. Zn toxicity occurs from self-supplementation or continued use of oral zinc additives for medical purposes. Excessive inhalation of Zn compounds causes such toxic indications as salivation, fever, cough, and sickness, but the effects are not lasting. Excess of Zn may also disturb Cu status with neutropenia, and anemia symptoms, decreased immune function and lower plasma HDL concentrations [206]. Breathing of molten Zn causes fume fever, which can be severe if the exposure is heavy. That is why, good ventilation is necessary in connection with the zinc-coated steel welding.

Organozinc compounds are widely used as reagents [3, 4]. Dimethylzinc CH_3ZnCH_3 and diethylzinc $(C_2H_5)_2Zn$ are used in the vapor deposition of zinc and

ZnO. Diphenylzinc $(C_6H_5)Zn$ is considerably less reactive. Zinc organometallic compounds are similar to the analogous magnesium compounds. Zinc forms various Grignard-type compounds, such as $(C_2H_5)ZnCl$, $(C_2H_5)ZnBr$, $(C_4H_9)ZnCl$, and $(C_4H_9)ZnI$. The combustion of highly flammable Zn organometallic compounds such as $(CH_3)_2Zn$ and $(C_2H_5)_2Zn$ produces finely divided particles of ZnO fumes:

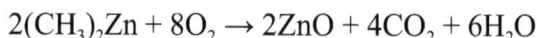

$$2(CH_3)_2Zn + 8O_2 \rightarrow 2ZnO + 4CO_2 + 6H_2O$$

Even though ZnO is used as a healing agent and food additive, inhalation of ZnO fume particles causes metal fever, manifested in high temperature and chills [3,4,206]. Diphenylzinc $(C_6H_5)_2Zn$ demonstrates the toxicity hazard that may be obtained from the organic fragment upon decomposition, releasing a toxic phenol:

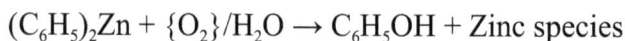

$$(C_6H_5)_2Zn + \{O_2\}/H_2O \rightarrow C_6H_5OH + \text{Zinc species}$$

Cadmium

The biological functions of cadmium have been studied very little. The physiological role of cadmium in the animal body is associated with its effect on the activity of certain enzymes and hormones and depends mostly on the binding of cadmium to sulfhydryl (-SH) groups that make up proteins, enzymes and other biologically active substances [207].

Unlike zinc, Cd is not a vital element for life. Instead, dissolved cadmium compounds are poisonous, and can enter the food chain in different ways [3, 4]. There are mixed views on Cd activity. While it is certainly supposed to not be vital for plants' and animals' life processes, some believe Cd is a trace metal with some required influence on the bioprocesses, although its necessity and usage are not presently established.

Toxicity: As a poisonous trace metal, Cd is very capable of producing environmental and professional hazards. Certain compounds of Cd are highly toxic and cumulative to humans [3,4,11]. Cadmium is widely used for many items, including electroplating for metals, solders, vapor lamps, control rods, and shields within nuclear reactors, and in Cd-Ni batteries and plastics industries. With growing industrial actions in the past years, the emissions of Cd into the environment have enlarged significantly above standard limits subsequently enriching the risk of exposure to this toxic metal. The exact mechanism of Cd toxicity is not very clear. However, free radical generation of ROS is suggested to be the main mechanism of its toxicity [207, 208]. In addition, the toxic cadmium interacts with some physiologically vital biogenic metals like Fe, Ca, and Zn and impairs their regular metabolic functions.

Cd^{2+} cation demonstrates high chemical resemblance with two biologically active metal ions: the lighter homologues Zn^{2+} and Ca^{2+}, close in size. Cd(II) ions can easily dislocate these cations and interfere with their biological functions. The toxicity of Cd is commonly explained by the fact that it replaces Zn(II) in significant enzymes, deactivating them. Cd(II), similar to Pb(II), shows a strong affinity to protein sulfhydryl groups, disturbing their bioactivity and it is known that cadmium is much more toxic than the toxic lead, which is very dangerous.

The most common in the industry and important, from the point of view of occupational health, is cadmium oxide CdO. In industry, it is formed during the smelting of zinc. It is used to make alkaline batteries and produce CdS (yellow paint). In the middle of the 20th century in Japan, the skeletal disease "itai-itai" was widespread because of cadmium pollution of water in rice regions when treated with fungicides. This bone disease is expressed in the strong fragility of the bones and extremely painful deformations of the skeleton [208].

Humans generally absorb Cd compounds by ingestion and inhalation. Its captivation through the skin is insignificant. Cadmium is absorbed through the gastrointestinal tract and by the lungs and is transported through the bloodstream to the liver and to other organs of the body [209]. In blood, Cd is found mostly in the blood cells. The enzyme metallothionein, seems to be responsible for protecting against the harmful Cd. Thanks to this enzyme, the body can withstand Cd to some extent. When the Cd(II) consumption is too great for this scavenging metalloprotein, the ion is further transported and binds to other vital proteins. The protective effect of metallothionein is due to the fact that it contains Cys, which forms a stable complex with cadmium cations, holding up to seven metal ions per molecule. The enzyme, saturated with Cd(II) ions, is further transported to the kidneys, concentrating a substantial portion of the body's concentration of cadmium. A small intake of Fe^{3+}, Zn^{2+} and Ca^{2+} rises the degree of cadmium absorption.

Cadmium may be distributed to many of the human organs, most of all in the kidneys, liver, and muscles with a predominantly long half-life of 10-30 years [210]. Nevertheless, the critical organ in Cd intoxication is the kidney, where Cd strongly accumulates and damages filtering mechanisms, which leads to proteins and sugars excretion from the body and additionally, kidney damage. Only negligible percentage of absorbed Cd^{2+} is excreted through the feces and urine.

In distinction to other toxic metals, Cd cannot easily pass into the CNS or into the fetus, because in biological conditions, cadmium cannot be bio-alkylated to produce membrane-penetrating organometallic complexes. It has good solubility in food organic acids and can form salts that are converted into $CdCl_2$ by gastric juices. Cadmium causes peroxidation of membrane lipids, deprivation of the antioxidant defense system, development of inflammation, protein structures disorders, and nucleic acid oxidation, affecting the DNA repair mechanism. Thus, Cd indirectly contributes to the production of free ROS [211]. Cadmium inhibits antioxidant enzymes which leads to increased OS resulting in membrane damage and loss of membrane-bound enzymes like ATPases.

Chronic cadmium exposure causes renal tubular dysfunction, disturbance of calcium metabolism, osteoporosis, and osteomalacia. Lasting inhalation of cadmium leads to pulmonary disorders such as chronic obstructive lung disease [210 - 212].

Acute cadmium exposure as a result of inhalation causes headaches, nose and throat dryness and lung edema. Acute intestinal symptoms are vomiting, nausea, and stomach irritation. Cadmium is also classified as a strong carcinogen in humans [212]. The liver and kidney are the main target organs in acute and chronic cadmium exposure. Other organs involved in cadmium toxicity are the heart, bone, testis, eyes and the brain.

There is no definite therapy for Cd intoxication. Due to slow excretion, Cd accumulates in the body over a lifetime and its biological half-life may be up to 38 years. Because it concentrates in critical organs such as kidneys, liver, *etc.*, primary prevention is crucial. Exposures to substantially higher Cd levels occur with smoking [213]. The smaller the Cd-carrying particles, the deeper the penetration into the lungs. In the cigarette fume, cadmium exists as very small particles, and the metal is deposited deeper in the lung tissues.

Due to the high toxicity, cadmium preparations are not used in medicine.

Mercury

Mercury is the only metal in the liquid state at normal conditions. Because of its high vapor pressure and slight water solubility, mercury is very poisonous. The mercury vapor absorbs through the lungs, dissolves in the bloodstream, and then passes to the brain, where produces irreversible impairment to the central nervous system. Elemental Hg easily crosses the blood-brain barrier and become oxidized to Hg^{2+}, which binds with protein -SH groups, particularly those of cysteine. The poisonousness of Hg compounds is principally based on the attraction of this metal ion to thiol-containing bioligands [214]. Hg compounds disturb the tertiary and quaternary protein structures and have a strong influence on their activities. The mechanism of toxic action of Hg compounds includes, in addition to binding to the carboxyl, amine, and sulfhydryl groups of proteins, irreversible inhibition of enzymes containing selenium (for instance, thioredoxin reductase, which plays a significant role in the fight against OS). Poisonous Hg compounds are speedily disseminated in the body. Their half-life is subject to the form of mercury and varies from days to months. Mercury accumulates mainly in the liver, kidney, and CNS, particularly in the brain. The Hg pollution of soil, water, vegetation, and animals is now typical in many regions. It is connected with the entry of a large amount of Hg into the biosphere as industrial products, transport exhausts, and toxic chemicals.

Toxicity: Widely distributed in nature, Hg is an extremely toxic metal with almost no identified physiological functions. Mercury is used in thermometers, barometers, dental amalgams, in the development of large-scale industrial processes (chlor-alkali plants, batteries and PVC production), in the manufacturing of mirrors, incandescent lights, x-ray machines, vacuum pumps, and is constantly released into the environment. Because of its widespread natural distribution through the atmosphere, Hg is considered a global contaminant, being deposited even in remote unspoiled aquatic systems, where it is biologically magnified through the food chain [215 - 217].

There are differences in the toxic effects of different forms of mercury (liquid Hg metal and Hg vapor), inorganic Hg salts, and organometallic (methyl-, ethylmercury) Hg compounds. Humans are exposed to all of these forms of Hg in a variety of ways. Lasting inhalation of Hg vapor leads to chronic intoxication. Metallic mercury Hg^0 is poorly captivated by the gastrointestinal tract, but with its high volatility mercury affects the lungs. An oral intake of liquid Hg poses a negligible risk for severe toxic conditions, as its intestinal absorption is small. Nevertheless, liquid Hg metal tends to vaporize, because of its vapor pressure. Inhaled Hg vapor concentrates particularly in the CNS, the location of the chief toxic effects of Hg [215]. Damage to the CNS by Hg vapor progressively disturbs the facial muscles and eyelids. Later the limbs can also be influenced. Moreover, metallic mercury has a high solubility in lipids, which enables its circulation across the alveoli, as well as its delivery to the body's lipophilic parts including the blood-brain barrier and the placenta, damaging fetal brains. Hg vapor has a short lifetime because it is quickly oxidized to mercury(II) in tissues, and then the processes are similar to intoxication by inorganic mercury compounds.

The degree of poisonous effects is dependent on the forms of mercury compounds, the exposure degree, the period, and the pathway of exposure. All Hg compounds induce toxic effects, especially the soluble ones. Inorganic mercury compounds are not a big problem because they are mostly insoluble. For the inorganic Hg salts, the common exposure paths of are the digestive tract and skin [216]. The poisonousness of inorganic salts rises with their solubility in water. Among the chlorides, $HgCl_2$ has a high water-solubility, whereas Hg_2Cl_2, called calomel, is low soluble. Hg_2Cl_2 was used in the past as a medication against syphilis. Exclusively toxic soluble Hg(II) salts like $HgCl_2$ do not easily cross the blood-brain or the placental barriers, nevertheless, they really accumulate in the placenta, amniotic fluid, and fetal tissues. The critical organs for inorganic Hg salts are the kidneys and the intestinal tract. The protein metallothionein to some grade prevents damage by low Hg intake as in the case of cadmium intoxication.

The most toxic and dangerous form of mercury is represented by organometallic compounds, which generally arise from biological sources, primarily freshwater or saltwater fish. Because of their specific lipid solubility, their absorption from the gastrointestinal tract is more complete than that of inorganic salts [217]. The body absorbs 90-100% of the oral doses. These compounds can easily be distributed and accumulated mostly in the kidney, brain, and liver. Organo mercury compounds readily cross the placenta leading to neuro logical and teratogenic effects. All Hg forms are toxic to the fetus, but $CH_3\text{-}Hg^+X^-$ is the most hazardous and leads to spontaneous abortion or retardation. Organic compounds of mercury are mainly of the aryl- and alkyl classes, which were broadly used, mostly as fungicides. The behavior of aryl derivatives, such as phenylmercuric acetate, is similar to that of inorganic mercury compounds. No fatal cases of aryl derivatives intoxication have been reported. Dangerous is the exposure to alkyl derivatives as they penetrate brain cells and are slowly excreted.

In chronic intoxication with Hg and its compounds, the typical symptoms are diarrhea, metallic taste, and severe salivation. Chronic exposure induces poisonous effects in the CNS (excitability, auditory and olfactory hallucinations, headaches, depression), and cardiovascular and renal systems. The symptoms of Hg intoxication "mercurism" are slowly generated (months to years) at working places with metallic Hg [214, 216].

Acute exposure caused by inhalation of metal Hg leads to respiratory symptoms (chest pain) and effects on the central nervous system (confusion, lethargy, tremor). Acute poisoning by inorganic Hg compounds causes serious damage to the mucous membranes of the gastrointestinal tract and the renal cells. Mercury compounds could be touched safely, but strict precautions must be taken to prevent inhalation, ingestion, or skin-contact absorption [214, 216].

For the treatment of Hg intoxication, thiol-based chelation agents like DMSA, DMPS, dimercaprol, and penicillamine are administrated (Fig. **8**), [215]. In severe toxic cases connected with renal functions, hemodialysis can be applied.

d-Elements of IIIB Group

Scandium

Although scandium is a comparatively widespread element in the earth's crust, until recently there has been little information on the biochemistry of this element. Published data on scandium are quite scarce. It can be concluded that scandium has an unknown biological role. It is a supposed carcinogen. Scandium radio nuclides have shown great potential in nuclear medicine [218]. Among the scandium radioisotopes, [43]Sc and [44]Sc are positron emitter radionuclides for PET imaging, while [47]Sc is of interest for radiotherapy.

Little information is available on Sc toxicity. Elemental scandium is considered non-toxic, although some of its compounds might be cancerogenic. Nevertheless, scarce *in vivo* testing of scandium compounds has been done. The major risk of scandium exposure could be aerosols and gasses within a working environment, because of some Sc-based damps and gasses in the air [219]. These emissions cause lung embolism, particularly in prolonged exposure. Sc is mostly dangerous for the liver at body accumulation.

Yttrium

Scandium and yttrium are typical rare earth metals. They are found in identical ores as lanthanide metals and show analogous properties. There are no significant functions of yttrium in living systems. However, it occurs in organisms and has a tendency to concentrate on many human organs. Normally, in tiny amounts, around 0.0077 g of this element is found in the body and about 4 ppm in the human breast milk [220].

Yttrium is usually dangerous in workplaces because of humidity and gases released into the air. This causes pulmonary embolism, particularly at longstanding exposure [220]. Yttrium can also enlarge the risk of lung cancer when it is inhaled. Exposure to 500 mg/m^3 if yttrium, is directly hazardous to life and health.

d-Elements of IVB and VB Groups

Titanium

Very little is reported on the functions of titanium in life processes. The element shows generally low toxicity [221]. Titanium is not thought to be essential and it has no identified application in humans, though it acts as a stimulant. In certain plants, Ti is useful for their energy production. Ti is considered as one of the most biocompatible metals. It is not damaging or poisonous to living tissues because of its resistance to body fluids.

Although it is not regarded as a toxic element, as a heavy metal, it has harmful health properties. This metal disturbs lung functions producing pulmonary diseases such as pleural illness, breathing difficulties, and coughing. Exposure to titanium can cause allergies including symptoms like urticaria, erythema, and eczema of the skin or eyes [221]. Titanium dioxide is supposed to be a human carcinogen. There are no safe levels of contact with this carcinogenic metal, so the exposure should be minimized. TiO_2 has a tendency to accumulate causing lung fibrosis. Some limits counting respirational tests and medical X-ray inspections are consequently prescribed for patients seriously exposed to titanium oxide at work.

Zirconium

Zirconium does not appear to be a vital element for living organisms. This element exhibits usually little harmfulness. In an average human body, there is approximately 4 mg of Zr, but this element does not have any identified biological functions. The usage of zirconium in medicine and dentistry has rapidly expanded [222].

Hafnium

Hafnium has no identified biological functions and the metal has no known toxicity. This element is an unreactive metal and cannot be affected by air, water, acids, and bases. The only ions known in aqueous chemistry are (4+) ions. Organohafnium chemistry is similar to organozirconium and organotitanium coordination chemistry [223]. Hafnium and its compounds are very rare and generally obtained as by-products of zirconium processing. Similar to cadmium, it absorbs neutrons and has mainly industrial use. Hafnium is not soluble in water, saline, and body fluids. Exposure occurs on ingestion, respiration or skin contact. Overexposure to this metal causes slight eyes, skin, and mucous membranes irritations.

Vanadium

The decomposition of V-based rocks under the environmental influence makes the metal accessible in soils. This is one of the essential elements for many species, including humans and is vital for good human health. Its exact biological function is poorly understood, although its content in the body is about 2.4 mg. Perhaps the capability to change between different oxidation states is important for its activity. The common oxidation states of vanadium are +III, +IV, and +V.

In vertebrates, predominantly humans, vanadium(IV) and vanadium(V) are likely to predominate [224, 225]. It is supposed that vanadium helps the body convert some food products into energy. It has also been suggested that diabetics may benefit from V when trying to stabilize the levels of blood sugar. Vanadium is also thought to help bone structures and teeth form properly.

Vanadium is definitely essential for some marine organisms and mushrooms. After Mo, V is the second most abundant transition metal found in seawater and in marine algae, fungi, and bacteria, where vanadium concentration reaches 100 mg/kg [224]. Bacteria, containing V, take part in the transfer of atmospheric N_2 to nitrogen compounds. Up to the present time, two classes of V-containing enzymes have been found in some nitrogen-fixing bacteria (*Azotobacter*): vanadium nitrogenases and V-dependent haloperoxidases (V-HPOs). Vanadium is a constituent of one of the central enzymes of N-fixing soil microorganisms, which restores the molecular N_2 to NH_3 - vanadium nitrogenase. Hydrated V(III) is existing in vanadocytes (blood cells) of sea squirts (*Ascidiacea*) at 350 mM concentration in a not clearly understood protein-based complex hemovanadin, supposed to serve in O_2 transport. Mushrooms of the genus *Amanita muscaria* hold amavadin where V(IV) is coordinately bound to two tetradentate N-oxyimino-2,2-dipropionate ligands. The oxidovanadium(V) core is found in vanadate-dependent haloperoxidases form, *inter alia*, marine algae, coordinated to the active center of histidine-N. The main function of haloper oxidases, V-HPOs, is to integrate halogens into bio organic molecules. Vanadate -dependent haloper oxidases can mimic enzymes responsible for the phosphate metabolism, where vanadate ions block the protein binding domain of phosphate ions. These competitive bonds may account for the insulin-mimetic/insulin-enhancing potential of V compounds. The vanadate-dependent enzymes, haloperoxidases and vanadium nitrogenases are the only naturally occurring V-based enzymes [225]. The blood of some ascidian and tunicate species contains vanabins (V(III) protein).

The most important feature of this element is its varying oxidation state. It is present as oxyanion at neutral pH values, a strong oxidizer which is chemically and electronically similar to phosphate anion. The similarity between V(V) in the form of vanadate and phosphate is possibly to be dominant to its biological functions [224, 225]. Remarkably, acid phosphatase enzymes, that use PO_4^{3-} as a cofactor, have evolved to accommodate VO_4^{3-} ion as a cofactor. In humans, V(IV) and V(V) species prevail and many vanadium complexes in these oxidation states are in clinical trials as antidiabetic agents, which are deliberated in the next sections.

There are no specific symptoms of V deficiency identified in humans [226]. Possibly not getting enough of vanadium affects the body capability to control the levels of blood sugar and contributes to developing diabetes and hypoglycemia. It is suspected that a deficiency of this element may cause kidney and heart diseases.

Vanadium inorganic compounds are not considered as a serious hazard. However, staffs exposed to vanadium peroxide dust have been observed to get severe eye, nose, and throat irritations. Vanadium has numerous health effects when the uptake is too high [227]. When vanadium acceptance takes place through air, it causes respiratory problems such as bronchitis and pneumonia. The acute V effects are irritations of the lungs, eyes, throat, and nasal cavities. Additional health effects of V acceptance are: cardiac, vascular disease, CNS damage, inflammation of the stomach and intestines, liver and kidneys hemorrhage, trembling and paralyzes, skin rashes, nose and throat pains, headaches, weakness, dizziness, behavior problems. The health dangers related to V exposure depend on the oxidation state. Metallic vanadium oxidizes to V_2O_5 during welding. The V(V) form is more toxic than the elemental V^0 form. Chronic exposure to V_2O_5 dust and fumes may cause eyes and skin irritations, systemic trachea and bronchi inflammation, upper respiratory tract problems, pulmonary edema. Symptoms of overexposure consist of conjunctivitis, nasopharyngitis, cough, chronic bronchitis, rapid heartbeat, changes in the lung, pallor of the skin, black tongue and allergic skin rashes.

The variety of biological applications of vanadium stimulated researchers to develop novel coordination vanadium-based antidiabetic and anticancer drugs with remarkable activity and low toxicity [228], discussed in the next section.

Niobium

Niobium is not an essential element. It has no known biological role and has not yet been discovered for possible therapeutic applications. Inhaled niobium is reserved mostly in lungs and bones. It interferes with Ca(II) as an enzyme activator. Niobium is one of the most inert metals, making it an ideal, safe, and hypoallergenic body material for jewelry production. The feasibility of using Nb-based films as coatings for implant materials has also been confirmed [229].

Tantalum

Metal tantalum has no known biological role. The metallic tantalum resistance to be attacked by foreign agents makes it compatible with human body tissue. That is why, the metal can be used in many biomedical applications, like Ti and Nb [230]. Tantalum is well known for its chemical and biological inertness and metal hardness. It is non-reactive, completely immune to body liquids, and non-irritating to body tissues. Tantalum is supposed to be the only material that is fully compatible with the human body. Because of that it is commonly used in lasting surgical implants and in the repairing of bone defects in humans due to its bioactivity, biocompatibility, exceptional corrosion resistance, and mechanical properties. The porosity of Ta affords a platform in medicine for bone ingrowth and mechanical bone attachments.

Tantalum may be moderately toxic by inhalation. Because of their low solubility, tantalum compounds are non-poisonous when taken orally. They are poorly absorbed and rapidly removed from the organisms of mammals [231]. Inhaling tantalum oxide (Ta_2O_5) has caused bronchitis and interstitial pneumonitis. Some skin irritations from tantalum have also been reported.

d Elements of VIB and VIIB Groups

Chromium

Chromium is a vital element and a constant component of plants, animals, and humans, although not enough studied. The entire content of chromium is around 0.006 g in an average adult ($10^{-5}\%$). There are no naturally occurring proteins that are known to contain chromium. Under normal conditions, the characteristic oxidation states of Cr are III+ and VI+, the latter as a chromate anion, CrO_4^{2-}, at pH 7. The biological activity of Cr is mainly due to the capability of Cr^{3+} ions to participate in complex compounds [3,4,11]. Cr^{3+} ions are involved in stabilizing the structure of nucleic acids. Chromium is an essential component of the biomolecules that work with insulin to stabilize the levels of blood sugar. This element can also help in the growth of muscle mass and reduce fat mass in the human body. It supports cells, such as heart muscle cells, to absorb energy to work properly. Chromium is a component of the digestive enzyme trypsin.

Many studies have reported the beneficial effects of trivalent chromium. Biosystems normally contain Cr^{3+} ions in minor concentrations. This microelement has an important role in plant and animal organisms as a nutrient. It is a component of some enzymes involved in the cellular oxidation-reduction reactions. Chromium is a constituent of pepsin, which splits proteins in the gastrointestinal tract of animals and is involved in the regulation of glucose absorption. Trivalent chromium is generally supposed to be a necessary trace element owing to its ability to strengthen the hypoglycemic activity of insulin and its influence on carbohydrate and lipid metabolism, perhaps by increasing insulin signalling [3, 4]. This stimulation of insulin activity happens without changing the insulin levels. It is also supposed that chromium is involved in glucose metabolism in the human body. Cr as a complex compound with nicotinic acid and aliphatic amino acids is regarded as an "impaired glucose tolerance factor".

The intake of chromium has a positive effect on humans and reduces the symptoms of diabetes in patients with glucose intolerance. After entering the body from exogenous sources, chromium(III) interacts with transferrin, a Fe-transporting plasma protein. The form of Cr(III) is the most stable naturally occurring form in living organisms but is not as biologically available as Cr(VI).

Chromium is the most contentious d-element in terms of its harmfulness and nutritional value since the Cr^{3+} ion is nontoxic while Cr(IV) is extremely toxic leading to oxidative damage to DNA. It has a bad reputation for its toxicity and carcinogenicity in the form of Cr(VI) in chromate CrO_4^{2-} and dichromate $Cr_2O_7^{2-}$ ions. Chromium(VI) compounds are poisonous and not used in medicine. Chromium is a human carcinogen mostly by inhalation exposures in working settings. There are many studies supporting the carcinogenic effects, so when Cr(VI) is used or obtained in technical processes, much consideration should be paid to the atmospheric conditions [232]. Chromium carcinogenic effects were first recognized a century ago. Chromium compounds with an oxidation state of +6, not formed in living organisms, were amongst the earliest inorganic compounds to be classified as strong carcinogenic agents that can easily penetrate through the biological cell membranes and cause damage. Lung cancer has been detected as a consequence of Cr(VI) exposure in smokers and nonsmokers as well as some cancers of other tissues such as CNS cancers.

Chromium(VI) ion as chromate CrO_4^{2-} is a strong oxidizer and can oxidatively damage DNA and proteins. Chromate ions can aggressively enter the cells through channels and transfer isoelectric and isostructural anions, such as sulphate and hydrogen phosphate channels. It reaches the nucleus of the cells if not reduced. In the cells, there are three main reducers for chromate ions: ascorbic acid, glutathione, and cysteine [233]. If the amount of the reducers is lower compared with the Cr(VI) levels, then Cr(V) and Cr(IV) intermediate products are obtained. These intermediates yield ROS radicals which attack the DNA leading to faulty gene expression.

The deficiency of chromium causes damage to glucose tolerance whereas toxicity leads to renal failure, skin dermatitis and lung cancer. Lack of Cr(III) in the body leads to insulin resistance. One of the consequences of this is a sharp increase in blood glucose - hyperglycemia. The risk of Cr(III) deficiency increases during pregnancy and malnutrition and is age-dependent. Nevertheless, chromium deficiency is difficult to achieve. People who exercise often have particularly higher chromium demands. Chromium is included in many supplements, but chromium is absorbed by the body from food much better [234]. A daily intake for adults of around 30 µg chromium per day is recommended.

Toxicity: Chromium is known as an important micronutrient, but it also is associated with several pathologies, including carcinogenicity [233]. Chromium is used in the manufacture of cars, linoleum, glass, and pottery, and is found in industrial wastes. Because of its widespread use in industry, Cr can pollute many of ecological systems. Exposure to too much chromium is a major concern because of the high risk of chromium-induced diseases in industrial settings.

The health risks associated with chromium exposure strongly depend on its oxidation state. The elemental metal form does not show substantial toxicity, but metallic dust can irritate lung tissues, which causes infections [235]. The hexavalent form poses a serious risk to human health, mainly to persons who work in the steel industry. The toxic Cr(VI) causes numerous health effects. When it is a component in leather products in textile industry, it causes allergic skin reactions, such as eruption, ulcerations, and dermatitis. Inhalation of Cr(VI) compounds causes nose irritation, nasal ulceration, and perforation of the mucous membranes, irritation of the larynx and pharynx, bronchospasms, asthmatic bronchitis, and edema. Other symptoms caused by Cr(VI) include respiratory problems, shortness of breath, upset stomachs and ulcers, kidney and liver damage, weakened immune systems, changes in genetic material, and lung cancer [233, 235]. Cr(VI) compounds are much more toxic than Cr(III) compounds.

Molybdenum

There are very scarce illustrations of the biological functions of elements with higher than 35 atomic numbers. The most important exceptions are Mo and iodine. Molybdenum is the only element from the II and III period of transition metals (4d, 5d) that is vital for most living organisms with a wide range of functions, although it occurs in the human body in a few-milligram amount (10^{-5}%). Molybdenum is an important trace element that occurs in nature in various chemical compounds and has a redox function, as evidenced by its extended oxidation state spectrum, ranging from II to VI among various forms and states of Mo oxidation. While it is comparatively rare in the environment, Mo is the most abundant metal ion in seawater in its most stable Mo(VI) form as molybdate MoO_4^{2-} anion, at pH 7. Mo does not form stable ions in its low oxidation states in biosystems [236]. In biological systems, it exists only in the form of complex ions in Mo(V) and Mo(VI) oxidation states. In complex compounds, Mo is connected typically with oxygen atoms. Although rare, molybdenum is biologically important because MoO_4^{2-} anion has a high solubility in water at pH≈7, which makes it easily transportable by biofluids. The negative charge of the ion makes it suitable for different surroundings compared to the other cations of 3d metals. It is suggested that the transport mechanism of MoO_4^{2-} is almost the same as that of SO_4^{2-}, which is an example of the resemblances of ions of VIA and VIB groups. Molybdenum has a wide variety of oxidation states (+4, +5, and +6), whit redox potentials overlapping with those of biosystems.

Molybdenum is found in all tissues of the body, but is the most concentrated in the liver, kidneys, small intestine, endocrine glands, skin, and bones [237]. In the blood, molybdenum is distributed evenly between the shaped elements and plasma in the form of complexes with proteins. In the liver and kidneys, Mo also forms protein complexes. Molybdenum is supposed to be significant in serving human cells to grow properly. Small volumes of nutritional Mo are connected with the promotion of healthy teeth. It is existing in tooth enamel and prevents its decay. Some evidence suggests that Mo reduces the risk of asthma attacks. It also activates the synthesis of hemoglobin.

Lots of enzymes are found to rely on Mo, which is typically absorbed as MoO_4^{2-}. Enzymes containing Mo are involved in the transition of oxygen group reactions. This is possible because of the affinity of molybdenum to oxygen and its ability to form solid oxygen complexes. The only identified form of Mo taken up by cells is the molybdate anion. This ion shows a close similarity to the biologically vital S-transporting SO_4^{2-}. The biologically relevant oxidation states of molybdenum lie between +IV and +VI [238].

Being a part of a number of enzymes in humans, molybdenum catalyzes redox reactions through xanthine oxidase (oxidation of xanthine to uric acid), xanthine dehydrogenase, sulfite oxidase (oxidation of sulfites to sulfates) and aldehyde oxidase. These enzymes are also essential in plant and animal organisms in the reactions associated with the transfer of oxygen. In these molybdenum enzymes, the transfer of O_2 to or from substrates is catalyzed by molybdenum (between Mo(IV) and Mo(VI) oxidation states) using water as an O-donor or O-acceptor atom. Mo also exists mainly as a cofactor of molybdopterin (MoCo) in xanthine oxidoreductase, nitrate reductase, CO-dehydrogenase and sulphite oxidase enzymes. This family of Mo-containing enzymes, named molybdopterins, has a core containing MoS_2 group and an organic ring structure identified as a pterin system (Fig. 7). MoCo consists of a tricyclic pterin that coordinates Mo through a dithiol group in the third pyranocircle. This group of enzymes frequently contain different metals, predominantly a Fe-S system, performing the vital roles of oxidants or reductants of poisonous species in the organism. For instance, sulfite oxidase oxidizes SO_3^{2-} to SO_4^{2-}, CO-dehydrogenase oxidizes CO to CO_2, and nitrate reductase reduces NO_3^- to NO_2^-. All molybdenum-dependent enzymes contain a pterin-type cofactor, except for bacterial nitrogenase. Molybdenum cofactor in molybdopterins is synthesized by means of a highly preserved multistep biochemical pathway. If this biosynthesis is lacking, then loss of human Mo-enzyme activity can occur [239]. The deficiency of molybdopterin biosynthesis leads to the deficiency of the Mo-enzyme activities, which causes rapid neurodegeneration and even early childhood death. Xanthine oxidase (XO) and aldehyde oxidase participate in the drugs and toxic substances metabolism. In fact, the physiological value of molybdenum in the body of animals and humans was first shown in 1953 with the discovery of the effect of this element on the activity of the enzyme xanthine oxidase. XO catalyzes the oxidation of xanthine by oxygen into uric acid. XO inserts hydroxyl groups into purine bases derivatives such as adenine and guanine, finally converting xanthine to uric acid, the final product of purine degradation, excreted by the urine. The lack of Mo in the body is accompanied by a decrease in the content of XO in the tissues. The absence of molybdenum affects the anabolic processes which lead to the weakening of the immune system. Sulfite oxidase catalyzes the oxidation of SO_3^{2-} to SO_4^{2-}, a process that is required for the metabolism of S-containing amino acids. Aldehyde oxidase participates in the metabolism of alcohols, it catalyzes the oxidation of aldehydes to carboxylic acids.

Molybdenum has an important role in the biological utilization of N_2 through the nitrogen cycle (nitrogen fixation). Nitrogen-fixing bacteria utilize enzymes that contain both molybdenum and iron, which can catalyze the reduction of N_2 to nitrogen compounds. Enzymes that contain molybdenum in their active sites catalyze the transformation of N_2 to NH_3 and other nitrogen-containing products. Consequently, molybdenum is important for plants. The most critical Mo-containing enzyme (which contains Fe additionally) is nitrogenase, used by bacteria to fix atmospheric N_2 into organically bonded nitrogen. These enzymes occur in bacteria which reduce the inert atmospheric N_2 to nitrogen-based products, which are used in the synthesis of proteins by plants [240]. Some of them have a symbiotic connection with leguminous plants. Another Mo-containing enzyme is nitrate reductase. This enzyme allows the reduction of NO_3^- to NO_2^- in vegetation and microorganisms. Nitrogenase and nitrate reductase are of great importance in nature since they are the most vital channels for the inclusion of N_2 in the bio-circulation for the variability between +4 and +6 molybdenum oxidation states.

In general, the toxicity of Mo compounds is relatively small. For humans, the toxic dose is 5 mg/kg and the lethal dose is 50 mg/kg. Some evidences of liver dysfunction with hyperbilirubinemia and signs of gout have been reported in working men chronically exposed to Mo compounds [241]. The main features observed are joint pain in the hands, knees and feet, articular abnormalities, erythema, and edema of the joint zones. The overload of molybdenum causes anemia, high concentrations of serum uric acid and impaired reproductive functions, as well.

Molybdenum is necessary, although in extremely small amounts. Per day, 75-250 µg of molybdenum enters the body of an adult with food, where cereals, legumes, dairy products, and meats are the richest and most important sources. The Mo amounts in plant food products vary and depend on the mineral content in the soil. Hard tap water can also add Mo to the nutrition. Molybdenum deficiency is rare and almost not found in living organisms because the dietary intake of manganese greatly exceeds its daily needs [242]. The biochemical irregularities in acquired Mo deficiency consist of very low levels of uric acid in serum and in urine (low xanthine oxidase action), low SO_4^{2-} levels in urine (low sulfite oxidase action) or molybdenum cofactor. Low levels of molybdenum may result in neurological complications and mental retardation. These anomalies appear to be caused by the harmfulness of inadequate quantities of sulfite available for the formation of sulfate compounds in the brain. A deficiency of molybdenum in human nourishments causes mouth and gum disorders and contributes to cancer diseases. XO and aldehyde oxidase may also be involved in the inactivation of certain toxic compounds, in so far as research has shown that Mo deficiency is a reason for the higher occurrence of esophageal cancer in people consuming food grown in Mo-poor soil [243]. Molybdenum deficiency has also been associated with tooth decay and cavities. Molybdenum has a Cu-antagonistic effect and excessive dietary Mo consumption induces a secondary Cu deficiency. A diet rich in refined and processed foods can lead to a deficiency of Mo, which may result in anemia, loss of appetite, loss of weight, and inhibited growth in animals.

Tungsten

Molybdenum and tungsten are the heaviest transition metals used in biology. Until now, tungsten was not included in the group of essential elements. Views are mixed about the necessity for this element in plants and animals, though it has been proven to have functions in some microorganisms [3, 4, 11]. This trace element has small functions in bioprocesses in the human body. The biological action of tungsten is due to its characteristic variable degree of oxidation (+4, +5, +6). Tungsten is most commonly encountered in biosystems as W(VI) in tungstate ion WO_4^{2-}. The biological role of tungstate in human health is not recognized. There are no tungsten-containing proteins known in humans.

Nowadays, it has become evident that tungsten is a constituent of many archaeal and bacterial enzymes [244]. W-containing enzymes are identified in some extremophile microorganisms, hyperthermal *Archaea*. Certain bacterial oxidoreductase enzymes use tungsten instead of Mo in the active sites of enzymes. Because these bacteria occur at very high temperatures (≈ 110 °C) it is claimed that W rather than Mo is utilized by the enzyme because tungsten forms stronger metal-ligand bonds, allowing the enzyme to function at high-temperature without decomposing. Connected to the bond strength, the rate of the reaction of the W-based enzyme at around 110 °C is analogous to that of the Mo-based enzyme at physiological temperature. Tungsten is used by some non-oxygen consuming bacteria in very hot ocean surroundings. The bacteria (*Clostridium*) in these environments use W to produce enzymes, which are required for some life processes. Precisely, how W is utilized by these unique anaerobic bacteria is relatively complicated. In these enzymes, W assists in oxidation-reduction reactions, for instance, the fixation of carbon dioxide. It is unidentified why nature uses W but not Mo in the mentioned processes.

The mononuclear Mo and W enzymes have the same defined metal center (Mo, W) coordinated by one or two pyranopterins. The presence of the same unstable complex, the molybdenum cofactor, that functions with both Mo and W in numerous organisms (from the earliest hyperthermophilic *Archaea* to human organisms) indicates the significance of molybdenum- and tungsten-containing enzymes in evolutionary processes [245]. It is supposed that before the presence of O_2 formed at photosynthesis, Mo and W were existing on Earth as WS_2 and MoS_2, rather than anions (MoO_4^{2-} and WO_4^{2-}). Since WS_2 has better solubility in water than MoS_2, most probably in the pre-oxygen era, W has been more accessible to microorganisms than Mo. That is why tungsten enzymes are found in strict anaerobic organisms, with few exceptions.

Tungsten is supposed to be used by a few enzymes in humans in a manner similar to molybdenum [244, 245]. Since tungsten possesses similar chemical properties as the vital plant microelement Mo, it is supposed that it inhibits the enzymatic activity of Mo by replacing the molybdenum ion in the cofactor.

The amount of W in natural water is very small and this metal is considered nontoxic. On the other hand, tungsten and its compounds are extensively used in many industrial applications and it is important to consider its potential health effects, particularly its possible involvement in the development of cancer and other deleterious health complications [246].

Manganese

The average human adult has around 15 mg of manganese, found mainly in nucleic acids. Around 43% of this content is found in bones, with the rest taking place in soft tissues of many organs (kidneys, liver, pancreas) and CNS [247]. Manganese level in the brain is not so much, however, the brain is the main target of manganese-induced toxicity. The daily requirement is around 2-5 mg per day. A small content of manganese in the body allows attributing it to trace elements. There is no doubt that manganese is a vital element, and that there are a variety of manganese enzymes with important functions in metabolism, immunological system, cell reproduction, regulation, and production of cellular energy as well as bone and connective tissue growth.

Manganese is an essential trace element for all living organisms [11, 247]. It regulates blood sugar levels. Additionally, manganese functions with vitamin K to help blood clotting. Vitamins B, and Mn help to control stress effects. Manganese enhances the synthesis of thyroid hormones. It is a contributor in the synthesis of vitamins C and B and in chlorophyll synthesis. In the body, it interacts with the ATP-ADP system by enzymatic reactions, in which the MnATP complex plays the role of the donor of phosphate groups, meaning that Mn participates in the processes of energy accumulation and transfer. Absorption of manganese from the digestive tract is connected inversely to the Ca, P, and Fe levels in the diet. Manganese is excreted through the bile.

The best-known role of manganese is in photosynthesis. It is an essential cofactor for the O_2-evolving complex (OEC) of photosynthesis [248]. The enzyme that oxidizes H_2O to O_2 holds a cluster of four Mn atoms and six O atoms (equivalent to Mn_2O_3). In the processes of formation of oxygen, this complex rearranges through multiple Mn oxidation states. When oxygen has left, a cluster of four manganese atoms with four oxygen atoms (equivalent to MnO) remains. The Mn content of soils varies widely. A deficiency in most crops is shown by complete chlorosis (deficiency of chlorophyll), with gray spots on the leaves. In these cases, $MnSO_4$ provides an effective remedy.

Manganese has been adopted by nature due to its different oxidation states (+2, +3, +4, +6, and +7). Manganese has three oxidation states of significance to biology: +II, +III, and +IV. In living matter, the commonly available oxidation states are Mn(II) and Mn(III). Mn(II) is the most stable form, while Mn(III) is a powerful oxidizing agent, which is usually disproportionated to Mn(II) and Mn(IV), or forms complexes with proteins, for instance, transferrin. The biogenic function of Mn^{2+} ions is to regulate the activity of enzymes and to support the immune system. In addition to this function, Mn^{2+} ions have a varied range of biological effects: they affect blood formation, mineral metabolism, reproduction, *etc.* Additionally, Mn^{2+} ions stabilize the structure of nucleic acids. Manganese as Mn^{2+} has analogous chemistry to Mg^{2+}, though unlike the latter it has an oxidation-reduction activity [3,4,247]. It has been proven that contributing to biochemical processes, manganese, in general, does not change its oxidation state. This is probably connected with the fact that there are no powerful oxidants in the body, and that the bioligands stabilize the status of manganese(II).

Manganese forms complexes *in vivo* with proteins, nucleic and amino acids [247]. These complexes are constituents of metalloenzymes (arginase, cholinesterase, *etc.*). As a component of these enzymes, manganese plays a role in oxidative phosphorylation, metabolism of fatty acids and cholesterol, mucopolysaccharide metabolism, urea cycle, *etc.* A number of Mn-containing enzymes are present in the human body (Table **13**).

Table 13. Manganese-containing enzymes.

Enzyme	Function
Mn-SOD	Dismutation of superoxide anion to H_2O_2
Glycosyltransferase and xylosyltransferase	Protein glycosylation, biosynthesis of glycosaminoglycans
Arginase	Urea cycle
Glutamine synthetase	Glutamine formation
Isocitrate dehydrogenase	Gluconeogenesis, maintenance of physiological concentration of oxaloacetate
Serine/threonine phosphatase	Cell cycle, apoptosis

Manganese is a cofactor and activator of many enzymes (transferases, lyases, hydrolases, isomerases, ligases, and oxidoreductases) involved in the protein, lipid and carbohydrate metabolism and in the ROS detoxification [249]. It is a vital cofactor of enzymes glycosyltransferases. They are essential for the synthesis of proteoglycans that are required for the formation of healthy cartilages and bones. Manganese is also part of enzymes like superoxide dismutase (Mn-SOD), arginase, and catalase. Arginase is involved in the transformation of L-arginine to L-ornithine and urea. In mammalians, hepatic arginase is the terminal enzyme of the urea cycle, which is the main end product of N-metabolism. Manganese in +3 oxidation state is easily accessible in the enzyme mitochondrial Mn superoxide dismutase. Mn-SOD is existing in eukaryotic mitochondria and in various bacteria. This enzyme catalyzes the two-step dismutation of $\cdot O_2^-$ to H_2O_2 and O_2 thus playing an important role in the protection of cells against OS conditions:

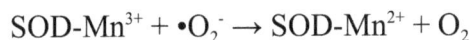

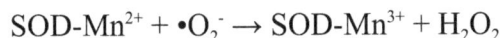

$$SOD\text{-}Mn^{3+} + \cdot O_2^- \rightarrow SOD\text{-}Mn^{2+} + O_2$$

$$SOD\text{-}Mn^{2+} + \cdot O_2^- \rightarrow SOD\text{-}Mn^{3+} + H_2O_2$$

The mechanism of Mn-SOD is equivalent to that of CuZnSOD, but manganese varies its oxidation states between +3 and +2.

The most plentiful manganese-binding protein in the body is glutamine synthetase, which has an important role in brain biochemistry (in astrocytes).

Manganese is essential to support the health of humans and animals. Due to its ubiquity, dietary Mn deficiency has been rarely reported. Mn deficiency causes many diseases, including decreased growth and low reproductive function [250]. Although it is very rare in humans, it is supposed that low levels of manganese in the human body result in skeletal anomalies, poor bone formation, reduced reproductive functions and growth, and altered metabolism of carbohydrates and lipids. Manganese deficiency in the body leads to a multitude of symptoms including impaired glucose tolerance, hypercholesterolemia, dermatitis, hair color changes, infertility, deafness, and decreased synthesis of vitamin K-dependent blood clotting factors. Congenital defects can occur when the expected mother does not receive enough Mn. There is a connection between poor manganese intake and higher skin cancer rates. Mn deficiency is quite rare, because the element is nutritionally critical only in small quantities. Humans can effortlessly get enough Mn from a good composed diet.

Toxicity: Although manganese is essential for various physiological functions, the accumulation of extremely high levels of Mn in the human body can result in severe toxicity [251]. Manganese is used as a purifying agent in the manufacture of some metals. Manganese intoxication can be caused by chronic inhalation and ingestion of Mn particles. The mechanism of its toxic effects is not clearly understood.

Excessive Mn results in ROS production, modifying mitochondrial ATP production, production of noxious metabolites and neurodegenerations like Parkinson's disease [251]. Bone, pancreas, liver, and kidney usually have higher Mn concentrations than other organs. The main tissue stored of Mn is in bones. Occupational exposure through inhalation results in diseases in the respiratory system or in the CNS. It is mainly the industrial use of MnO_2 that is dangerous, affecting mainly the respiratory tract and brain. Mn toxicity upon overexposure is connected with inhalation in professional settings (alloy production, mining, welding) and can result in neuro-behavioral and neurological effects (hallucinations, forgetfulness, and nerve damage), tremors, postural instability and rigidity. A high occurrence of pneumonia and other respiratory infections is found in workers exposed to dust or Mn compound fumes. Industrial manganese toxicity is well recognized, known as manganism, a typical neurodegenerative syndrome that leads to dopaminergic neuronal death and Parkinson-like indications. This process results in overexposure and production of ROS and toxic metabolites as well as the exhaustion of cellular antioxidant defense mechanisms. Chronic Mn toxic conditions can result from continued inhalation of Mn dust and fumes. The CNS is the main site of damage from the disease, which results in constant disability. The typical symptoms include emotional disturbances, weakness, sleepiness, repeated leg cramps, spastic gait, and paralysis.

The naturally existing and the most stable manganese isotope is ^{55}Mn, and 18 isotopes have been discovered, with a different half-life ranging from seconds to million years. In medical practice, given its paramagnetic properties, manganese serves as a contrast agent in magnetic resonance imaging (MRI) [252]. Manganese inorganic compounds and complexes are experimental ambiguous cancerogenic agents. Permanganates are poisons for the body.

Technetium

Technetium is the first human-made element in 1937. It is the lightest radioactive element in the periodic table, having no stable isotopes. Artificially obtained technetium is a slightly reactive metal, slowly reacting with air and acid. Technetium has no known biological role and is not typically found in the body. It is mainly used in medical radiation imaging as a tracer. This element does not occur naturally in the biosphere (it has only unstable isotopes and is very rare on Earth) and so generally never presents a risk [11 - 13]. All technetium compounds are considered as highly toxic, mainly because of their radiotoxicity. Technetium has 26 unstable and 11 metastable isotopes-isomers and all of them are radioactive.

Technetium has significant medical applications. The metastable radioisotope ^{99m}Tc, a strong γ-emitter with a half-life of 6 h, is used in single photon emission computed tomography (SPECT) allowing rapid diagnosis. Technetium-99m is useful in the examination of the metabolic process without significant harm to the patient. The diagnostic procedures are non-invasive on the brain, heart, kidneys, and thyroid. This radioactive isotope is used in radiation treatment of cancers. Since 1964, a diagnostic procedure is used in which the radioisotope ^{99m}Tc is injected in the body. This isotope is absorbed mainly in tumors that can later be detected. The choice of ^{99m}Tc is justified because the half-life of this γ-emitting isotope is low. The radioisotope can therefore perform its medical function with minimal adverse effects on the patient. Technetium-99m, the most widely used radioisotope in nuclear medicine, is currently applied in more than 80% of all nuclear medicine procedures [253].

When enters the body, technetium-99m can pose a health risk. It usually concentrates on the thyroid gland and the digestive tract. Nevertheless, the body constantly gets rid of this radioisotope in feces. Technetium-99m is a γ-emitter, making it a very negligible risk of toxicity. Most commonly, ^{99m}Tc causes rash, fever, angioedema, and anaphylaxis due to hypersensitivity reactions [253]. The short 6-hour half-life and quick excretion from the body minimize the toxic effects and give enough time to complete diagnostic imaging, with minimal radiation exposure to the patient.

Various radiopharmaceuticals have been labeled with ^{99m}Tc nuclide. In medicine, different technetium compounds are used. One of them is the salt sodium pertechnetate $Na^{99m}TcO_4$. Intravenously applied ^{99m}Tc-pertechnetate is loosely bound to plasma proteins and quickly moves out of the intravenous compartments [253]. After the intervention, this substance is removed from the body *via* the kidneys with the urine.

Rhenium

As rhenium is a very rare microelement, it gives no ecological problems in nature and appears to have no known biological functions in living systems. There is no information on the metal or its compounds being toxic. Rhenium is the last discovered stable metal and it is one of the rarest elements on earth. Rhenium has one stable isotope, rhenium-185, which, however, occurs in very small abundance in nature. It is less reactive to air than manganese, which is located in the same group of the periodic table [254]. Rhenium is readily soluble in water, and by this interaction, the colorless perrhenic acid $HReO_4$ is formed. Its salts ($MReO_4$) contain a tetrahedral ReO_4^- ion. Ammonium perrhenate NH_4ReO_4 is the most important for the production of other Re compounds.

Many rhenium coordination complexes with potential antineoplastic properties have been synthesized in recent years with the purpose to overcome the clinical limitations of Pt-based agents [255]. Among other metals, rhenium merits special consideration, due to its varied range of oxidation states (from -1 to +7), giving the opportunity for great structural diversity of the complexes and for the ability to modify the redox status of cancer cells. Re(I) complexes constitute the most distinguished group of anticancer rhenium compounds and the Re(I) tricarbonyl subunit $[Re(I)(CO)_3]$ is the most commonly used organometallic fragment for the synthesis of Re coordination compounds. Many Re(I) complexes were found able to reduce free radicals' production even at low concentrations [254, 255]. Re has some biological properties that are similar to that of technetium. Thus, it is being used frequently to replace technetium or in conjunction with technetium.

d-Elements of the Iron Group VIIIB

Iron

Iron is present in large amounts all over the Earth and is available to a great degree in the plant kingdom [3, 11]. Among the biogenic elements, iron is one of the most important elements for the vital activity of all living beings and is the most abundant metal in the body (10^{-5}%). An adult man has about 4 g iron, distributed to 3 g in the respiratory pigment of erythrocytes - hemoglobin, 0.15 g in myoglobin, and the rest in different Fe deposits (ferritin, hemosiderin, oxidoreductases, *etc.*).

In an oxygen atmosphere, Fe is present in various oxidation states (+2, +3, and +4). The most stable oxidation state is +3, forming $Fe(OH)_3$ with very low solubility, the reason for the decrease in the accessibility of soluble Fe^{2+} salts for uptake [3, 4]. Iron in the oxidation states +2 and +3 very easily forms complex ions with biomolecules, the coordination number being mostly 6.

In mammals, the functions of iron are reduced to the following three main ones: oxygen transport, electron transport, and the structural organization of enzymes [256]. Iron seems to play a dominant role, being an activator of many catalytic processes in the body and being involved in the transport of gases into the blood. Around 70% of the total iron content in the body is concentrated in hemoglobin, which carries oxygen from the lungs to the muscles.

Iron is part of the structure of many significant body constituents, *e.g.,* hemoglobin, muscle protein myoglobin, enzymes like cytochromes, peroxidases, xanthine oxidase, aldehyde oxidase, catalases, mitochondrial α-glycerophosphate oxidase, and a number of other enzymes necessary for the metabolism of all known biological species [256]. In all of them, iron is present as heme form or porphyrin form (Fig. **5**). Iron-based structures can be classified as mainly found in hemoproteins and other Fe proteins, examples of which are given in Table **14**.

Table 14. Iron-based proteins.

Hemoproteins		
Protein	**Redox state**	**Function**
Hemoglobin	Fe^{2+}	Transport of O_2 from the lungs to tissues, tetramer, 4 Fe^{2+}
Myoglobin	Fe^{2+}	binding and storage of O_2 in muscles, monomer, 1 Fe^{2+}
Cytochromes	$Fe^{2+} \rightleftarrows Fe^{3+}$	electron transfer in the terminal respiratory chain
Catalase	Fe^{3+}	decomposition of H_2O_2
Peroxidase	Fe^{3+}	hydrogen peroxide detoxication
Other proteins containing iron		
Transferrin	Fe^{3+}	Transport of iron in blood plasma
Ferritin Hemosiderin	Fe^{3+}	storage of iron in tissues, mostly in the liver
Lactoferrin	Fe^{3+}	storage of iron, degradation product of ferritin
FeS-proteins	Fe^{3+}	antimicrobial effect
	$Fe^{2+} \rightleftarrows Fe^{3+}$	transfer of electrons in the respiratory chain

Over 500 human metalloproteins contain Fe and many of them have either a heme prosthetic group or Fe-S cluster [257]. Organisms bind Fe to organic molecules suitable for life functions like the heterocyclic compound pyrrole. The most important pyrrole derivates represent macrocyclic rings with 4 pyrrole molecules, porphyrins. There are many groups, such as methyl, vinyl, or acetyl, bound to the peripheral C atoms. Hemoproteins contain heme as a prosthetic group. Heme is a chelate where Fe^{2+} or Fe^{3+} ions are bound to a porphyrin ring.

The best-known and perhaps most important is hemoglobin. Hemoglobin is a complex protein, the molecule of which consists of two parts: protein (globin) and iron-containing (heme) [11,256,257]. Heme is a complex of iron with substituted porphyrin (a closed cycle of four pyrrole rings). In the composition of the hemoglobin molecule, there are four hemes, in each of which there is an iron atom. And although these atoms account for only 0.35% of the mass of a large molecule, it is iron that gives it a unique property - the ability to capture molecular oxygen and give it where it is needed. Iron(II) ion localizes in the center of the porphyrin molecule between the four N atoms, bonded to all of them in the plane of the porphyrin ring. This is a typical example of chelation. This is the iron-porphyrin complex, named heme (after Greek haima blood), that binds oxygen. The fifth iron orbital forms a bond with the N atom of the imidazole groups of histidine. The sixth orbital of iron(II) ion in the heme is used for the hemoglobin-oxygen (or hemoglobin-carbon monoxide) binding. Iron in the heme group can vary its oxidation states between Fe^{2+} and Fe^{3+} and thus give an O-binding and an O-releasing effect. The porphyrin traps iron, which does not dissociate from heme. Binding to O_2 molecules is weak enough that upon reaching the site of oxygen utilization, such as muscle, O_2 can be released. Heme generally donates the proteins in which it is an ingredient, with the ability to transport and store O_2. The main biological function of hemoglobin is the ability to bind O_2 from the lungs and transfer it back to the tissues. Hemoglobin, which attaches oxygen, is named oxyhemoglobin and hemoglobin which gives oxygen is dezoxyhemoglobin.

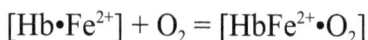

$$[Hb \cdot Fe^{2+}] + O_2 = [HbFe^{2+} \cdot O_2]$$

Oxyhemoglobin-Fe ions are in the plane of the porphyrin ring (Fig. **5**). In oxyhemoglobin, Fe(II) is in the diamagnetic, low-spin state. Once O_2 is lost, iron in the deoxyhemoglobin molecule shifts below the plane of the porphyrin ring and away from the vacant coordination site, because it has become a larger, paramagnetic, high-spin Fe(II) ion. Throughout the cycle, iron stays in the Fe(II) state, only varying between its high-spin and low-spin forms [3,256,257]. It is only when exposed to air that the red Fe(II)-based hemoglobin is oxidized to the brown Fe(III) species, which reaction is irreversible.

In the same way, hemoglobin reacts with carbon monoxide, when CO intoxication occurs, thus forming the macrocyclic complex - carboxyhemoglobin:

$$[Hb \cdot Fe^{2+}] + CO = [HbFe^{2+} \cdot CO]$$

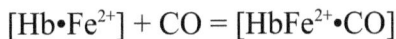

CO is extremely toxic because the carbonyl ligand binds very strongly to the Fe ion of hemoglobin, preventing it from carrying O_2 [4, 256]. The obtained carboxyhemoglobin disrupts the transport of O_2 from the lungs to the tissues and causes CO-intoxication. Much research has been done to understand how CO and molecular O_2 bind to the heme proteins myoglobin Mb and hemoglobin Hb. It has been observed that the selective binding of O_2 rather than CO in biosystems is complicated by the fact that naturally occurring metalloproteins including Mb and Hb produce CO during their degradation.

Hemoglobin is existing in large quantities in red blood cells and gives the red color of blood. The Hb molecule has developed according to the different needs of nature [5]. Hb in animals living in thin air has a particularly high capacity for O_2 uptake. In human blood, the Hb content is usually 135-160 g/l (for men) and 115-140 g/l (for women). Newborns have a significantly higher content, 150-250 g/l, during the first days of life.

A significant part of iron is found in myoglobin, which is a structural relative of hemoglobin [256, 257]. Myoglobin, the muscle oxygen storage heme protein, contains a heme group that is also able to reversibly bind O_2 in muscle cells and is used to temporarily store O_2 in tissues. The functional units of myoglobin and hemoglobin in deoxygenated form contain a pentacoordinate iron center where Fe is in the +2 oxidation state in which the metal ion lies out of the plane of the porphyrin's four pyrrole-nitrogen donor ligands. After binding O_2, the oxidation state of Fe changes to +3 and the ion forms hexacoordinate octahedral complexes. Although both myoglobin and hemoglobin have the same functional unit for O_2 binding, hemoglobin shows the phenomenon of cooperativeness for O_2 binding, whereas myoglobin does not exhibit such properties, which helps transport oxygen from hemoglobin to myoglobin. Some classes of invertebrates use non-heme iron, hemerythrin as a storage and transport of O_2. Hemerythrins, used for O_2 transportation by some marine invertebrates, ligate Fe through protein side-chain ligand atoms only and do not bind with O_2 in a cooperative manner. The quantity of myoglobin in animal muscles varies and influences the meat color. Beef meat has a high amount of Mb (0.50%) and is dark red, while pork meat, with 0.06% of Mb is paler.

There is a group of Fe-containing enzymes which are able to catalyze the electron transfer processes in mitochondria, named cytochromes (CCh). Altogether, more than 50 cytochromes are recognized. The most studied cytochrome is the extremely multifunctional protein - cytochrome *c* [258]. It intermediates electron-transfer in respiration, works as a ROS detoxifying agent, and participates in cell apoptosis. The electron transfer in a redox chain involving this enzyme is carried out by changing the oxidation states of iron:

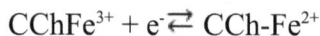

$$CChFe^{3+} + e^- \rightleftharpoons CCh\text{-}Fe^{2+}$$

Cytochromes' oxidized forms with Fe^{3+} (ferri-form) are changed to reduced Fe^{2+} (ferro-form) by accepting electrons. Cytochromes are proteins that are red in color as a result of their content of heme. Taking part in oxidation-reduction reactions, they are included in the respirational structures of mitochondria, and power stations of the cells. Hemes of cytochromes are electron transporters in contrast to hemoglobin and myoglobin. Cytochrome P-450, found in animals, plants, fungi, archaea, protists, and bacteria, contains heme-based Fe in the active sites, plays an essential role in the oxidation of most compounds, and acts as a monooxygenase. Cytochrome P-450 can affect the toxicity and efficacy of many medications and is critical for the metabolism and biotransformation of drugs, synthesis of hormones, and the detoxification of xenobiotics [259].

Depending on the characteristic enzymatic activities, heme-containing peroxidases are classified into four classes, *viz.,* peroxidase-catalases, peroxidase-cyclooxygenases, peroxidase-chlorite dismutases, and peroxidase-peroxygenases. This enzyme peroxidase family mainly quickens the oxidation of organic substances by H_2O_2. They are frequently used in many medical applications [260].

In addition, iron is present in a non-heme form named non-heme iron [261]. Non-heme iron proteins contain a wide variety of iron sites that have numerous chemical and structural properties. Non-heme iron is present mainly as ferritin and transferrin. Iron is transported in the plasma as Fe^{3+} form and is taken up by protein transferrin (an iron-carrying protein present in human serum at concentrations of 2.5-3.5 mg/mL). The transfer of iron to transferrin is catalyzed by a Cu-containing protein, *viz.,* ceruloplasmin. Transferrin tightly binds and transports ferric iron ions. Released from the blood serum transferrin Fe(II) ions are used for the synthesis of Fe-dependent proteins and enzymes (hemoglobin, cytochrome c-oxidase, cytochrome p-450, *etc.*) or stored by conjugated protein ferritin in the reticuloendothelial cells and hepatocytes. Ferritin is a ubiquitous protein found throughout the animal, plant, and microbial kingdoms. It stores highly concentrated Fe(III), releases it as Fe(II) when required, and thus keeps the iron regulation in the body. The protein family, ferritins, represents a shell of linked peptides surrounding the core of Fe(III) oxohydroxophosphate. This core is a cluster of Fe(III) cations, oxide, hydroxide, and phosphate ions of average empirical formula $[FeO(OH)]_8[FeO(OPO_3H_2)]$, similar to the mineral ferrihydrite. The molecule is very large, hydrophilic, water-soluble, and concentrated in the spleen, liver, and bone marrow. The genes for human transferrin and ferritin receptors have been revealed and the mechanisms of regulation of expression of transferrin receptors and intracellular ferritin in response to the Fe supply have been widely studied and recognized [262]. When Fe is in excess, the synthesis of transferrin receptors is reduced and ferritin production is enlarged, which favors Fe storage.

Plants and bacteria use an electron transfer chain, a family of Fe(III)-sulfur structures (Fe-S clusters), as the core of their redox proteins, ferredoxins. These proteins hold covalently bonded Fe and S, and act as exceptional electron transfer agents for the transfer of electrons from the oxidized unit to the reduced unit and vice versa in the oxidation-reduction reactions. Iron-sulfur (Fe-S) clusters are highly conserved and ubiquitous prosthetic groups of proteins, made of iron and sulfide (S^{2-}) ions, of which the [2Fe2S] and [4Fe4S] clusters are the most common in biosystems [263]. The reversible variations in the oxidation states of iron +II or +III permit the quick electron transfer to the required catalytic site. The metal-sulfur clusters are a vital part of the complex enzyme nitrogenase. They are numerous, varied, and typically involved in oxy-reduction processes carried out by the protein in which they constitute prosthetic centers. Most of them are characterized by the number of Fe ions in the prosthetic center like rubredoxin with one iron ion, ferredoxins with two or four Fe ions, aconitase with three iron ions.

Iron is introduced into the body through nourishment [257]. Bread and meat are significant Fe-rich foodstuffs. In food, iron is existing in the ferric form either as Fe(III) hydroxide or in combination with ferric organic compounds. The acidity of gastric juice results in the release of ferric Fe(III) form. Fe(III) form is reduced to the ferrous Fe(II) form by reducing agents such as glutathione, vitamin C, and cysteine. Low phosphate intake rises Fe absorption, whereas high phosphate food reduces Fe absorption by forming insoluble iron phosphates. Oxalates also decrease iron absorption by forming low soluble iron oxalate. The biological availability of iron is affected also by phytate (inositol hexaphosphate), polyphenols, and tannins. Acidic conditions promote the solubility of iron ions either in Fe(III) or Fe(II) forms. Iron in Fe(II) form is more soluble and is more easily absorbed than the Fe(III) form.

Microorganisms have found an alternative route for iron uptake by siderophores [264]. Siderophores (ferrichrome, enterobactin) represent organocyclic compounds containing catecholate, hydroxamate, and carboxylate groups for binding Fe^{3+} and formation of very stable Fe^{3+} complexes (Fig. **10**). This enables the dissolution of any Fe(III) compound and takes it inside of microorganism cells, where iron is released as Fe^{2+}. Therefore, siderophores help to acquire the necessary amount of iron from the surrounding environment.

Iron overload includes several disorders characterized by iron accumulation in cells, subcellular compartments, tissues, and organs [265]. Iron causes conjunctivitis, choroiditis and retinitis if it contacts and remains in tissues. Chronic inhalation of excessive levels of iron oxide fumes or dust may result in the progress of pneumoconiosis (siderosis). No physical damage of lung function has been related to siderosis. Inhalation of excessive amounts of iron oxide may enhance the hazard of pulmonary cancer development in workers exposed to respiratory carcinogens. If iron is taken in abnormally large quantities, the excess is placed in the liver. Excessive accumulation of Fe in the liver, pancreas, lung, heart, and other tissues results in hemosiderosis and hemochromatosis. Elevated Fe levels appear to play a significant role in neurodegeneration.

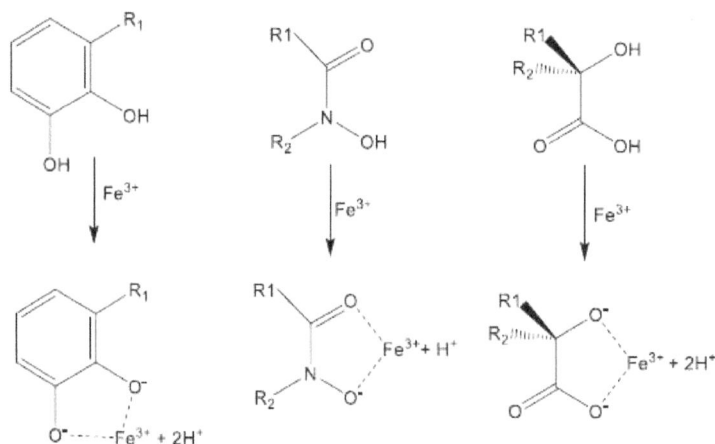

Fig. (10). Modes of Fe^{3+} binding with catecholate, hydroxamate, and carboxylate groups of siderophores for iron transportation.

When iron is deficient, then opposite changes occur, which leads to a decreased ferritin production that decreases iron storage so that iron can be maximally used in the body [266, 267]. There are many actors inhibiting iron absorption: malabsorption syndrome, diarrheal diseases, excess of phosphates and oxalates, subtotal gastrectomy, surgical removal of the upper small intestine, antiacid therapy, chronic infections, *etc*. With a lack of iron in the human body (or a large loss of it), iron deficiency hypochromic anemia occurs, causing serious damage to organs and tissues. In addition to the symptoms which are common to all anemias, the patient shows some characteristic indications such as abnormal nail growth, glossitis, fissures around the corners of the mouth, *etc*. syndromes. Food enrichment with iron is becoming more common. The enrichment material may be Ferrum reductum, a finely dispersed, porous, metallic Fe. Different types of bonded Fe, which is more easily absorbed by the body, can be also used.

Cobalt

Cobalt is an essential element for life and most importantly is required as a trace element for humans, plants, and animals. The average human adult contains about 1.1 g of cobalt with a daily requirement of 0.0001 mg per day. Co^{2+} ions act as a coenzyme of a number of enzymes: arginase, carboxylase, polypeptidase, lecithinase, *etc.* Cobalt is very important biochemically for the homeostasis of DNA, heme, amino acids, and fatty acids. While cobalt has no specific function by itself, the Co^{3+} ion forms the core of vitamin B_{12} (cobalamin), (Fig. **6**). Vitamin B_{12} with a composition $C_{63}H_{90}N_{14}O_{14}PCo$ is a bioinorganic complex compound, in which complexing ion is Co^{3+} with a coordination number equal to 6, where cobalt(III) is at the core of the molecule, surrounded by a macrocyclic ring structure, called corrin, which is similar to the porphyrin ring. Cobalt, contained in vitamin B_{12}, is strongly bound in a corrin ring and the oxidation states +1, +2, and +3 are important in its activity. It is the first recognized man organometallic complex which readily forms Co−C bonds (to deoxy-adenosyl and methyl groups). Cobalt ion is the only metal ion that is a part of the structure of vitamins. Vitamin B_{12} is necessary for normal hematopoiesis and maturation of red blood cells. Vitamin B_{12} helps vitamin C perform its biofunctions and is required for the proper ingestion of food. In addition, vitamin B_{12} prevents nerve damages by contributing to the formation of a protective sheath that insulates nerve cells. Vitamin B_{12} appears to possess antioxidant properties [268]. Certain anaerobic bacteria use a related molecule, methylcobalamin, in a cycle to produce CH_4. The same biochemical cycle converts elemental Hg and insoluble inorganic Hg compounds in Hg-contaminated waters to soluble, highly toxic methyl-Hg(II), $[HgCH_3]^+$, and dimethyl-Hg(II), $Hg(CH_3)_2$. There are enzyme systems, in which vitamin B_{12} acts not in the free state but in the form of B_{12}-coenzymes. A cofactor is an active part of the enzyme, which can be easily separated. It participates in two processes - transfer of the propellent CH_3-groups (methylation reactions) and transfer of hydrogen ions. Vitamin B_{12} can be produced only by microorganisms (bacteria and archaea). Bacteria in the body may produce it. Nevertheless, in humans this process is unproductive because it occurs only in the colon, from where very small uptake into the blood is possible. Consequently, a daily supply of cobalamin in the human diet is necessary. The best sources are meat, fish, eggs, and dairy products [269]. In animals, vitamin B_{12} is obtained more efficiently in the gut, and ruminant animals like cows and sheep can produce it for their own usage.

Lack of vitamin B_{12} in the body leads to the blood illness pernicious anemia with deterioration of the bone marrow cells responsible for replacing blood [270]. Anemia is caused by the inactivation of one of two enzymes in humans where vitamin B_{12} is the vital coenzyme (methionine synthase and methylmalonyl-CoA mutase). A deficiency of vitamin B_{12} can prevent the red blood cells from carrying enough O_2 from the lungs to the different organs of the body, consequently causing anemia. The typical symptoms include loss of energy, loss of appetite and moodiness. An absence of vitamin B_{12} may also lead to disturbances in the CNS causing nerve cells to work wrongly and finally resulting in irreversible nerve injury with symptoms like eye disorders, delusions, dizziness, confusion, and loss of memory. Different from other B complex vitamins, vitamin B_{12} can be deposited in the body. Because of this, it is very easy to get sufficient amounts of this vital vitamin in the human diet. Vitamin B_{12} deficiencies are rare in young people, but do sporadically occur in adults due to gastrointestinal conditions. As vitamin B_{12} is found only in animals, vegetarians are at risk of this deficiency. As said, certain animals may produce their own vitamin B_{12}. This, obviously, implies the intake of enough Co in the diet. When there is a deficiency in soil and animals show symptoms of anemia, they should be given salts containing 0.1% cobalt as sulphate.

Toxicity: Cobalt has both positive and damaging effects on human health [271]. High amounts of cobalt can damage human health producing a variety of adverse health effects. Cobalt and its compounds are widespread in nature. Occupational cobalt exposure is considered to be most prevalent in grinding, mining, paints, cobalt processing plants, and hard metal industry.

Professional Co poisoning can be caused mainly by inhalation of dust. Continued exposure to Co powder can produce allergic sensitization, chronic bronchitis, and asthma-like diseases with indications varying from cough, breath shortness, and dyspnea to reduced pulmonary functions, nodular fibrosis and lasting disabilities. Co-metal and its compounds (oxides and sulfides) have not been categorized as carcinogenic agents although some experiments with animals indicate that. Excessively high Co amounts in the air cause lung effects (asthma and pneumonia). This mainly occurs with persons who work with Co compounds.

Inorganic compounds of Co are poisonous to humans, and the longer they remain in the body, the more negative effects they cause in the cells [272]. Cobalt compounds are absorbed orally, by inhalation and through skin contact. The degree of digestive absorption depends on the concentration. Very low doses are absorbed practically completely, while higher amounts are less well absorbed. Co is stored in the plasma, liver, kidney, spleen, and pancreas. It is excreted quickly by urine and feces, independently of the route of exposure. The excess level of cobalt in the body may cause hypothyroidism and overproduction of erythrocytes, fibrosis in the pulmonary systems and asthma. Soils near mining and smelting facilities contain very high quantities of Co and its compounds so the consumption by humans through plants causes health effects like heart problems, thyroid damage, vision problems, vomiting and nausea. Higher concentrations of cobalt lead to numerous dysfunctions in the plant systems as well. These mainly include the production of ROS, hydroxyl radicals' generation, formation of H_2O_2, increased content of proline, and alteration of antioxidant activity of the enzyme [273].

Naturally occurring Co consists of one stable isotope [59]Co. By irradiation of [59]Co with neutrons in nuclear reactors the radioisotope ^{60}Co can be obtained. The radioactive isotope ^{60}Co is a powerful gamma-ray emitter with a half-life of 5.27 years. This radioactivity is of the same type as that of X-rays, and for this reason, ^{60}Co is used as an anticancer agent in the so-called cobalt therapy, a specific form of radiotherapy for the treatment of malignant tumors [274]. This radiation can also be used for sterilizing medical equipment, supplies, and medical waste. In radiation therapy, the energy destroys cancer cells that are later substituted by fresh tissue. Two different methods of radiotherapy are available: cobalt therapy and treatment with X-rays. The latter is technically very sophisticated, and complicated and can be used only in large clinics with innovative medical and technical expertise. In contrast, Co therapy is simple and appropriate for small hospitals in developing countries. For Co therapy, the active strong ^{60}Co radiation is directed against the tumor location through an aperture. The ^{60}Co radiation is also used for the testing of materials, *viz.,* to show the pores in the welds, which is cheaper than the corresponding X-ray technique. Radiation from ^{60}Co has found many other technical applications. The suitable characteristics of the other cobalt radionuclide, [57]Co, make it interesting for application in brachytherapy. The radioactive isotope [57]Co combines the high specific action with the emission of comparatively low-energy photons and its short half-life of 272 days [275]. [57]Co decays by electron capture to the stable [57]Fe. The health effects of cobalt may also be caused by the radiation of Co radioisotopes. Cancer patients suffer from sterility, bleeding, diarrhea, hair loss, and sickness, leading to coma and even death. Exposure to high doses of cobalt radiation has been shown to result in damage to nervous tissues, especially peripheral nerves.

Nickel

Nickel is known to be a vital trace element. Nevertheless, compared with Fe and Co, nickel plays a more modest role in the human body and its biochemistry is the least understood of all 3d transition metals [276]. However, nickel was a crucial element in the earliest age of Earth's life, when the atmosphere was composed of methane, hydrogen and hydrogen sulphide. The simple functions of archae bacteria in such an environment required Ni-containing enzymes as a catalyst. The appearance of oxygen in the atmosphere changed its composition to oxygen, nitrogen, and carbon dioxide. This transformation fundamentally reduced the Ni requirement as a catalyst and its role was taken over by the other transition metals Fe, Cu, and Mn, although anaerobic bacteria are still active in O_2-free environments. They get their energy supply by metabolizing H_2 and releasing methane, a reaction catalyzed by Ni.

The transition metals Fe, Co, and Ni, representing a triad in the middle of the periodic table, are similar in their chemical properties but quite different in their impact on the atmosphere and their implications for life. Iron is extremely significant for human life, being essential for hemoglobin and thus for O_2 uptake in the lungs. Cobalt, present in the form of vitamin B_{12}, is required to prevent anemia. Although it is widespread on the Earth, the role of Ni in mammals and humans is very limited and restricted to its presence in a single enzyme urease, which catalyzes the decomposition of urea to NH_3 [277]. However, no Ni-based enzyme or cofactor has been identified in high animals, but they do occur in bacteria, archaea, some plants and unicellular eukaryotes, the typical example being *Helicobacter pylori*.

The body of an adult contains between 5 - 13.5 mg of nickel and is found in all biological materials. The most common oxidation state of Ni in biosystems is +2. Although the biofunctions of nickel are still rather unclear in the body, nevertheless, Ni can be found in the highest amounts in the structures of nucleic acids, predominantly RNA, and is supposed to be involved in protein structure or function. There are indications that Ni, like Co, participates in the blood formation, affecting carbohydrate metabolism [278]. Nickel cations Ni^{2+} are able to form complex compounds with amino acids, carboxylic acids, and other bioactive compounds that contain N- or O-donor atoms. Obviously, because of its complex-formation ability, Ni stimulates cellular amino acid synthesis, quickens the regeneration of blood plasma proteins and regulates the hemoglobin content in the blood. Nickel cations are existing in some enzymes in the form of porphyrin-type metal complexes.

Nickel can enter the body through inhalation, ingestion, and dermal contact [276, 278]. The amount of Ni absorbed by the digestive tract is dependent on the type and the content of Ni species in the food products, and on the absorbent capacity. Usually, only 1-2% of consumed nickel is absorbed. The daily intake of Ni is around 35 - 300 µg per day.

In the human body, its deficiency causes inhibition of several liver enzymes (urease, Ni-superoxide dismutase (Ni-SOD), glucose-6-phosphate, isocitrate, lactate and glutamate dehydrogenase), disruption of respirational processes in the mitochondria, lipid content changes in the liver. Natural deficiencies of nickel practically do not occur [279]. Nickel is normally only one of the numerous components of enzymes, which may contain several different coenzymes and other inorganic components. The requirements for Ni were clarified when it was found that most of hydrogenase enzymes contain Ni together with Fe-S clusters. Although from a chemical point of view, the +3 is a very rare oxidation state, nickel(III) is involved in the enzyme redox cycle.

Nickel is vital for several species of animals and is found in some plants that accumulate metals [280]. Bacteria also use nickel for the production of enzymes and to function properly. Nickel-dependent enzymes are found and well-characterized in bacteria and some eukaryotes. Because of the human symbiotic existence with microbes, it is likely that Ni is important for the survival of some microorganisms [281]. Despite the scarcity of Ni-based enzymes, they are often essential, playing crucial functions in various metabolic processes, such as the metabolism of energy, virulency and functioning in redox or non-redox enzyme systems. Enzyme urease catalyzes the urea hydrolysis, forming NH_3 and CO_2. The molecule of urea is very stable that typically hydrolyzes very slowly and the enzyme catalytic activity strongly increases the hydrolysis rate. Numerous methanogenic bacteria contain the enzyme CO-dehydrogenase, which catalyzes the oxidation of carbon monoxide and carbon dioxide. The process is enzymatically reversible and may consequently serve as an alternate method of carbon dioxide fixation (assimilation) by photosynthetic bacteria. Ni-superoxide dismutase (Ni-SOD) catalyzes disproportionation of $\cdot O_2^-$ to molecular O_2 and H_2O_2. Nickel can also make some microbes infectious. It is a virulence determining factor for the gastric pathogen *Helicobacter pylori* in humans, which possesses two critical for *in vivo* colonization, Ni enzymes, Ni/Fe hydrogenase and urease. These two nickel enzymes are potential new therapeutic targets for the therapy of *Helicobacter pylori* infection conditions, which can prevent ulcers from healing. In microorganisms, Ni/Fe hydrogenase catalyzes the transformation of H^+ to H_2 and *vice versa*.

It has to be mentioned that the essentialness of Ni in humans has not been confirmed. In small amounts, nickel is vital, but when the acceptance is too high, it can be a hazard to human health [282]. Patients with some liver and kidney illnesses are identified to have low amounts of Ni in the body. Excess Ni in the human body is connected with a high risk of heart diseases, thyroid disease, and cancer, although the significance of the nickel amount in the body is unidentified. Most probably, Ni affects cellular membranes, hormones, and enzymes.

Actually, small amounts of nickel are important for the body. The biologically available Ni^{2+} ions dictate the human health noxiousness and ecological toxicity of metal Ni and its compounds [283]. Nickel has a universal toxic effect, and at higher concentrations may cause the nasopharynx and lung diseases, malignant neoplasm formations, dermatitis, eczema *etc.* Nickel allergy is definitely well known. It is one of the most common allergies in humans. Nickel contact dermatitis and nickel allergy are well-recognized among women. Persistent eczema occurs after sensitization to some nickel-based nickel-plated earrings. Recent investigations have indicated that such sensitizations can be avoided by the use of corrosion-resistant alloys [283].

Peoples exposed to Ni-based compounds show a higher risk for the respirational tract, development of nasal cancers, and allergic contact dermatitis. Humans are exposed to Ni by breathing air, drinking polluted water, consuming contaminated food or smoking cigarettes. It has been established that acute exposure to Ni carbonyl, an oncogenic gas that is produced from the reaction of Ni with heated CO, can cause indications such as frontal headaches, nausea, sickness or vertigo. Prolonged Ni inhalation and uptake of too large amounts of nickel may cause serious health problems, including a higher risk of progress of nose, larynx, lung, and prostate cancer [284]. Nickel fumes are respiratory irritants that cause pneumonitis. Nickel and certain nickel compounds are reasonably anticipated to be carcinogens. That is why nickel and its compounds are almost not used in medical practice.

Platinum Metals

The platinum metals are located in groups VIIIB-XB and periods 5 and 6 of the periodic system. Platinum metals are six transition noble metals, which include light metals (ruthenium, rhodium, and palladium) and heavy metals (osmium, iridium, and platinum). They possess analogous physicochemical characteristics and occur in the same mineral ores. Their melting points decrease in the period (Ru to Pd, Os to Pt). Os has the highest melting temperature of all metals after W and Re. The hardness characteristics of the metals vary in the same way but more evidently. All platinum metals are noble and thus cannot be attacked by O_2 of air and water at all [11, 285]. At high temperatures, Ru and Os form volatile RuO_4 and OsO_4, while Pt compounds of the type diammonium hexachloroplatinate $(NH_4)_2PtCl_6$ do not produce oxides but a very finely pulverized metal, platinum sponge, which has a huge specific surface and possesses good catalytic properties.

The contents of Pt group metals are extremely low in the earth's crust. It is not known that these elements have any biological role in life. The platinum-group metals' coordination compounds belong to conventional chemotherapeutics. According to the structure, most of these substances are non-electrolytes, cis-isomers, derivatives of two- and tetravalent platinum, the most effective of them being cis-di chloro diammineplatin $[Pt(NH_3)_2Cl_2]$ and cis-tetrachloro diammineplatin $[Pt(NH_3)_2Cl_4]$. The success of Pt(II) and Pt(IV) complexes sparked new research to design metal coordination compounds with other platinum elements [285]. The obtained metal-based drugs, like all effective drugs, are toxic. The oxides RuO_4 and OsO_4 are very toxic. Alloys of platinum-iridium, platinum-gold, as well as palladium alloys are used in dental prosthetics. Iridium in an alloy with platinum is used to make electrical stimulators of the heart.

Ruthenium

Ruthenium has no identified biofunctions, but this metal is present in the human body at a higher amount than the essential biogenic metal Co. Very little information is available on Ru impact on plants, although algae appear to concentrate it. No negative ecological effects have been reported so far. Ru compounds are encountered comparatively rarely by people. All Ru compounds should be regarded as highly poisonous and carcinogens [285]. Compounds of ruthenium stain the skin very strongly. It appears that ingested Ru is retained mostly in bones. Ruthenium tetroxide RuO_4 is highly noxious and volatile, thus has to be avoided.

Ruthenium has seven stable isotopes. Apart from these stable isotopes, 34 radioactive isotopes of Ru have also been found. The most stable radioisotopes are [106]Ru, [103]Ru, and [97]Ru. The nuclear separation products [103]Ru and [106]Ru are minor ingredients of nuclear power plant effluents. The potential for microbes to accumulate ruthenium radioisotopes has been widely studied [286]. Ruthenium-106 is one of the radioactive nuclides involved in atmosphere testing of nuclear weapons. It is between the long-lived radioisotopes that have caused and will continue to cause increased cancer risk for years and centuries to come.

Ru complexes are presently objects of great attention in medicinal chemistry, as anticancer agents with selective antimetastatic effects and low systemic toxicity [285, 287]. Ruthenium complexes appear to penetrate rationally well the tumor cells and bind efficiently to DNA. Ru approved drugs are particularly important in clinical practice due to their small toxicity. This is partly due to the capability of Ru to mimic the binding of Fe to certain biological molecules (serum transferrin, albumin), taking advantage of the mechanisms that the body has evolved for nontoxic Fe transport. The proteins serum transferrin and albumin are used by animals to solubilize and transport Fe, thus reducing its toxicity. Quickly dividing cells, for instance, microbially infected or cancer cells, have greater requirements for Fe and increase the number of transferrin receptors positioned on their cell surfaces. The anticancer Ru complexes are widely discussed in the next sections.

Additionally, ruthenium is unique amongst the Pt group elements because it can exist in various oxidation states, the most common being the oxidation states +2, +3, and +4, which are accessible under biological conditions. The redox potential between the different available oxidation states occupied by Ru allows the body to catalyze different oxo-reduction reactions, depending on the biological environment. These two characteristics combine to give Ru drugs lower toxicity compared to other Pt group metal compounds and consequently make Ru compounds promising for clinical applications. Ruthenium and its complexes have important applications in therapy and diagnostics [287]. Ruthenium is used for the characterization of calcitonin level in blood. This Ca determination is helpful in the diagnosis and therapy of diseases associated with the thyroid and parathyroid glands. Ruthenium plays a significant role in many other medical assays, which are important for therapy. Ruthenium also has been applied in treatment as an immunosuppressive agent (Ru(III) complex of Cyclosporin A) [288], antimicrobic agent (Ru(III) complex of Chloroquine) [289], antibiotic agent (Ru(III) complex of Thiosemicarbazone) [290], an inhibitor of NO (Ru polyamine carboxylates) [291]. The most important are the applications of Ru compounds in anticancer research as anticancer agents (bind and inhibits the replication of DNA, inhibits protein synthesis) [292], in radiation therapy (Ru radio sensitizers) [287], in photodynamic therapy [293], as well as activity on cancerous mitochondria effect and on metastasis. The mechanism of action of Ru as an antitumor agent is that it causes apoptosis of cancer cells by acting at DNA level. In radiation therapy, the radio sensitizers Ru complexes are used because of the affinity of ruthenium to bind to DNA easily. Ruthenium finds application in photodynamic therapy because it increases the access of chemical compounds to malignant cells. Ruthenium red, which has tumor inhibiting activity, is a type of Ru that is used to stain cancerous mitochondria. Ruthenium complexes (NAMI-A and derivatives) possess anti-metastatic activity by interacting and binding to mRNA and producing a denatured protein which becomes accumulated on the tumor surface producing a hard film and stops any blood supply to the cancer cell which inhibits the metastasis.

Rhodium

Rhodium has no known biological use and has been comparatively little used in biological or medical life processes. Rhodium's main usage is in catalytic converters of automobiles, where it reduces the quantity of exhaust nitrogen oxides NOx released into the environment. Interactions of rhodium cations with the protein casein were reported for the first time in 1958. Subsequently, many rhodium(II) complexes were studied as antineoplastic agents or enzyme inhibitors [294].

Rhodium compounds have desirable characteristics for use in complex biological processes. Rh complexes at all common oxidation states (0, +1, +2, +3) display low oxophylicity and, subsequently, broad functional-group tolerance, kinetical inertness, and aqueous stability. This functional group tolerance is crucial to the progress of rhodium in catalytic organic synthesis and in emerging fields such as organometallic frameworks [295]. The therapeutic applications involve acting as antineoplastic and antimicrobic agents in the Rh(I), Rh(II) and Rh(III) oxidation states due to their tunable chemical and biological properties as well as distinct mechanisms of action [296]. In fact, rhodium complexes have a limited history and there are a small number of reports about their biological activity documented in the scientific literature.

There are almost no reported cases of human beings affected by rhodium in any way. All rhodium compounds should be considered highly poisonous and carcinogenic [295]. While some rhodium compounds are carcinogenic, there is no sufficient evidence of their toxicity, which may be due to the fact that rhodium compounds are so rare. Rhodium is hypoallergenic in contrast to nickel. It actually guards against other metals alloyed with nickel to keep the skin safe.

Palladium

Palladium has no identified biological role. It is not toxic. Palladium is considered as low toxic, being poorly absorbed by the human body at ingestion. It may cause skin, eye, or breathing tract irritations and skin sensitization. Solutions of its compounds may cause burns to the skin and eyes. Palladium is the least dense metal in the Pt group. It is widely used in dental medicine where Pd is a very used component of dental casting alloys, and its usage has increased over the past years in response to the increased cost of Au [297]. By alloying Au with Pd, the dental Au can become harder and more wear resistant. The inclusion of more gold plating of porcelain crowns has enlarged this Pd use. At sufficiently high concentrations of the ionic forms of palladium, the metal shows poisonous and allergic effects on biosystems. Pd allergy almost always occurs in persons sensitive to Ni. The oncogenic potential of the palladium ions is still not clear, although there are some indications that it is able of acting as a mutagen. However, there are no known cases of adverse bioreactions to the metallic Pd. Furthermore, in spite of the possible adverse bioeffects of palladium cations, the risk of using Pd in dental casting alloy materials appears to be very low because of the small dissolution rate of palladium cations from its alloys.

Pd compounds are encountered comparatively rarely by humans. All Pd compounds should be considered as highly noxious and oncogenic. Palladium chloride is very toxic, harmful if swallowed, inhaled, or absorbed through the skin contacts. It causes liver, bone marrow, and kidney damages. However, $PdCl_2$ was formerly prescribed as a therapeutic agent for tuberculosis without too many bad adverse effects. Palladium has little environmental impact although there is no information as yet available to evaluate the effects of its exposure [298]. It is present at low amounts in some soils. Most plants tolerate it.

Palladium complexes are closely associated with their Pt analogs, because the physicochemical properties of Pt and Pd are similar to each other. Pd, like Pt, is contained in its structures in elemental or ionic forms (Pd^{2+} or Pd^{4+}). Palladium is used in radiotherapy, as the radioisotope [103]Pd. Comparable physicochemical properties of Pt and Pd suggest that they can be used interchangeably in corresponding compounds with anticancer [299] and antimicrobial [300] properties. Organopalladium complexes are interesting candidates due to their good stability in physiological environments. Many of these compounds have revealed promising *in vitro* and *in vivo* antineoplastic activity against some cisplatin-sensitive and cisplatin-resistant tumor lines with different modes of action compared to platinum-based drugs [301]. In contrast to the drug cisplatin, Pd derivatives bind to the oligonucleotide $[d(CGCGAATTCGCG)]_2$, which leads to blocking the replication of DNA. Due to the bypassing resistance of tumor cells, it has been observed that they can also enter into non-covalent, electrostatic, and H-bond interactions with DNA. Introducing monoethylphosphine or diethylphosphine groups is advantageous, as it allows for increasing the solubility of the complex compounds. Despite some resemblances between Pd(II) complexes and their Pt analogs, both with regard to chemistry (electronic structure and coordination interactions) and mechanisms of action, there are some differences between them. First of all, these complexes have different stability constants. Secondly, their mechanisms of action are slightly different. Pt(II) analogs, the same as Pd(II) complexes, intercalate into DNA, cause OS, and induce apoptosis *via* the extrinsic and intrinsic pathways. The difference between them is possible only in the phase of the cell cycles in which the cells are arrested [302]. Novel palladium compounds show potent action in the treatment of resistant cancer cells. It has been demonstrated that the complexes with thiosemicarbazone are more selective and powerful chemotherapeutics than the current standard cisplatin. Toxicological examinations have shown ten times lower toxic activity of some Pd compounds than their Pt-based analogues *in vivo*. The decreased toxicity of Pd complexes to normal tissues may be explained by the impossibility of -SH groups to substitute for the strongly bound chelate bioligands of Pd(II) when the compounds interact with proteins inside the cells.

Osmium

Pure metal Os does not occur in nature, it exists in a combined state in Cu and Ni alloys. It is the densest metal identified, although only by the narrowest limits. Os is unaffected by H_2O and acids, but dissolves in molten bases. Of the Pt metals, Os is the most quickly attacked by air [11 - 13]. The metal, even at normal temperature, shows the specific odor of its poisonous volatile oxide OsO_4 in detectable amounts. Because the solutions of OsO_4 can be reduced to the black dioxide OsO_2 by some biomaterials, this oxide is used to stain the tested tissues for microscopic examination.

Os has a very wide variety of oxidation states ranging from -2 to +8 in its inorganic compounds, except for +1. The element contains well-characterized and stable compounds in +2, +3, +4, +6, and +8 oxidation states [3,4,303]. It has also carbonyl-based and organometallic compounds in its lower oxidation state −2, 0, and +1. Ru is the only other element known to have an oxidation state of 8 because the chemistry of Ru and Os is typically comparable. Although +8 is very high, the highest oxidation state goes to its analogue iridium with a remarkable +9.

Osmium has no known biological functions but is existing at a very low background level in the body [303]. The metal is poorly absorbed, non-toxic and does not normally cause problems as it is comparatively not reactive, but all Os compounds should be considered as highly toxic. The metallic Os dust is a strong skin irritant and represents a fire and explosion danger.

The most common compound of Os and the main compound of toxicological interest is osmium oxide [304]. OsO_4 is volatile and very toxic, causing lung problems, skin and severe eye damage. OsO_4 can be absorbed into the body by inhalation of its vapor aerosols, and by ingestion. A harmful pollution of the air can be reached very rapidly on its evaporation at room temperature. Extremely toxic, chronic exposure to low amounts can cause fatal lung edema. Acute inhalation exposure can lead to headache, burning sensation, tearing, cough, wheezing, shortness of breath, lung edema, and death at high concentrations. The oxide particularly should only ever be handled with caution. Osmium oxide is a strong oxidizing agent which reacts with flammable and reducing materials. It interacts with HCl to form toxic Cl_2 gas. No information can be found about its ecotoxicity. It is probably very small because of its strength as an oxidizing agent that makes it be readily converted to OsO_2, which is reasonably innocuous. The oxide OsO_4 improves the effect of contrast in electron microscopy. It is the ease of reduction of oxide to metal that is used in this application. The capability of Os cations to exchange electrons at high rates is also the base for the medical usage of Os-containing sensors. They can be implanted in diabetics and are used to check the blood glucose levels continuously.

Osmium complexes of oxidation state +2 and +6 are used as antitumor and antimicrobial agents. Many of these complexes are isostructural and isoelectronic with the equivalent Ru-based analogues. Depending on the metal-ligand location, various modes of action are possible including redox activation, DNA targeting, or protein kinase inhibition. One major benefit of Os over Ru is the relative stability of the coordination sphere with regard to ligand exchange or hydrolysis and consequent deactivation of the complex. Some of Os(II) complexes demonstrated comparable to cisplatin cytotoxicity against cancer cells [305]. Some of the coordination compounds of osmium have prospective benefits in luminescent cellular imaging and photodynamic therapy because of their good photophysical and photochemical characteristics. Osmium nanomaterials also show promising features for applications in catalysis, sensing, and medicine [306].

Iridium

Iridium is one of the rarest elements on the Earth. It is found in an uncombined state in nature in sediments, in the form of iridium-osmium alloys (osmiridium and idrosmine) and is commercially recovered as a byproduct of Ni refining [307]. Iridium has no identified environmental impact because it does not allow products to reach groundwater, water bodies, or sewage systems.

Iridium has variable oxidation states varying from −3 to +9 and the most stable are +1 and +3. The common coordination numbers in its complexes are 4 and 6. The inactive and stable nature of Ir(III) ions is a suitable characteristic for the formation of organo iridium co ordination complexes with many bio active ligands. The organo metallic Ir(III) complexes proved to have the potential for anti neoplastic [308] and anti microbial [309] activity. Additionally, the combination of Ir(III) complexes with nanomaterials, such as polymer and up-conversion nanoparticles, has contributed to drug delivery, intracellular sensing and photodynamic therapy applications [310].

Iridium has no known biological functions. The metal has low toxicity and does not normally cause complications as it is comparatively unreactive. Nevertheless, all iridium compounds should be considered extremely toxic [311]. The potential health effects are connected with possible ingestion. Its compounds may cause eye problems or irritation of the gastrointestinal tract. They have low ecological hazards for common industrial handling and low ingestion hazard.

All of the iridium isotopes are either radioactive or relatively stable, meaning that they are predicted to be radioactive but no actual decay has been detected. Iridium-192 is a radioactive isotope that can permanently injure persons who handle the radioactive substance for minutes to hours, and it causes dead in close proximity within hours to days [312]. External exposure to ^{192}Ir can cause burns, acute radiation conditions and even death. Internal exposure to ^{192}Ir radioisotope can cause stomach and intestines burns if the high-energy manufacturing pellets are accepted.

Platinum

Platinum has no known biological functions. This element is highly biocompatible, meaning that it is safe to use inside the body. It is non-toxic and does not normally cause problems as it is unreactive. Platinum metal is found uncombined in alluvial deposits. Human health effects from Pt at low environmental doses or at biomonitored levels from low ecological exposures are not known. The toxicity is dependent on the type of the compounds (metallic, inorganic or organometallic), on the route of the exposure (intravenous therapeutic use, by inhalation, dermal contacts, oral application), and on the duration of exposure [313]. Pt as a metal is biologically inactive and is not very dangerous, nevertheless, almost all platinum compounds should be considered as extremely toxic which can cause several health effects, such as DNA modifications, allergic skin and mucous membrane reactions, damage to some organs, like intestines, kidneys, and bone marrow, and hearing damages. Pt can also cause toxicity potentiation of other dangerous chemical components in the human body, for instance, Se. Soluble Pt compounds (halogenated salts), encountered in professional settings, can cause Pt salt hypersensitivity with indications that include bronchitis and asthma after inhalation and contact dermatitis after skin contact. Animals exposed to chloroplatinated salts, widely used in industry, have shown severe hypersensitivity with asthma-like signs and anaphylactic shock. Metallic Pt and its insoluble salts produce eye irritations. At ingestion or inhalation, Pt metal and its insoluble salts are very poorly absorbed and cleaned from the body very quickly. Most amounts of absorbed Pt accumulate in the kidneys and are excreted by the urine.

Currently, the most widely used drugs for cancer chemotherapy are Pt complexes, now constituents of nearly 50% of all treatments. The pharmaceutical drug cisplatin has been determined as an animal and human carcinogen. The carcinogenicity of other platinum compounds remains unclear. The fast development of nanobiotechnological studies enables the possibility of targeted delivery of bactericide and antitumor Pt agents [314]. Combined with good biocompatibility and photoluminescence, Pt nanoclusters have demonstrated exciting potential for biological applications such as biological imaging, enzyme-like property, and cancer treatment [315].

There are 6 Pt isotopes in nature. The most abundant are platinum-194 (33%), platinum-195 (34%), and platinum-196 (25%). The others account for around 8% (^{198}Pt, ^{192}Pt and ^{190}Pt). The latter isotope is weakly radioactive, while the other five are non-radioactive [316]. In medicine, Pt metal is also used to produce dental crowns and dental medicine instruments.

F-ELEMENTS (LANTHANIDES AND ACTINIDES)

f-Elements occupy a unique position in the periodic table and exhibit a variety of interesting optical, luminescence, fluorescence, magnetic, *etc.,* properties and applications. Lanthanide elements are all metals with chemical reactivity similar to that of group IIA elements. Actinides are all radioactive elements. The lanthanide series (Ln) includes 15 f-block elements from lanthanum to lutetium. Lanthanides along with Sc and Y belong to the group of rare earth elements (REEs). f-Elements, commonly called "rare earths", are in fact more abundant than gold and relatively abundant compared to other biologically relevant metals (cerium is the 25th most abundant element), which make them potentially biologically accessible [317]. The concentration of rare earth metal cations in natural water is very low, as their minerals are almost insoluble in water. It is generally supposed that these elements have low toxicity.

The compounds of lanthanides and actinides are potentially dangerous to human health and there is a need to clarify their bioeffects on tissues. Due to their low solubility in water solutions, lanthanides and their compounds have a low availability in the biosphere and are not identified to naturally form parts of any biologically active molecules. Recently, Ln^{3+} ions have arisen as enzyme cofactors of methanol dehydrogenases of the XoxF type. The xoxF gene, encoding a pyrroloquinoline quinone-dependent methanol dehydrogenase, is found in all known proteobacterial methylotrophs. It is now clarified that XoxF enzymes can functionally replace the alternative, Ca-dependent, MxaFI-type methanol dehydrogenases, when Ln^{3+} ions are available [317]. Compared to other heavy metals, non-radioactive lanthanides are classified as having relatively low toxicity [318]. They may represent an accumulation risk which may affect their metabolism. Lanthanide elements and their compounds can affect numerous enzyme activities. The reported toxicology studies showed that lanthanide chlorides tend to accumulate mainly in the liver, bones, and spleen, while the other organs comprise much smaller concentrations. In the liver, they react with proteins, which affect enzyme activity and physiological functions causing morphological changes. The lanthanide accumulation has been systematically studied in the spleen where it was found that metal levels showed regular variation with different degrees of infection of the organs in alcoholic persons. Solutions injected into the peritoneum cause hyperglycemia, spleen degeneration, reduced blood pressure and fatty liver. If injected into a muscle, a high amount of the rare-earth element remains at the site, moving to the liver and bones. When consumed orally, only a small amount of the rare-earth element is absorbed by the body. Cerium is responsible for Mg deficit, which may be a cause of cardiac fibrosis that could result in cardiomyopathy. Gadolinium chloride $GdCl_3$ is a selective inhibitor of phagocytosis in liver macrophages and simultaneously contributes to the selective eradication of these cells, since it blocks the channels, competing with the Ca membranes because of the similarity of the gadolinium radius to that of Ca. Other lanthanides possess a protective liver effect. However, the observed poisonous effects of lanthanides in some cases may represent a combination of the hepatotoxic action of the active metabolite produced and the effects of Ln(III) ions that selectively block the cells by Ca channels. Long-period inhalational or intratracheal exposure to lanthanides could result in pneumoconiosis in humans and acute pneumonitis with neutrophil infiltration in the animal lungs. The mechanisms mediating the toxicologic effects of lanthanides on cell functions have not been fully established.

Organically complexed lanthanides are to some extent more toxic than inorganic solids or solutions [319]. As is right for most chemical compounds, dust and vapors should not be inhaled, nor should they be ingested.

All actinide elements are toxic, with toxicity comparable to that of lead. Large amounts of them ingested over a long period cause serious diseases. The real danger with actinides is connected with their radioactive properties, except for the long-lived uranium and thorium radioisotopes. They are strong emitters of tissue-destroying and cancer-producing α-, β-, or γ-rays. Once ingested, they have a tendency to remain in the body. Plutonium and americium have been found to migrate to the bone marrow, where their radioactivity affects the production of the red blood cells. Plutonium is known to be extremely toxic *in vivo*. It can displace Fe internally and is transported to the liver by transferrin, a Fe transporting protein. Exposure to plutonium and other trans-uranium elements, such as americium, has to be treated by chelation therapy [320].

Lanthanides and actinides have relatively similar physicochemical properties. These are elements with vacant f-orbitals. In comparison to main-group elements and transition metals, the chemistry and chelation properties of lanthanides and actinides are exceptionally interesting for many reasons. These 4f and 5f elements are stereotypically defined as highly oxyphilic, hard cations with a strong Lewis acid character. The 4f and 5f valence electrons are shielded by s and p electrons and have little impact on bonding, subsequently, the interactions between Ln(III) ions and ligands are mainly electrostatic in nature and the metal−ligand bonding is highly ionic [321]. The trivalent lanthanide ions are hard acceptor agents, making them perfect to form coordination complexes with ligands containing O-donor. They possess a strong affinity for H_2O and the preferred chelating ligands are monodentate ligands as it is difficult for them to displace H_2O molecules from the inner coordination sphere. Thus, the common complexes of lanthanides often contain hard carboxylate bioligands and a flexible, sterically-driven coordination geometry. Being hard Lewis acids, Ln(III) ions powerfully coordinate ligands having high electronegativity (hard Lewis bases), in the next direction: $F^- >$ HO$^-$ > H_2O > NO_3^- > Cl$^-$. The inherent strong oxyphilicity of Ln(III) ions causes preferred interactions with binding sites such as COOH, OH (phenolic), OH (hydroxylic), O (carbonyl), N (amino, imido, imino), and S (sulphydryl). N-S donor sites of biological molecules also enter into complexation when Ln(III) undergoes chelation. That is why the coordination chemistry of f-elements differs significantly from the chemistry of d-block elements, where covalent binding is preferred. Combined, the above properties render the bonding in lanthanides and actinides nondirectional because of the weak covalent bonding interactions. These behaviors, along with the large ionic radii, allow lanthanide(III) ions to accommodate high coordination numbers, which are rarely encountered with other common metal cations. The high charge of these cations results in poor solubility of their hydroxide and phosphates.

The aqueous chemistry of lanthanides and actinides is dominated by the +3 oxidation state, although other less prevalent oxidation states are possible. Though other oxidation states are reachable, most particularly Ce(IV) and Eu(II), under normal biological conditions, it is generally supposed that lanthanides would be limited to the +3 oxidation state, Ln(III) [321]. Lanthanide(III) ions are the largest ions in the periodic table, therefore exceptional in many respects. Consistently, depending on the steric demand of the ligand, their coordination numbers are regularly much higher than those observed for the other elements (typically 6, 8, and higher), and chelation is determined by the requirement to sterically saturate the coordination sphere of the respective f-element. The ionic radius decreases across the series from La(III) to Lu(III), the so-called lanthanide contraction. Chelating of actinides is additionally complicated because of the numerous oxidation states. Actually, actinide coordination chemistry has not been as seriously studied as that for lanthanides, due to their limited accessibility and radioactive effects.

The biological utilization of lanthanides is very reasonable from a chemical viewpoint. The lability of Ln(III) complexes, very fast water exchange reaction, strong oxyphilicity, non-directionality of Ln-ligand bond, and varying coordination numbers all contribute towards Ln interaction with biomolecules. The smaller size of the chelating bioligands can even suit larger Ln with lowered coordination number. Correspondingly, small lanthanides can expand their coordination number and can produce stable chelates with larger biological molecules. This can explain the different coordination power and different biological behavior of the respective lanthanides under different biological conditions. The lanthanides are divided into two primary groups, light REEs (La-Eu) and heavy REEs (Gd-Lu). The first lanthanides (La, Ce, Pr, Nd) primarily used in biology are relatively abundant in the environment with the abundances, similar to other metals like Cu and Zn. They perform similar chemistry to other biologically useful metals (Ca(II), Mg(II), and divalent first-row transition metal ions), thus they are accordingly more efficient catalysts due to their higher Lewis acidity. Their functional and size similarities with biogenic metal cations facilitate the evolutionary linking to the corresponding pathways concerning these metals. It has been proven that the primary site of Ln interaction with the living cells is only on the external surface, thus the molecular mechanism of binding of lanthanides to the cellular membranes is of great importance. Undoubtedly, cell membranes are extremely complex in structures where the major constituents are phospholipids. The chelating ligands (phospholipids) capture the Ln(lll) ion and then the process is followed by a passage of the captured Ln(lll) ions into the cell. The strong attachment to the external surface of the cell membranes can be because of the phosphate constituents, which form strong complexes with Ln(III), where the complexation of Ln(lll) with the cell surface active center represents a predominantly electrostatic interaction. These conclusions have been found very effective in discovering lanthanide compounds (salts, complexes, and coordinated chelates) and their usage in drug development as well as in the diagnosis, prognosis, and therapy of many diseases, like atherosclerosis, multiple-sclerosis, cerebrospinal, cardiovascular diseases, and cancer. The observed differences between light and heavy REEs might provide the biology an opportunity for more selective uptake and utilization of lanthanides [322].

Although their similar chemistry, lanthanide ions possess sufficiently distinct coordination chemistry from that of other metals used in biology, which allows for selective uptake, transferring, and incorporation into enzymes. The biological coordination chemistry of lanthanides is analogous to that of other biogenic metals, predominantly Ca(II) and Fe(III), but with some differences [321, 322]. Their low solubility in water ($Ksp \approx 10^{-21}$) somehow hinders their uptake, transportation, and storage in living systems. Ligands, such as carboxylate, aspartate, and glutamate, may bind and stabilize lanthanides in living systems. Although, the high coordination number of lanthanide ions results in a compact and highly negative binding site, which is difficult to be achieved with biological ligands. However, the effect of lanthanides on biosystems has been understudied. Although displacement of Ca^{2+} ions by lanthanide ions in tissues and enzymes has long been detected, only a small number of recent investigations suggest some biological functions for lanthanides.

Lanthanides have many properties that make them very suitable for a variety of therapeutic applications. Lanthanide chemistry has been widely studied over the past decades due to the recognized unusual chemical characteristics of these elements including fluorescent and potent magnetic properties as a consequence of their unique 4f electrons. Lanthanides have been rapidly and efficiently integrated into numerous compounds and materials for sophisticated applications. Although the chemical differences between the various Ln(III) ions are small, their physical distinctions are dramatic. This can be attributed to the presence of different numbers of unpaired electrons (between 0 and 7), which leads to specific paramagnetic properties as reflected in magnetic resonance. Lanthanide ions are unique in their luminescent properties. The exploitation of these special optical properties in medical diagnosis and therapy requires a multidisciplinary chemical, physical, and biological approach [323].

The strong Lewis acidity of Ln(III) chelates makes them very effective catalysts for the hydrolytic cleavage of phosphate esters in RNA and DNA with the use of antisense technology. Photochemical properties of Ln(III) chelates can be exploited in the photodynamic therapy of tumors and arterial plaque. Correspondingly, other Ln(III) chelates have been tested as radiation sensitizers in cancer therapy and appear to be very promising. An additional new technique is the neutron capture therapy with lanthanide chelates of the stable isotopes $^{155/157}$Gd, ^{149}Sm and ^{151}Eu. To make this technique clinically applicable, it will be necessary to localize a large number of metal ions at the tumor site, possibly with dendrimer structures [324].

Lanthanides can be mediators in many degenerative diseases based on their antioxidant properties and their function as scavengers of ROS (mainly oxygen-derived free radicals and peroxides). The involvement of lanthanides in ROS elimination is rather different from the inhibition of ROS by bio organic substances, which scavenge ROS by single electron exchange and thus transform themselves into radicals, consequently acting as pro-oxidants [325]. Lanthanide (lll) cations interact very easily with ROS and peroxide without turning into radicals. The controlled modulation of the redox activity of Ce(III), Sm(III), Eu(III), and Yb(III) may be expected to allow the development of selective oxidants and reductants.

Novel lanthanide and actinide chelators find widespread applications in MRI, PET imaging, targeted radionuclide therapy, and especially in cancer chemotherapy [326]. As a result of their different degree of stabilization, experienced by the 4f, 5d, and 6s orbitals, taking place at the ionization of the neutral Ln atoms, lanthanides exist almost entirely in their +III oxidation state in coordination complexes and supramolecular assemblies. Moreover, covalency plays only a negligible role in Ln-ligand coordination bonds with small exceptions. The coordination sphere is controlled by electrostatic interactions and inter ligand steric constraints.

Brief conclusions on the reviewed B groups' elements of the periodic table are listed in Table **15**, a list that includes the essential elements.

Table 15. Examples of the biological role of d-block elements.

Atomic number	Element	Biological role	Deficiency	Excess
25	Mn	Mn-based protein glutamine synthetase; MnSOD in mitochondria	Bone and cartilage defects; depressed reproductive functions [247].	Psychiatric conditions - manganism. Influences memory and speech. Gives hallucinations [247].
26	Fe	A component in hemoglobin and enzymes important for respirational functions; non-heme Fe proteins ca 1% of the human proteome	Anemia; overall weakness [266, 267].	Hemochromatosis, is an inherited syndrome that causes the body to absorb and store too much Fe in the liver, heart, and pancreas [265].
27	Co	Component of vitamin B_{12} and involved in the synthesis of hemoglobin uptake and carrier proteins for vitamin B_{12}	Anemia; anorexia; growth reduction; White liver disease (in sheep) [270].	Heart failure; hypothyroidism [271, 272]
29	Cu	A component of oxidative enzymes involved in heme synthesis; Cu proteins ca 1% of the human proteome.	Anemia; ataxia; defective melamine production and keratinization [196, 198].	Liver necrosis, in Wilson's disease; hypertension [196, 199].
30	Zn	A component in numerous enzymes; Zn^{2+} proteins ca 10% of the human proteome.	Anorexia; growth reduction; sexual immaturity; depression of the immune responses [205].	Relatively non-toxic except at high doses [206].
42	Mo	Mo enzymes from xanthine oxidoreductase and sulfite oxidase families; may be taken up only as molybdate	Growth reduction; defective keratinization [242]	Anemia; persistent dysentery (in grazing animals) [243].
Potentially essential elements				
23	V	Vanadate competes possibly with phosphate in important biological processes, role in phosphate biochemistry	Growth depression; failure of reproduction [225]	Unknown except at high doses [226, 227]

(Table 15) cont.....

Atomic number	Element	Biological role	Deficiency	Excess
24	Cr	Influence on glucose metabolism	Impaired glucose tolerance; elevated serum lipids; corneal opacity [234]	Hexavalent chromium, CrO_3, CrO_4^{2-} can give lung cancer. Cr may cause contact dermatitis, mostly in men [233, 235].
28	Ni	Ni may replace other metals in their ordinary sites in enzymes; essential for some microorganisms; allergenic: MHCII-Ni-peptide recognition by T cells.	Growth reduction; Impaired reproduction; prenatal mortality (in animals) [279]	Lung cancer; contact dermatitis, mostly in women [283, 284].

CHAPTER 4

Application of Main Group Elements and Their Compounds in Medicine

THE USE OF S-ELEMENTS AND THEIR COMPOUNDS IN MEDICINE

Hydrogen

In medical practice, distilled water is used to prepare solutions and water for injection (a pyrogenic). A 30% hydrogen peroxide solution is used for the treatment of purulent wounds [22]. The 3% solution of hydrogen peroxide is used as a disinfectant for wound washing and rinsing in inflammatory diseases of the mucous membranes (stomatitis, sore throats), for the treatment of purulent wounds, stopping nosebleeds, *etc.*

Even though most of the naturally occurring hydrogen is protium ^1H (99.9885%), with a small quantity of the heavier isotope deuterium ^2H (0.0115%) in almost everything people consume and drink. The deceleration of biochemical reactions including the heavier isotopes of elements has been studied [327]. Organisms can integrate lighter isotopes favorably, which may have significance for evolution processes [328]. Deuterium ^2H is widely used in the pharmaceutical industry [329]. In medicine, the isotope of hydrogen (deuterium) is used as a label in studies of the pharmacokinetics of drugs [16, 329]. Radioactive isotope tritium ^3H with a half-life of 12.3 years is used in radioisotope diagnostics as a radiotracer, being a β−emitter. Tritium is also used in the study of biochemical metabolic reactions. Apparently, elemental hydrogen H_2 is not utilized by human bodies, but it is used by various bacteria species (nitrogen-fixing bacteria, cyanobacteria, *Salmonella* and *Escherichia coli*, photosynthetic bacteria species, *etc.*) as a significant reducing agent in enzyme hydrogenase.

Lithium

Lithium ions Li^+, affecting the activity of certain enzymes, regulate the ionic Na^+ - K^+ balance of cells of the cerebral cortex. The symptoms of Li deficiency in humans are supposed to be manifested mainly as behavioral anomalies [24 - 26]. A connection between low Li intake and changed behavior and aggressiveness has been elucidated [330]. That is why lithium-containing drugs are widely used in psychiatric clinics in the therapy of manic depression (bipolar disorder) [331 - 333]. For example, lithium carbonate Li_2CO_3 is used to treat manic arousal in various mental illnesses. Lithium salts are orally administered in some controlled doses per day. Problems in the treatment result from the toxicity of Li at higher amounts. Solutions of lithium chloride or lithium bromide are used in air conditioning installations, because the solutions of these salts are able to absorb ammonia, amines, and other impurities from the atmosphere.

Sodium

In the body, sodium comes primarily in the form of NaCl (table salt). The daily need of the body for sodium is 1 g. Depending on the concentration of sodium chloride, isotonic (physiological), and hypertonic solutions are known. Isotonic is a 0.9% solution of NaCl, since its osmotic pressure corresponds to the osmotic pressure of the blood plasma (7.7 atm) [28]. Isotonic solution is used as a plasma-substituting solution for dehydration of the body, for dissolving medicinal substances, *etc.* Hypertonic solutions (3-, 5-, 10%) are used externally in the form of compresses and lotions for the treatment of purulent wounds.

Sodium hydroxide NaOH (caustic soda) is used in soap, tannery, pharmaceutical, textile industry, and agriculture. A 10% solution of NaOH is part of the silamine used in orthopedic practice for casting refractory models.

Sodium bicarbonate $NaHCO_3$ (drinking soda) is used for increased acidity of stomach juice, peptic ulcer of the stomach, and duodenum. The introduction of sodium bicarbonate into the stomach leads to the rapid neutralization of hydrochloric acid in gastric juice:

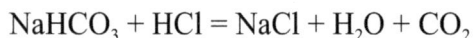

$$NaHCO_3 + HCl = NaCl + H_2O + CO_2$$

Too large doses of $NaHCO_3$ lead to alkalosis, which is no less harmful than acidosis.

$NaHCO_3$ is used in the form of rinses for inflammatory diseases of the eyes, and mucous membranes of the upper respirational tract [3, 4, 10]. The action is based on hydrolysis, as the solution has a slightly alkaline environment:

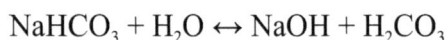

$$NaHCO_3 + H_2O \leftrightarrow NaOH + H_2CO_3$$

When alkalis are exposed to microbial cells, cellular proteins are deposited and, consequently, the death of microorganisms occurs.

Sodium sulfate decahydrate ($Na_2SO_4.10H_2O$, Glauber's salt) is used as a laxative [3, 4, 10, 12 - 15]. This salt is slowly absorbed from the intestines, which leads to an increase in osmotic pressure and the accumulation of water in the intestine, its contents are liquefied, and feces are quickly excreted from the body.

Sodium tetraborate decahydrate $Na_2B_4O_7 \cdot 10H_2O$ (borax) is used externally as an antiseptic agent for douching, rinsing, and lubrication [3, 4, 10, 12-15]. In aqueous solutions, borax is easily subjected to hydrolysis:

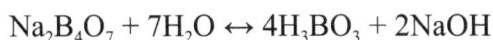

$$Na_2B_4O_7 + 7H_2O \leftrightarrow 4H_3BO_3 + 2NaOH$$

Formed during hydrolysis, boric acid has an antiseptic effect.

Sodium and potassium iodides (NaI and KI) are used as iodine medications for thyroid diseases [3, 4]. Sodium and potassium bromides (NaBr, KBr) are used as sedative agents [3, 4, 10]. Sodium fluoride (NaF) is used in dentistry (2% solution) and for the prevention of dental caries in children.

Sodium nitrite $(NaNO_2)$ is prescribed orally, subcutaneously, and intravenously (in the form of 1% solution) as a coronary dilator agent for angina pectoris [3, 4].

Sodium thiosulfate $(Na_2S_2O_3)$ is used as an antidote and a desensitizing agent [3, 4, 10, 193]. In case of cyanide poisoning, less toxic thiocyanates are formed after ingestion of sodium thiosulfate:

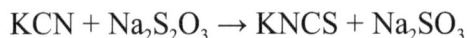

$$KCN + Na_2S_2O_3 \rightarrow KNCS + Na_2SO_3$$

Solutions of sodium citrate are used for blood preservation purposes [3, 4, 10].

The complex sodium nitroprusside $Na_2[Fe(CN)_5NO]$, (Fig. **11**), serves as an agent for lowering blood pressure, since it relaxes the muscles of blood vessels [334, 335].

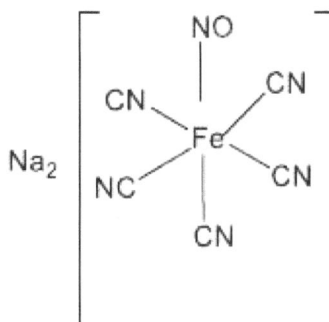

Fig. (11). Structure of sodium nitroprusside.

Radioactive ^{24}Na is used as a label for the determination of the blood flow velocity and for the treatment of some forms of leukemia [28].

Potassium

Potassium chloride (KCl) is used in conditions accompanied by a disorder of the electrolyte metabolism in the human body (uncontrollable sickness, profuse diarrhea), and for the relief of cardiac arrhythmias [33]. Application of KI after silver diamine fluoride (SDF) has some potential for reducing the staining of tooth structure. Potassium permanganate ($KMnO_4$) is an antiseptic substance used externally in aqueous solutions for washing wounds, rinsing, lubricating ulcerative and burn surfaces, and for douching and washing in gynecological and urological practice.

The natural radioisotope of potassium ^{40}K (β-emitter, $T_{1/2} = 1.3.10^9$ yr.) has an abundance of 0.012%. There is around 0.017 g of ^{40}K present in the body. While in the body, potassium-40 constitutes a health danger from the β-particles and γ-rays [33].

Rubidium

Similar in its biochemistry to K, rubidium exists in great amounts in the muscle tissues, red blood cells, and intestines. Rubidium salts can be used as antishock agents, antidepressants, and in the treatment of epilepsy and thyroid disorder. There are two natural isotopes of rubidium, ^{85}Rb and ^{87}Rb, of which ^{87}Rb is radioactive. The radionuclide rubidium-82, decaying by electron capture, is used in positron emission tomography (PET). It has fast serial imaging because of its short half-life ($T_{1/2} = 75$ s). It is used for PET myocardial perfusion MPI imaging [34, 336, 337]. ^{82}Rb is a valuable tool for identifying myocardial ischemia by using PET imaging. Once in the myocardium, ^{82}Rb becomes an active participant in the Na^+-K^+ exchange pump of the cells because of the similarity with K^+. The short half-life of ^{82}Rb allows for lesser radioactivity experienced by the patient.

Cesium

Radionuclide ^{131}Cs, with electron capture decay and $T_{1/2} = 9.7$ days, is used in oncology in the treatment of prostate cancer and brain tumors, as well as for Cs therapy of depression and schizophrenia [34, 338]. The optimum combination of its half-life and radiation energy makes ^{131}Cs an attractive radionuclide for brachytherapy of malignant tumors (in lungs, brain, prostate gland, mammary gland, *etc.*), where radioactive seeds are implanted in or near the tumor, exposing it to high radiation while reducing the radiation exposure of the normal tissues.

Magnesium

Preparations of biogenic magnesium, together with complex compounds, are popular antacid agents, some of them being well-known drugs [45, 339-341]. In medical practice, magnesium oxide MgO (burnt magnesia) is one of the main representatives of antacids used to reduce the increased acidity of stomach juice; when injected into the stomach, it neutralizes hydrochloric acid of gastric contents.

Magnesium sulfate heptahydrate $MgSO_4.7H_2O$ (bitter salt, Epsom salt) is used as a laxative, choleretic, and analgesic for spasms of the gallbladder [45]. The absorption of $MgSO_4$ from the intestines is limited, it binds H_2O and acts as a strong osmotic laxative. The solution of magnesium sulfate is administered parenterally as an anticonvulsant agent for epilepsy, as an antispastic for urinary retention, bronchial asthma, and hypertension. Depending on the dose, the salt solution can cause hypnotics or narcotic effects.

Magnesium carbonate $MgCO_3$ is an antacid and anti-ulcer agent [45, 339-341]. To compensate for magnesium deficiency, oral application of $MgCO_3$, Mg(II) citrate or lactate is initiated to replenish the deficiency of Mg^{2+} in the body. In an acute deficiency of Mg(II), intravenous administration of magnesium aspartate is suitable. Mineral-vitamin complexes of magnesium with lactate, orotate, and aspartate are good additives. Dolomite $MgCO_3.CaCO_3$ is a magnesium micro fertilizer.

Calcium

Calcium salts are widely used in medicine [53, 342]. Calcium chloride hexahydrate is used in allergic diseases (serum sickness, urticaria), and allergic complications associated with medication, in case of poisoning with magnesium salts and HF acid as an antidote.

Calcium sulfate semi-hydrate $2CaSO_4 \cdot H_2O$ (burnt gypsum, semi-aqueous gypsum) can be obtained by calcination of natural gypsum by lasting heating to 110-120°C:

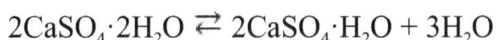

$$2CaSO_4 \cdot 2H_2O \rightleftarrows 2CaSO_4 \cdot H_2O + 3H_2O$$

When soaked in water, the calcium sulfate hemihydrate $CaSO_4 \cdot 1/2H_2O$ hardens quickly. This property is based on its use in the manufacture of plaster dressings. In dentistry, it is used as a blinding material for dental prosthetics [53, 342].

Freshly precipitated calcium carbonate $CaCO_3$ has a strong antacid activity, enhances the secretion of gastric juice, and is a part of tooth powders [53].

The mixture of solid calcium oxide and sodium hydroxide (soda lime) serves as an absorbent of exhaled CO_2 in respirators and in anesthetic applications [53, 342].

Calcium salts (oxalate, lactate, pangamate, pantothenate, gluconate) are used as antiallergic, hemostatic, and replenishing the deficiency of Ca^{2+} ions [342].

Organic di- and tricarboxylic acids react with Ca^{2+} ions to form chelate complexes [193, 194]. Compounds that form chelates with Ca^{2+} ions like sodium citrate and Na_2-EDTA are the common anticoagulants used for obtaining noncoagulating blood plasma.

The beta emitters ^{45}Ca ($t_{1/2}$ = 162.6 d) and ^{47}Ca ($t_{1/2}$ = 4.54 d) have been the starting point of research on alkaline earth radionuclides for human applications. The Ca isotopes have been mainly used for the investigation of Ca metabolism in humans and also applied as therapeutic agents for palliative care and pain treatment of bones. The radioactive isotope of calcium ^{45}Ca is extensively used in biomedicine in the study of the processes of mineral metabolism in the living organism, and the processes of calcium absorption by plants [53].

Strontium

Some of the strontium effects seem to be positive. Sr(II) salts are good toothpaste additives. Consistent tooth brushing with Sr-accompanied toothpaste rises Sr(II) amount in the enamel, which is beneficial in cariogenesis prevention and possibly hardens tooth enamel [343]. The medication Sr(II) ranelate supports bone growth, rises bone density, and reduces the frequency of fractures in osteoporotic patients [344, 345]. This drug has a polymeric structure where each Sr(II) ion binds carboxylate and O-atoms of water. The detected increase in bone density is supposed to be a consequence of the strontium's higher atomic mass compared with that of Ca.

It has been observed that the usage of Sr(II) salt additives in topical preparations decreases the symptoms of irritant dermatitis, a type of allergy [346].

Several interesting radioisotopes of strontium like ^{85}Sr, ^{87m}Sr, ^{89}Sr, and ^{90}Sr are known. Strontium-89 is a permitted β-emitting radionuclide ($T_{1/2}$ = 50.5 d), often applied as a Sr(II) chloride for the therapy of breast and metastatic prostate cancer [347 - 350]. Its accumulation into osteoblastic bone metastases is about quintuple greater in comparison to normal bones. Strontium-89 is active in calming relief of pain from metastases of bones, prostate, and breast cancer. Radioactive ^{85}Sr is used to treat severe bone pain, consequential from bone cancer. Like the other radioisotopes of Sr, the extremely radioactive ^{85}Sr accumulates in the bones of the patients. Radiation, in particular, kills the surrounding nerves that cause extreme pain. ^{90}Sr provides the possibility of preparing a ^{90}Sr/^{90}Y radionuclide generator, thus delivering ^{90}Y, a therapeutic beta emitter of high importance for medical use.

Strontium concentrates in the bones, partially replacing calcium. The radioactive isotope ^{90}Sr causes radiation sickness. It affects bone tissue and especially bone marrow. The accumulation of ^{90}Sr in the atmosphere and in the body contributes to the development of leukemia and bone cancer. Using EDTA to remove ^{90}Sr results in additional leakage of Ca from the bones. Therefore, it is not acid EDTA that is used, but a complex $Na_2CaEDTA$ [193, 194].

Barium

Except for beryllium, divalent cations of every alkaline earth metal are characterized by their Ca-mimetic behavior, accumulating in bone tissues. The comparatively low soluble barium sulphate meal is applied as a radiopaque contrast agent for the gastrointestinal tract's X-ray imaging, providing radiographs of the stomach, oesophagus, and duodenum. $BaSO_4$ has very low water solubility and is non-volatile making it not dangerous and practically safe to the body [59, 351]. Barium radioisotopes can be ascertained as useful imaging agents and possible diagnostic analogues for theranostic approaches.

Radium

The radioisotopes of the elements Ca, Sr, Ba, and Ra have been investigated, but to date, only Sr and Ra radioisotopes gained importance for applications in nuclear medicine, mainly for pain-reducing and palliative treatment of bone metastases. All of the isotopes of Ra possess radioactivity. There are ultra-trace quantities in the human body with no positive role. The radioactive Ra-223 dichloride is an α-emitting radiopharmaceutical with a half-life of 11.4 days. It is permitted for the therapy of symptomatic bone metastases and prostate cancer. ^{223}Ra^{2+} is a typical Ca(II) mimetic that selectively targets the bone metastases with α particles (with short range and high energy) which causes double-strand breaks in DNA displaying great local cytotoxicity, with insignificant myelosuppression [352, 353]. The activity of ^{223}Ra isotope *in vivo* has led to the estimation of its effectiveness and protection in clinical trials of patients suffering from bone-metastatic and prostate cancer, as well as for palliation of bone pain [354 - 357]. None of the presented Ca, Sr, and Ra radioactive isotopes is suitable for imaging purposes using PET or SPECT techniques.

The biological role, medicinal applications, and toxic effects of s-elements are collected in Table **16**.

Table 16. The biological role, medicinal applications, and toxic effects of s-elements.

Element	Location and functions in the body	Drugs	Toxic effect, antidotes
H	Element organogen	H_2O_2 - 3%-antiseptic, 30% - for treatment of purulent wounds; a local hemostatic; HCl - 8,2-8,3% - with reduced gastric acidity; deuterium - a label for pharmacokinetics of drugs, tritium is used in radioisotope diagnostics [22, 327-329]	-
Li	Regulate the ionic Na^+ - K^+ balance of the cerebral cortex cells	Li_2CO_3 - in treatment of manic-depressive illness [24 - 26, 330-333]	Low abundance, its influence is insignificant
Na	Extracellular cation, in buffer systems, osmosis, K/Na - pump	NaCl - 0,9% - isotonic solution (saline) for simple blood substitution; NaCl - 4-10% - hypertonic solution; $NaHCO_3$ - baking soda, antacid; Na_2SO_4-lenitive; sodium nitroprusside [28, 334,335]	Hypernatremia [30]
K	Intracellular cation, osmosis, K, Na - pump	KCl - for the relief of cardiac arrhythmias; $KMnO_4$ - antiseptic for washing wounds [33]	Hyperkalemia [32]
Rb	In the soft tissue; slight stimulatory effect on metabolism	Probes for studying cell membrane channels; Rubidium-82 - radionuclide for PET in myocardial perfusion imaging [34, 336,337]	Low abundance, its influence is insignificant
Cs	^{134}Cs and ^{137}Cs - responsible for the continued radioactive pollution	Probes for studying cell membrane channels; ^{131}Cs - application in oncology for treatment of prostate cancer, in brachytherapy [34, 338]	Low abundance, its influence is insignificant
Be	Allergic and carcinogenic effect, inhibits the activity of many enzymes activated by the Mg^{2+}	Due to the toxicity of beryllium compounds, they are not used as drugs [37, 40]	Berylliosis [36 - 42], beryllium rickets; antidotes - excess of Mg^{2+} salts
Mg	Intracellular ion; osmotic pressure inside cells; transport of calcium and potassium ions; action against the spasm	$MgSO_4$ - 25%-solution - strong purgative; MgO -antacid effect; $MgCO_3.Mg(OH)_2.3H_2O$-antacid effect; $3MgO.4SiO_2.H_2O$- talcum powder, adsorbing agent for powders; $MgSO_4 \cdot 7H_2O$ (bitter salt, Epsom salt) - laxative, choleretic, and analgesic for spasms of the gallbladder [45, 339-341]	Hypermagnesemia [52] is reversed by intravenous injection of a corresponding amount of Ca^{2+}

(Table 16) cont.....

Element	Location and functions in the body	Drugs	Toxic effect, antidotes
Ca	Bone and dental tissues in the form of: $Ca_5(OH)(PO_4)_3$ or $CaCO_3$. $3Ca_3(PO_4)_2.H_2O$; blood clotting	$CaCl_2$- antiallergic, anti-inflammatory, increases blood clotting; Ca(II) gluconate - anti-inflammatory effect; $2CaSO_4.2H_2O$- burnt plaster casts; $CaCO_3$ - pronounced antacid activity, enhances the secretion of gastric juice, part of tooth powders [53, 342]	Hypercalcemia [57], magnesium deficiency
Sr	Accumulates in bone tissue and affects bone formation; ^{90}Sr disrupts bone marrow hematopoiesis	Sr salts - toothpaste additives; Sr(II) ranelate supports bone growth and density; Strontium-89 is a permitted medical radionuclide, applied as a Sr(II) chloride for the treatment of breast and metastatic prostate cancer [343 - 350]	Brittle bones, strontium rickets, impossible to extract Sr from the bones [344, 345]
Ba	Retina	$BaSO_4$ — radiopaque contrast agent for gastrointestinal tract's X-ray imaging [59, 351]	Soluble salts Ba^{2+} are toxic [59]; antidotes - Na_2SO_4, $MgSO_4$
Ra	$^{223}Ra^{2+}$ is a typical Ca^{2+}-mimetic	Ra-223 dichloride (α-emitter) is permitted for treatment of symptomatic bone metastases and prostate cancer [352 - 357]	Ultra-trace quantities in the human body

where: dimercaprol - 2,3-dimercapto-1-propanol, DMPS - 2,3- dimercapto-1-propanesulfonic acid, DMSA - 2,3-dimercaptosuccinic acid [193, 194].

THE USE OF P-ELEMENTS AND THEIR COMPOUNDS IN MEDICINE

Boron

Various boron-based preparations are used in medical practice [61 - 65]. Ortho boric acid H_3BO_3 and sodium tetraborate $Na_2B_4O_7 \cdot 10H_2O$ (borax) have long been used as antiseptic agents. Orthoboric acid is a part of various ointments. In the form of solutions (1-3%) it is used for rinsing the oral cavity and in ophthalmological practice. In combination with potassium iodide, copper sulfate, and vitamins, boric acid is used to treat hypotrophy. In addition, boric acid as a filler is part of the formulate, which is used in the dental prosthetic practice when casting steel teeth. Sodium borate with aluminum hydroxide is part of dental pastes used as a glue layer for dentures. Sodium tetraborate (borax) is an antiseptic, used externally as an antimicrobial and anti-inflammatory agent for douching and rinsing lotions.

Boromycin is a polyether-macrolide antibiotic with bactericidal properties isolated from gram-positive *Streptomyces antibioticus* bacteria [358]. It is known for being the first natural product that contains boron. It is effective against the majority of gram-positive bacteria, nevertheless, it is not active against gram-negative bacteria. Recent investigations have shown that boromycin has anti-HIV activity [359].

Boron-containing drugs are in the study as therapeutics for many disorders [61, 62, 360]. Boronic acid picolinate ester (AN0128) possesses antimicrobial and anti-inflammatory action for the treatment of acne and atopic dermatitis [361]. Kerydin (AN2690) is an oxaborale antifungal medication for the therapy of onychomycosis of the toenails caused by *Trichophyton rubrum* or *Trichophyton mentagrophytes*.

One of the numerous perspectives under study against cancer is boron neutron capture therapy (BNCT) [65, 362]. Boron isotope ^{10}B, along with other stable isotopes, such as ^{97}Ru and ^{157}Gd, has a good radiotherapeutic effect. The main principle of such therapy is to have a radioactive source selectively within malignant cells. Radioactivity destroys only cancer cells, leaving healthy cells uninjured. This method is particularly interesting in the cases of inoperable brain tumors or as a means of killing any tiny clusters of tumor cells that remain following surgical removal of tumors. Borate ions, boron hydrides, and boranes of complex ion composition $(B_{12}H_{11}SH)^{2-}$ (BSH) are commonly used for this purpose. The stable B compound infiltrates into the tumor and irradiates with neutrons, transforming it into a radioisotope, and then the radiation destroys the malignant cells:

$$^{10}_{3}B + ^{1}_{0}n \rightarrow ^{7}_{3}Li + ^{4}_{2}He$$

Boron neutron capture therapy is a simple, promising binary disease-targeted technique but difficult to turn into reality.

Boron is an essential micronutrient in plants [64, 363]. It has a specific effect on carbohydrate metabolism in plants and is necessary for normal growth and cell division. Boron is supposed to play a chief role in the synthesis of one of the bases for RNA formation and in cellular activities, such as carbohydrate synthesis. With boron starvation, plants do not form seeds or there are few of them. Boron is the most common soil deficiency worldwide after zinc. The introduction of boron fertilizers increases the plants' yield. Fertilization is carried out through the soil or spraying (foliar fertilization). Pre-sowing feeding of seeds with aqueous solutions of boric acid is effective. Magnesium borates, boro-superphosphate, and thermal borates are the main fertilizers.

Aluminum

Aluminum-potassium alum $KAl(SO_4)_2 \cdot 12H_2O$ is used externally as an astringent in aqueous solutions (0.5 - 1%) for rinsing, washing, lotions, and douching in inflammatory diseases of the mucous membranes and skin [71, 364, 365]. It is also prescribed for cauterization with trachoma and as a hemostatic agent for cuts. Aluminum hydroxide $Al(OH)_3$ has an adsorbent and enveloping effect, lowers the acidity of the gastric juice, and is a part of the combined drug "Almagel". The phosphate $AlPO_4$ is used as an antacid, enveloping, and anti-ulcer agent [71]. Aluminum sulfate $Al_2(SO_4)_3$ is most commonly used in the chemical method of water purification. This salt reacts with calcium bicarbonate $Ca(HCO_3)_2$ contained in water:

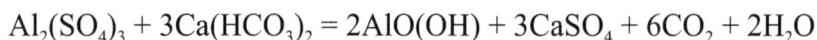

$$Al_2(SO_4)_3 + 3Ca(HCO_3)_2 = 2AlO(OH) + 3CaSO_4 + 6CO_2 + 2H_2O$$

As a result of this interaction, aluminum meta-hydroxide $AlO(OH)$ precipitates in the form of a flaky substance that captures impurities in water, including small suspended particles, as well as most bacteria.

Salts of aluminum are applicable as vaccine adjuvants which facilitate immune responses [364]. Alum $KAl(SO_4)_2 \cdot 12H_2O$ (hydrated potassium Al sulfate), although is one of the most common adjuvants applied, is nowadays being reevaluated in vaccine preparations as there are issues about its toxic effects [365]. Al^{3+} cations can complex with O-donor ligands, particularly phosphates, found in the gastrointestinal tract and in cells. In the presence of inorganic phosphate, the permitted free Al^{3+} is decreased, through formation of insoluble $AlPO_4$, which facilitates the elimination of Al^{3+} from the body. In contrast, citrate solubilizes Al^{3+}, and may pass through cell membranes and provide Al^{3+} absorption into the body.

Aluminum is relatively benign and is still used in dietary supplements and indigestion pills. It is usually connected to Alzheimer's disease and the body has a hard time ridding itself of excess Al [68, 69]. Al is slightly more toxic to plants then to humans because it is a soil-forming element. The greatest amount of Al stimulates the germination of seeds. Excess of Al reduces the intensity of photosynthesis, disrupts phosphorus metabolism, delays the growth of the root system. The presence of Al^{+3} in the soil causes the exchange acidity of the soil solution harmful to plants. Al^{+3} ions are absorbed by soil colloids, but under the action of salts like KCl are displaced from the soil.

Gallium

The low melting point has made gallium alloys non-toxic replacements for Hg in some applications that require a liquid metal at normal temperature. Gallium is useful in high-temperature thermometers, barometers, pharmaceutical, and nuclear medicine tests. Gallium inorganic and coordination compounds are used in therapy and in diagnosis [72, 366]. Gallium nitrate $Ga(NO_3)_3$ (Ganite) has been reported to inhibit the growth of subcutaneously implanted tumors [367]. Ga(III) nitrate, when administered intravenously, is effective for the treatment of certain cancers, Paget's bone disease, and hypercalcemia. It is useful for treatment of patients with brain tumors, rhabdomyosarcoma, neuroblastoma, non-Hodgkin's lymphoma, and refractory solid tumors. Studies of gallium nitrate antitumor activity have shown that blood Ca levels decrease in many patients, motivating research to manage elevated blood Ca levels connected with cancer [72, 368]. One of the common problems in cancer patients is hypercalcemia, the disproportion between the net resorption of bone and urinary excretion of Ca. Through infusions of $Ga(NO_3)_3$, Ca resorption from the bones is reduced, as Ga(III) exerts a hypocalcemia effect.

With regard to ionic radius, oxidation states, and coordination numbers, Ga^{3+} closely resembles Fe^{3+}. Similar to Ru(III) complexes, Ga(III) complexes are able to compete for Fe-occupied sites in biomolecules. This ionic mimicry is central for the bioactivity of gallium(III) compounds [369]. $Ga(NO_3)_3$ is useful for the treatment of patients suffering from cystic fibrosis, where redox-inactive Ga^{3+} inhibits redox-active Fe^{3+}-dependent pathways, including Fe pathways in bacteria [370]. Ga(III) appears to be related to iron biochemistry, as most of the Ga(III) ions in the blood are absorbed by transferrin. Rapidly spreading malignancies have high metabolite activity and need substantial Fe intake. Lots of forms of cancer show overexpression of transferrin receptors. Ga(III) ions compete with Fe(III) ions for transferrin binding which allows it to penetrate Fe-hungry cancer cells and display its biological effects - damage of DNA synthesis, disturbance of mitochondrial function, complete inhibition of Fe-dependent enzymes, ROS formation, and finally apoptosis. One of the promising new agents is the octahedral complex [Ga(III)(maltolate)$_3$]. Oral plasma absorption of this compound is fast, followed by an almost complete transfer of Ga(III) to transferrin. For the similar gallium complex with 8-hydroxyquinoline, [Ga(8-hydroxyquinoline)$_3$] (KP46), clinical trials have been conducted for its usage as an oral anticancer drug [72]. The complex KP46, tris(8-hydroxyquinolinato) gallium(III), (Fig. **12**), contains the chelating agent 8-hydroxyquinoline, which itself has antineoplastic activity [72, 371].

Numerous cytotoxic Ga(III) complexes with different bioactive ligands have recently been obtained. Unlike the most predominant 6-coordinated complexes, the complexes with planar tetradentate ligands or tridentate ligands tend to block reactions between the metal cation and bioligands to a lesser extent. In these cases the vacant coordination sites may possess labile solvent molecules that would theoretically allow for improved reaction with bioligands by means of solvent ligand exchange. The best-known candidates, synthesized in the last decade are presented in (Fig. **13**), [372 - 379].

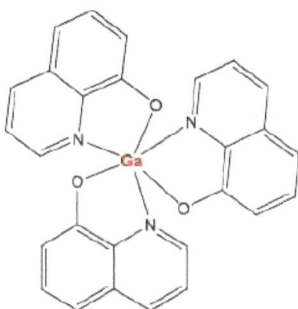

Fig. (12). The structure of tris(8-hydroxyquinolinato) gallium(III) (KP46).

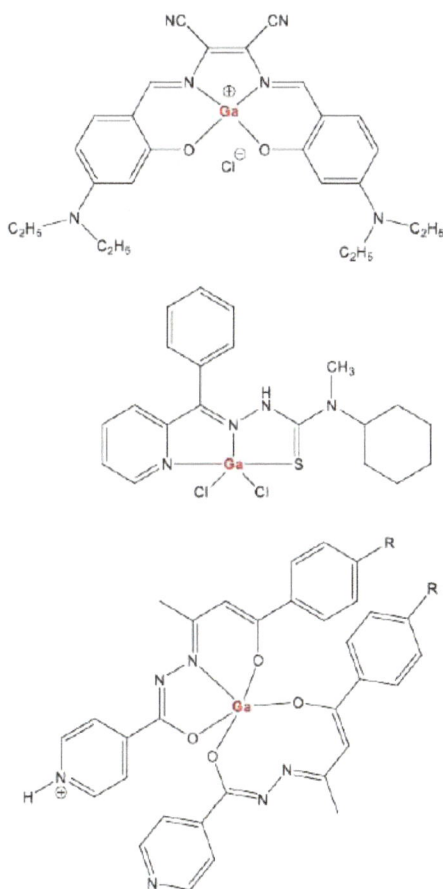

Fig. (13). Recently synthesized gallium(III) complexes.

Gallium with its isotopes ^{67}Ga for SPECT and ^{68}Ga for PET imaging is a good alternative to technetium-99m. The radionuclide ^{68}Ga, which decays by electron capture, can be efficiently produced by ^{68}Ge/^{68}Ga generator [380]. Its short half-life (1.1 h) makes ^{68}Ga-labelled radioactive pharmaceuticals prevalent for clinical usage as tumor imaging agents [381]. The many advantages of ^{68}Ga radioactive pharmaceuticals and particularly its simple formation have been discussed and questioned for many years. ^{68}Ga pasireotide tetraxetan (SOMscan) has been developed for the use in PET imaging for gastro-entero-pancreatic neuroendocrine tumors. The product consists of a radioactive ^{68}Ga, attached to pasireotide tetraxetan, a synthetic substance which is similar to a natural hormone called somatostatin. The isotope ^{67}Ga with a half-life of 3.3 days, which decays by electron capture followed by γ-emission is a widely used radionuclide. ^{67}Ga scintigraphy is utilized in oncology for the detection of malignant tumors, as well as Hodgkin's and non-Hodgkin's lymphomas [382].

Indium

Gallium-67, gallium-68, and indium-111 share the same group in the periodic table and can be harnessed for a range of applications in nuclear medicine, including scintigraphy, SPECT, PET, and targeted radiotherapy. Indium-111 (^{111}In), is a readily available γ-emitting radionuclide, which is used in clinical diagnostic imaging [383]. ^{111}In can be used as a label for red cells, platelets, and leukocytes. Similar to Ga, In exists in +3 oxidation state in water solutions, however, it is significantly larger in size than gallium ion. Indium(III) ion is considered a softer acid than Ga(III) ion. It usually forms bonds with hard acid donors, such as N or O, but it can also form bonds with thiol groups, therefore, it can interact with many chelators. Open-chain CHX-A″-DTPA and macrocyclic DOTA are the leaders for In(III) chelation, because of their obtainability and stable coordination to In(III) ions [384]. They perfectly coordinate In(III) with its preferred coordination number of 8. DTPA and its derivatives form very stable square-planar structures with In(III) and have been exploited in a number of radioactive pharmaceuticals approved for clinical practice, for prostate and neuroendocrine cancers. DOTA is very suitable for indium-111 labeling of proteins, *e.g.,* peptides and ESPs. Because of its larger size, In(III) fits the DOTA macrocycle and forms a complex with high stability [385].

Thallium

Thallium is a very poisonous element that concentrates in tissues with high amounts of K^+ ions. It inhibits the activity of potassium-activated enzymes containing thiol-groups -SH. Ions Tl^+ and K^+ are synergists (acting together in the same direction). Thallium is preferred over K by the same cell transport mechanism. On the other hand, Tl(I) is a soft acid, so it interacts with the soft base S of thiol-amino acids in mitochondria and blocks oxidative phosphorylation. Tl intoxication causes degenerative changes in all the cells, but predominantly with that of the CNS and hair follicles [386, 387].

Naturally occurring Tl, the heaviest of the IIIA group elements, consists almost completely of a mixture of two stable isotopes: ^{203}Tl (29.5%) and ^{205}Tl (70.5%). The isotope thallium-205 is useful for NMR detection. Thallium-201 is a potentially valuable radioisotope for various medical applications including myocardial visualization and possible assessment of physiology, as a renal medullary imaging agent, and for tumor detection. Tl-201 with a half-life of 73 h decays by electron capture. It is used extensively in radio-diagnostic imaging (SPECT) and in particular for perfusion tests of the myocardium. Thallous chloride Tl-201 injection is applied in adults for the diagnostics of heart diseases (coronary artery disease and heart attacks) [388].

Carbon

Carbon is one of the basic elements of life [6 - 10, 78 - 80]. Activated charcoal (carbo adsorbents, carbolene) and modified activated carbons are widely used in medical practice as a non-toxic intestinal adsorbent, *e.g.,* during diarrhea or intoxication. Preparations that have a large surface activity, are capable of adsorbing gases, alkaloids, salts of heavy metals, and various non-polar toxins, and are used in hemo- and lymphosorption. In overdosing on some medications, activated charcoal limits their absorption, though it should be administered in high doses (around 50 g, dispersed in water).

The salt of carbonic acid - sodium bicarbonate $NaHCO_3$ (baking soda) lowers the acidity of gastric juice, and neutralizes hyper-acidic gastric secretion although it is not very appropriate for this purpose. Solutions of $NaHCO_3$ in infusions are used in the therapy of some types of acidosis or some kinds of intoxication (salicylates). $NaHCO_3$ is applied orally in chronic complications accompanied by acidosis or for the alkalization of urine. Aqueous solutions of $NaHCO_3$ are used for rinses and lotions. The bicarbonate buffer system (HCO_3^-/H_2CO_3) is one of the most important buffer systems for maintaining the pH of the blood [3, 4, 6-10].

Many drug molecules based on carbon monoxide have been developed for therapeutic purposes [78 - 80]. Carbon dioxide interacts with strong hydroxides to form carbonates. This interaction is used for removing CO_2 from mixtures of gases, for instance, from the exhaled air in the respirators or anesthesia apparatuses with a closed cycle [6 - 10]. The gas passes through the solid granulated mixture of NaOH and $Ca(OH)_2$, which captures CO_2:

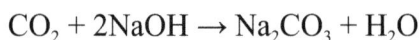

$$CO_2 + 2NaOH \rightarrow Na_2CO_3 + H_2O$$

CO_2 is used for medical purposes in minimally invasive surgery (laparoscopy) to broaden and stabilize body cavities. In the liquid state, it can be used to provide temperature down to -76°C for cryotherapy or for local skin surface analgesia by external application. Solid CO_2, so named dry ice, which sublimes at -79 °C is used as a cooling medium for the transport of biomaterials [6 - 10]. These properties are used in the freezing of tissues in histology. In dermatology dry ice is applied locally in the treatment of lupus erythematosus, neurodermatitis, leprosy, warts, *etc.*

The radioactive isotope ^{14}C with a period of 5,730 years is commonly used for the dating of archaeological objects [3, 4, 6-10]. The radionuclide ^{11}C has a period of only 20 minutes. This short period and the relative convenience of substituting ^{11}C for the stable ^{12}C make it a suitable radioisotope used in nuclear medicine, predominantly in PET.

Silicon

Dietary Si is beneficial to bones and connective tissues [82, 83, 86]. Inorganic silicon compounds are used in medicine. Aluminum silicate $Al_2(SiO_3)_3$ - white clay - is used as an enveloping and adsorbing agent in the form of powders, pastes, ointments, *etc.* Magnesium trisilicate $2MgO \cdot 3SiO_2 \cdot nH_2O$ is used as an enveloping, adsorbent, and antacid agent. Talc $3MgO \cdot 4SiO_2 \cdot H_2O$ is applied in the form of powders, pastes, and tablets. In dental practice, Si(IV) carbide SiC is used for fillings and plastic prostheses. SiO_2 is a component of silicate dental cement. These cements are used in dental practice as a permanent filling material for filling teeth under crowns, for fixing single crowns, bridges, fixed prostheses, *etc.* In an amount of 2.5%, silicon is part of the stainless chromium-nickel steel, which is used in orthopedic practice. Organosilicon compounds are useful for sterilizing surgical instruments. They are part of ointments, creams that are used in the treatment of skin diseases, burns, *etc.* Liquids containing silicon compounds are injected into divers after deep dives for rapid decompression.

A silicon-based phthalocyanine (Pc4) is a second-generation photosensitizer in clinical practice. It kills tumor and lymphoid cells through apoptosis [389, 390]. Pc4 is useful in photodynamic therapy of skin cancer, actinic keratosis, Bowen's disease, mycosis fungoides, and non-Hodgkin lymphoma [391]. Silicon phthalocyanines have been extensively used in light-dependent medical applications, mainly as antitumor, antibacterial, and antifungal agents [392]. Photosensitive Si phthalocyanines have been utilized in PDT, photo-immunotherapy (PIT), photo-uncaging techniques, and photothermal therapy (PTT) [393].

Germanium

There is no suggestion to support the essentialness of this element for humans. However, Ge-based medications are sold as nutritional supplements and with requested benefits for some diseases, including malignancies and AIDS [394]. Taking Ge supplements is effective in treating allergies, arthritis, high blood pressure, elevated cholesterol levels, and cancer. Germanium can stimulate the immune system against cancer in humans [395]. Ge has anticancer activity but is not toxic to normal cells. As it acts as a stimulator of the immune system, it does not damage the rest of the body's tissues like the other anticancer agents. Some cases of renal failure, nephropathy, anemia, myopathy, and digestive disorders have been described after Ge intoxication [396], though the carcinogenicity, mutagenicity, and teratogenicity of Ge compounds seem to be normally low [397]. Organo-germanium containing medicine has been recently used for special treatments of *e.g.,* cancer and AIDS. 3-Carboxyethylgermanium sesquioxide delays the development of some malignant tumors, prevents the appearance of metastases, lowers blood pressure, acts as an anesthetic, to a certain extent protects against radioactive radiation. It is also beneficial in the treatment of burns, hepatitis, and certain cardiovascular diseases [398, 399].

In the human body, germanium binds to oxygen-donor molecules, thus showing efficiency at getting O_2 to the body tissues. The enlarged oxygen supply in the body improves the functions of the immune system and excrete the damaging toxins. The study of the biological role of this element continues. Testing of new germanium-based anticancer compounds is ongoing, and possibly new, less harmful, cancer treatments using this element would be developed [86, 394, 397, 399]. On the other hand, germanium is able to interact with SH-groups of proteins, and therefore such compounds have bactericidal properties, so they are used in medicine as astringents, cauterizing, and antiseptic agents.

Tin

Inorganic tin compounds are less toxic than organotin compounds [400]. Tin in the amount of 28% is part of the powder (an alloy of silver, copper, and tin), which is used in dentistry to obtain silver amalgam (AC-2), used for metal fillings. In addition, tin is an integral part of the cement and liquid "Gallodent-M" (eutectic alloy of thallium-tin), which are used to obtain mercury-free metal fillings in pediatric stemmatological practice.

Organotin(IV) compounds are used worldwide as stabilizers, catalyzers and biocidal agents. Many organotin compounds have been reported to have antiparasitic, antimicrobial, antihypertensive, anti-hyperbilirubinemia, anticancer and antiviral activity, although none of them has got clinical trials because of their high toxicity, despite their multiple biological activities. Some examples include tri-n-butyltin(IV)lupinyl sulfide hydrogen fumarate that possesses *in vitro* and *in vivo* activity against leukemia and melanoma [400 - 402]. Compounds such as hydroxotributyltin, $(C_4H_9)_3SnOH$, are active against fungal infection in many plants [403]. The organotin compounds, used in the paints of ships' hulls, kill the larvae of mollusks, attached to the hull of ships. However, the organotin compounds are very toxic and their marine use has been curtailed.

Tin is used in clinical practice in the composition of the PDT agent purlytin (Sn(IV) ethyl-etiopurpurin). Purlytin experienced clinical trials for various cancers, like Kaposi's sarcoma in AIDS patients, cutaneous basal cell cancer, and for breast metastases [404].

Lead

Lead and its compounds are highly toxic and cause chronic poisoning [91 - 96]. In medicine, lead compounds such as lead(II) oxide, lead(II) acetate, lead water (2% solution of the lead hydroxy acetate $(CH_3COO)(OH)Pb$), and lead patches are used. Their usage is only external in dermatology for lotions, along with antiseptics, astringents, and anti-inflammatory, and antimicrobial agents. Lead oxide PbO is part of the lead patch used in inflammatory skin diseases, and furunculosis. Lead acetate $Pb(CH_3COO)_2$ is used as an astringent. Lead materials are used in the production of clothing for the medical staff of X-ray rooms because Pb absorbs X- and γ-rays [405]. Organolead compounds such as alkyl-Pb(IV) compounds are metabolized to neurotoxic metabolite derivatives.

The β^- emitting radioisotope ^{212}Pb with a half-life of 10.6 h, which quickly generates the α-emitting ^{212}Bi, is useful for targeted α-therapy and radioimmunotherapy [406]. Its decay results to the emission of two short-lived α-particles which show powerful therapeutic action on cell nuclei [407]. The radiolabeled compound ^{212}Pb-TCMC-trastuzumab, a humanized monoclonal antibody carrying ^{212}Pb, shows promising pre-clinical antitumor activity. The antibody trastuzumab transports and delivers ^{212}Pb with a short range for more precise irradiation and killing of cancer cells without affecting healthy tissue. It binds to the extracellular area of human epidermal growth factor receptor 2 (HER-2), a tyrosine kinase receptor, overexpressed on the cell surface of many different cancer cells. Thus, ^{212}Pb delivers α-radiation upon internalization [408].

Nitrogen

Nitrogen and its compounds are widely used in medicine [80, 99, 101, 334, 335]. Liquid nitrogen is an effective tool for the therapy of a number of skin and mucous membranes diseases, including warts, vascular birthmarks, papilloma, *etc.*

The endothelium of blood vessels uses NO to signal the surrounding smooth muscles to relax, leading to vasodilation and raised blood flow [80, 99 - 101, 334, 335] Nitric(II) oxide in a mixture with oxygen creates a light anesthesia without the stage of excitation. Nitric oxide does not irritate the respiratory tract and is used in surgical operations, for the prevention of traumatic shock and as a therapeutic anesthesia for myocardial infarction (inhalation anesthesia). Among other nitrogen-containing compounds in medicine, nitric(I) oxide N_2O and ammonium hydroxide NH_4OH are used. Nitric(I) oxide or "laughing gas" in a mixture with oxygen is used in surgical gynecology and dentistry, as well as for anesthesia of childbirth. It possesses weak narcotic activity, and thus it should be used in large amounts. An aqueous solution of ammonia NH_4OH (ammonium hydroxide, $NH_3.H_2O$) is used to excite breathing and remove patients from fainting, for which a small piece of cotton wool or gauze moistened with ammonia is carefully brought to the nasal openings. In high concentrations, ammonium hydroxide can cause reflex respiratory arrest.

Nitric acid is used externally to cauterize warts and calluses. In the practice of laboratory clinical trials, nitric acid is used to quantify protein in urine and other biological fluids. In medical practice, some inorganic and organic nitrites containing groups -O-N=0 and organic nitrates containing groups -O-NO_2 are widely used. Compounds of nitrogen are used in the form of nitric acid esters nitroglycerin, nitrosorbide, *etc.* These are coronary drugs that are used to treat heart diseases. Nitroglycerin $C_3H_5(ONO_2)_3$ is used as a medication in the therapy of angina pectoris. It has the capability to broaden the coronary arteries. The simple molecule NO has complex biofunctions. It diffuses through cell membranes and takes part in blood pressure regulation, as it influences muscles that are outside conscious control [409]. Various dosage forms of nitroglycerin are arranged for the prevention of angina attacks, particularly long-acting drugs. Amyl nitrite is representative of organic nitrites and is not currently used as a cardiovascular agent. The drug has found application as an antidote to poisoning with hydrocyanic acid and its salts, which is explained by the ability of nitrites to form methemoglobin in the blood, which binds the CN^- ion and prevents these lesions of tissue respiratory enzymes.

Nitrates perform various biological functions, including blood pressure decrease, platelet aggregation inhibition, and vessel protecting effect, similar to the functions of NO [97]. Sodium nitrite $NaNO_2$ is a spasmolytic (coronary dilator) agent. It is prescribed for chronic coronary insufficiency. Sodium nitrite in very rare cases is used orally as a vasodilator for angina pectoris, sometimes for spasms of cerebral vessels. It is known as an antidote for poisoning with methemoglobin-forming substances (cyanide, carbon(II) monoxide, *etc.*). Apart from this, nitrites have inhibitory effects on some microorganisms (*Clostridium botulini*) [410]. Ammonium chloride NH_4Cl is used as a diuretic for edema caused by cardiovascular failure. In some cases, it is prescribed to enhance the action of mercury diuretics. In addition, ammonium chloride is used as an expectorant. The anion of HSCN is part of the blood and saliva. Recent studies have shown that rhodanide ions SCN^- inhibit the ability of the thyroid gland to produce the hormone and reduce gastric secretion. Salts KSCN and NaSCN are used in medicine to treat hypertension.

Radioactive nitrogen nuclide ^{15}N is used in biology and medicine. By using the heavy nitrogen nuclide ^{15}N, the ability of an animal organism to use ammonia compounds for the synthesis of protein molecules was established. The nitrogen nuclide ^{13}N is a positron-emitting radioisotope used in PET imaging. It has a very short half-life of 10 min. ^{13}N-ammonia has long been used for cardiac PET imaging [411]. It is applied by injection and is present as an equilibrium mixture of $^{13}NH_3$ and $^{13}NH_4^+$ in the bloodstream [412]. The neutral ^{13}N-ammonia can easily diffuse across plasma and cellular membranes and once inside myocytes re-equilibrates with its protonated form which is then trapped in glutamine *via* the enzyme glutamine synthase. Toxic NH_3 is converted into urea which is excreted *via* the urea cycle by the kidneys.

Phosphorus

Phosphorus-based compounds are involved in vital processes or functions ranging from biochemistry, biogeochemistry, ecology, and agriculture, to industry. One of the most popular agricultural and industrial applications is dichlorvos (DDVP), which used to be a broad-spectrum insecticide and acaricide. Phosphorus and calcium salts are commonly included in toothpaste because they perform an important function in keeping teeth, gums, and jaws strong [107]. As $Ca_{10}(PO_4)_6 F_2$ is more resistant to acidic attacks than $Ca_{10}(PO_4)_6(OH)_2$, toothpastes usually contain F^- ions (NaF or Na_2PO_3F), which tolerates the exchange of F^- ions for OH^- ions in $Ca_{10}(PO_4)_6(OH)_2$ in the teeth. The high content of F^- ions results in dental or skeletal fluorosis. Numerous phosphorus-based drugs have been designed as prodrugs in the form of phosphotriesterase, phosphinates, phosphonates, and phosphine oxides possessing higher selectivity and bioavailability.

Of the phosphorus compounds that are used in medicine, sodium adenosine triphosphate (salt of adenosine triphosphoric acid, ATP) is used for muscular dystrophy, muscular atrophy, myocardial dystrophy, angina pectoris, mild hypertension, *etc.* ATP and creatine phosphate are used as energy preparations which are prescribed for spasms of peripheral vessels, atony of internal organs, and chronic coronary insufficiency [3, 4, 109]. Calcium glycerophosphate enhances anabolic processes, and normalizes the function of the nervous system. It is prescribed for neurasthenia, overwork, dystrophy, *etc.*

In addition, phosphorus preparations are used in dentistry, for example, ammonium phosphate is an integral part of cobalt-chromium alloy, which is used to cast hard dental products. Phosphoric acid, as well as phosphate salts, are part of the filling fluids used in dental practice [107]. Zn phosphate cement is used in dental practice for the cementation of crowns, inlays, and other stomatology reconstructions. It is prepared from the solution of H_3PO_4 (40%), ZnO, and MgO.

The phosphate buffer system ($H_2PO_4^-$/HPO_4^{2-}) is one of the major buffer systems in biology which controls the acidic-base balance of animal fluids [6 - 10].

Phosphorus nuclides are used in biological research as labeled atoms. Phosphorus-32 ($T_{1/2}$= 14.3 d) is a radionuclide with β-emission, used in biochemical tracing. It is explored for the detection of malignant tumors, because cancer cells accumulate more PO_4^{3-} ions than healthy cells. A solution of sodium phosphate Na_3PO_4 for injection, labeled with phosphorus-32, is used in oncological therapy and diagnostics, for instance, chronic leukemia therapy and malignant tumors diagnosis [413]. Phosphocol P-32 (chromic phosphate) is a ^{32}P radiolabeled therapeutic radiopharmaceutical that is used for the treatment of malignancies and tumor-related side effects.

Arsenic

In small doses, arsenic compounds have therapeutic effects [111, 112]. They have stimulant effects, arousing the Hb synthesis and development of erythrocytes, and inhibiting leukopoietic processes. As-containing drugs have long been used. In spite of the As toxic character, its compounds do have certain beneficial efficiency. As-based drugs have been employed starting from the XVIII century when $NaHCO_3$-containing solution of As_2O_3 (Fowler's solution) was given for various diseases [414]. This solution represents KH_2AsO_3 and was mainly used as a restorative agent. Arsenic iodide was used against leprosy.

In medicine, arsenic(III) oxide, or white arsenic, As_2O_3 is applied externally for the treatment of skin diseases. In stomatology, it is used for pulp necrotization. The body can get used to As_2O_3 if it is introduced gradually, increasing the dose. Arsenic trioxide has been approved by FDA for the treatment of the rare and lethal leukemia named acute promyelocytic leukemia (APL) [415], and for other malignancies like unresectable hepatocellular carcinoma and non-small-cell lung cancer [416] with almost complete remission in most of the cases. In water solution, arsenic(III) oxide forms arsenic(III) hydroxide which enters cells *via* glycerol transport pathways (aquaglyceroporins). In an aqueous medium at a physiological pH value, As_2O_3 exists in the form of hydroxide. $As(OH)_3$ is a weaker acid than phosphorous acid $P(OH)_3$. In cells, arsenic(III) is easily exposed to oxidative methylation:

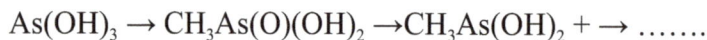

$$As(OH)_3 \rightarrow CH_3As(O)(OH)_2 \rightarrow CH_3As(OH)_2 + \rightarrow \ldots\ldots$$

Bacteria have protein-coding genes (ArsB and ArsAB) that yield As(III) (arsenite). Arsenic(III) is transported as a conjugate to GSH, and the reductase (ArsC) converts AsO_4^{3-} to As(III) ions.

Inside As_2O_3 is prescribed in micro-doses for anemia, exhaustion, and neurasthenia [111, 414, 416]. Solutions of As(III) oxide can be administered until the concentration of 1-2 µmol/l in the blood plasma without hematopoietic noxiousness. Treatment of cells with As_2O_3 causes collapses of mitochondrial membrane potentials, a release of cytochrome *c* from mitochondria into cytosol and apoptosis. In the same diseases (anemia, neurasthenia), solutions of potassium arsenite K_3AsO_3 and sodium hydroarsenate Na_2HAsO_4 are also used in clinical practice. Crystalline sodium arsenate, a disodium salt of arsenic acid, and 1% sodium arsenate solution for injection in small doses, stimulate the erythrocytic function of the bone marrow, enhance anabolic processes, improve skin trophism, and suppress leukopoiesis in large quantities. They are also used for neurosis and in large doses - for leukemia.

Arsenic is part of many organic compounds that are well known drugs. Melarsoprol, 2-(4-amino)-(4,6-diamino 1,3,5-triazin-2-yl)-phenyl-1,2,3-dithi-arsolan-4-methanol (Mel B, Arsobal), (Fig. **14**), is an organoarsenic compo-und that is used for the therapy of trypanosomiasis or human African sleeping sickness, in spite of its adverse encephalopathic effects [417].

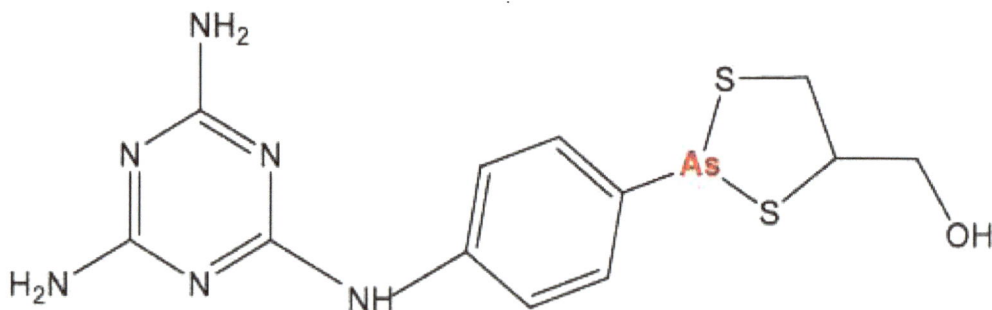

Fig. (14). Melarsoprol, 2-(4-amino)-(4,6-diamino 1,3,5-triazin-2-yl)-phenyl-1,2,3-dithiarsolan-4-methanol (Mel B, Arsobal).

Darinaparsin, S-dimethylarsino-glutathione with potential antineoplastic activity induces greater accumulation of intracellular As and cellular death *in vitro* with lesser general toxic effects compared to As_2O_3 [418]. Darinaparsin, S-di methyl arsinoglutathione (ZIO101), (Fig. **15**), is an arsenic-based anticancer agent, active against myeloma.

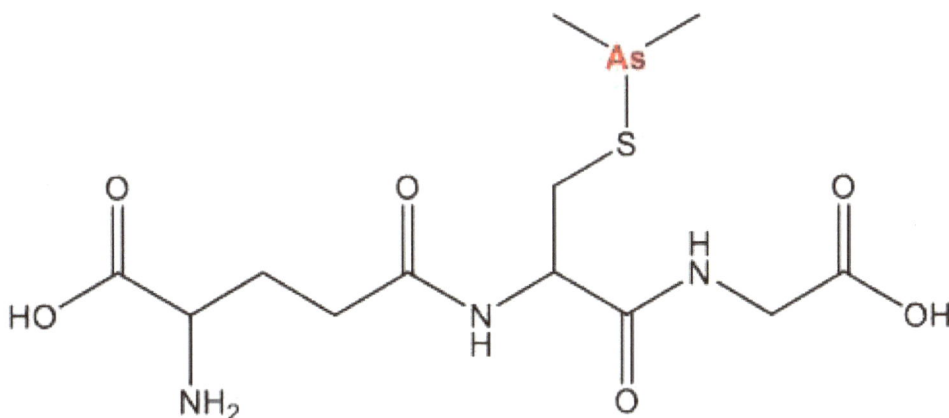

Fig. (15).   Darinaparsin, S-dimethylarsinoglutathione (DAR, ZIO101).

Certain of the firstly explored metal-based drugs in therapy indeed were As-based antimicrobic and antiparasitic agents.

Salvarsan (3,3'-diamino-4,4'-dihydroxyarsenobenzene dihydrochloride) and Neo-salvarsan (sodium 2-amino-4-[4-hydroxy-3-(sulfenatooxymethylamino) phenyl] arsanylidenearsanylphenol) (Fig. **16**) were introduced at the beginning of the 20th century as the primary efficient therapies for syphilis as antibiotics. Salvarsan is one of the first therapeutic arsenic-based metallodrugs. Salvarsan was supposed to have As=As double bonds. However, recently, the As-As bonds in Salvarsan have been revealed to be single but not double bonds. Salvarsan was observed to contain mixtures of cyclo-(RAs)₃ and cyclo-(RAs)₅ species, in which R is 3-amino-4-hydroxyphenyl [419]. Although the structures of salvarsan have been clarified, their precise composition remains unknown. In spite of that fact, it is extensively used in humans. With the addition of Hg and Bi, this compound remained the standard medication for syphilis treatment until its replacement by penicillin. It is supposed that As could almost totally be excluded from the pharmacopoeia.

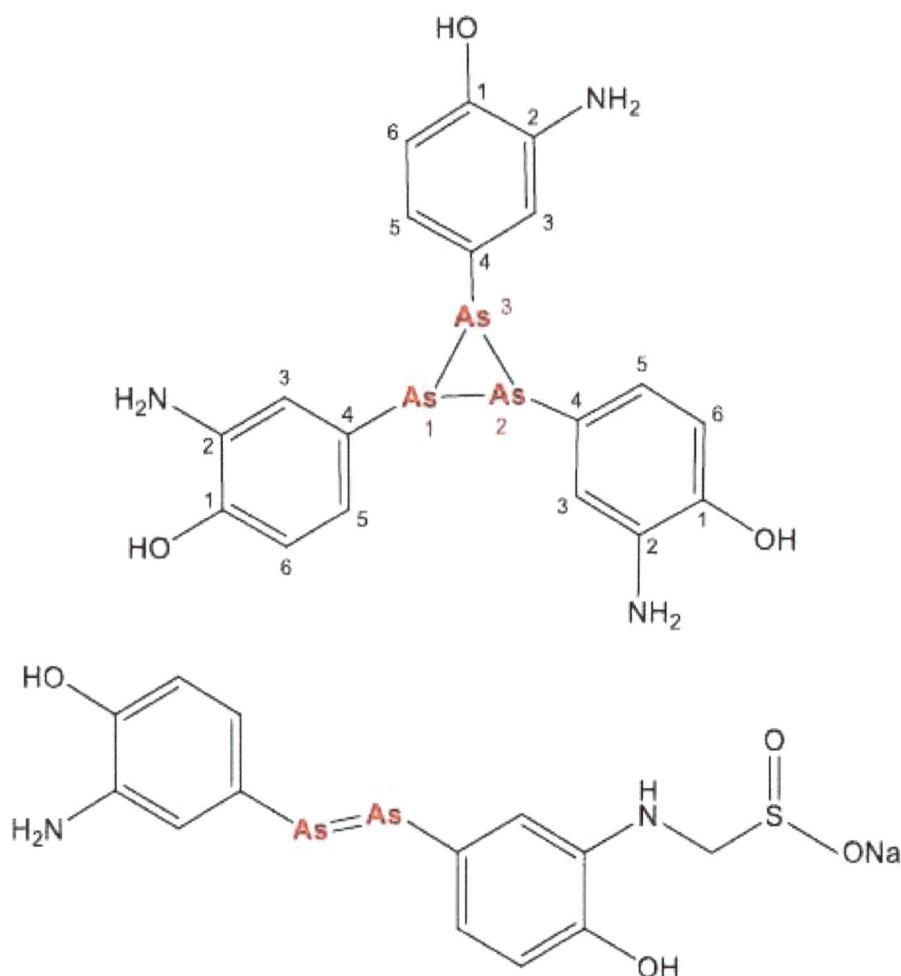

Fig. (16). Salvarsan and Neosalvarsan.

There are some radioisotopes of As appropriate for diagnostic imaging and radiotherapy emissions. Arsenic nuclides, such as the radioactive nuclides ^{71}As and ^{74}As, have been used in biology and medicine. They have been applied in blood diseases, as well as for diagnostic purposes to clarify the localization of brain tumors. Although As is popular as a radio-diagnostic agent, the absence of suitable chelator agents and problems with its toxicity have blocked its use in radiotherapy [420].

Antimony

Antimony-based compounds have been used in medical practice for many years [421 - 425]. The mineral antimony sulfide (antimony glance) was recognized in ancient times for the preparation of ointments. Antimony(V) sulfide is used as an expectorant. Polynuclear metal oxyanions, named polyoxometalates (POMs), such as HPA-23 (ammonium-21-tungsto-9-antimonate) have been administrated to AIDS patients with reduced levels of human immunodeficiency virus (HIV).

The most important application of antimony is the use of organoantimonial compounds against microbes and parasites, particularly for the treatment of cutaneous and mucocutaneous leishmaniasis [421]. The parasitic transmission of this tropical illness has been clarified in the early XX century, when Sb(III) potassium tartrate was given for mucocutaneous and visceral leishmaniasis [422]. The hydrated potassium antimonyl tartrate $K_2Sb_2(C_4H_2O_6)_2$, (Fig. **17**), the so-called "tartar emetic" has been used in medicine as a diaphoretic, expectorant, and emetic. Shortly thereafter, the bioactivity of As against visceral leishmaniasis was established, which resulted in the preparation of a variety of As-based antiparasitic agents along with the antimonyl compounds. Actually, the use of Sb(III) compounds for medicinal purposes was temporarily forbidden, since there were serious side effects observed with such compounds.

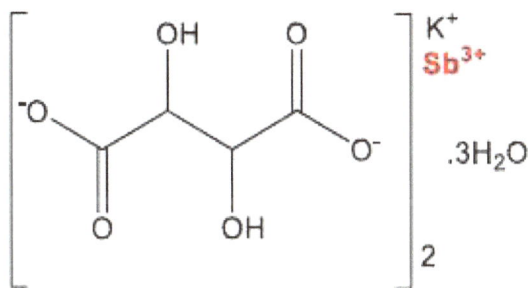

Fig. (17). Hydrated potassium antimonyl tartrate $K_2Sb_2(C_4H_2O_6)_2$.

The less poisonous antimonial Sb(V) substances were first reported in the 1940s, such as Stibosan, Neostibosan, and Ureastibamine. Two forms are still used for leishmaniasis therapy, antimonitae N-methylglucamine or meglumine antimoniate (MA, Glucantime, Glucantim) and sodium stibogluconate (SSG, Pentostam), but the relative potency of these treatments is not clear due to the growing antimony-resistance of the parasites. The targets for Sb(V) compounds are probably white blood cells (macrophages), where the parasites are eliminated. It has been predicted that Sb^{+5} is a typical prodrug, reduced to Sb^{+3} by the parasites or host cells [423]. The target of the organoantimonial compounds is supposed to be trypanothione, a thiol with low molecular weight, occurring in the *Leishmania* parasite. Together with the enzyme trypanothione reductase, trypanothione provides an intracellular reducing site to bypass the OS and thus ensures the parasites' survival. Investigational studies have indicated that the intracellular reduction of Sb^{+5} to Sb^{+3} is followed by the interaction of Sb^{+3} with trypanothione to produce a complex compound that may inhibit the enzyme trypanothione reductase through thiolate exchange [424, 425].

Bismuth

Bismuth salts and coordination compounds are widely used in medicine [123 - 125]. Bismuth(III) ions, whose ionic radius is close in size to Ca(II), may have coordination numbers from 3 to 10, and form compounds with different types of geometry. The free electron pair $6s^2$ occasionally exhibits a stereochemical effect, the so-called inert pair effect. Bismuth(III) ion is hydrated by water molecules producing strongly acidic aqueous solutions. The first step of deprotonation of the aqua-cation has a pKa 1.5:

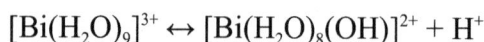

$$[Bi(H_2O)_9]^{3+} \leftrightarrow [Bi(H_2O)_8(OH)]^{2+} + H^+$$

Additional deprotonation to form coordinated hydroxides and oxides proceeds easily, and clusters with bridged oxygen atoms are quickly formed in the aqueous solution, such as $[Bi_6O_5(OH)_3]^{5+}$ and $[Bi_6O_4(OH)_4]^{6+}$. Bi(III) complexes often contain bismuth(1+), oxo-ion (BiO$^+$), and hydroxide ligands along with other types of ligands [426]. Such compounds are usually referred to as basic or oxysalts.

Bismuth-containing medicines have been applied to humans for more than 200 years mainly in cosmetics, medications (antacids, antimicrobial agents, *etc.*), and in some therapeutic procedures. Consequently, trace levels of Bi can be found in almost all human organisms. Biologically, it is present in ionic form in the body. The very common and popular ingredient in traditional and mineral cosmetic formulations bismuth oxychloride BiOCl, which gives a pearlescent make-up sheen, has been approved by FDA as a safe product for the eyes, face, lips, and nails. However, skin irritation from its use is not unusual. Especially for those with sensitive skin, acne, rosacea, BiOCl can aggravate and irritate the condition and enlarge pore size permanently. Sulbogin is a topical ointment for the treatment of wound healing. It contains bismuth subgallate (Fig. **18**) as one of its main constituents [426]. Bismuth subgallate accelerates coagulation.

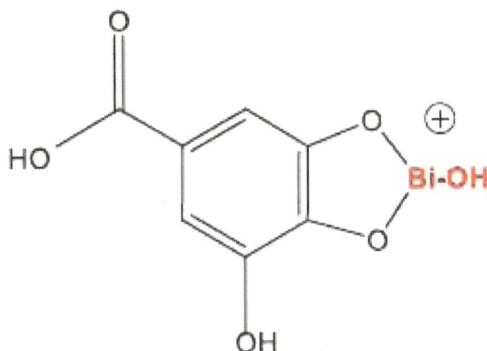

Fig. (18). Structure of bismuth subgallate.

Bismuth-based drugs have been described to exert antimicrobial activity against digestive tract pathogenic microorganisms, *e.g., Helicobacter pylori, Vibrio cholera, Campylobacter jejune,* and *Yersinia enterocolitica* [123 - 125]. As bismuth has low toxicity to humans, though insoluble Bi(III) salts are neurotoxic, interest in oral Bi treatment has recently increased owing to the results gained in gastritis and peptic ulcer action associated with *Helicobacter pylori* infection. *Helicobacter pylori* are gram-negative bacteria which are the contributing agents in gastrointestinal diseases like peptic ulcers, gastritis, and gastric cancer [427]. The best candidates as remedies for gastrointestinal disorders are Bi(III)-based compounds with hydroxycarboxylate ligands (salicylate, citrate). Bismuth salts eliminate bacteria that cause stomach problems. They also act like antacids for the treatment of problems like indigestion. Bi may also accelerate blood clotting.

Bismuth shows direct antibacterial effects through different modes of action. It can form complexes in the bacterial wall and periplasmic space. It also can inhibit various enzymes, ATP synthesis, and adherence of the bacteria to the gastric mucosa [428]. The effectiveness of bismuth as an antibacterial agent relates to its unique chemistry. The main oxidation state of bismuth is +3, but free Bi^{3+} cations do not exist, and thus the covalent interactions dominate. The only available ionic bismuth types are the bismuthyl ions BiO^+, which form basic, oxy-, and sub-compounds. Actually, the chemistry of Bi in aqueous solutions is dominated by the production of clusters, for instance, $[Bi_6O_4(OH)_4]^{6+}$. That is why the stoichiometry of Bi bactericides is variable. The main drugs which contain bismuth are: Bismatrol, Diotame, Pepto Bismol, Kapectolin, Kaopectate, Kola-Pectin, BisBacter, *etc.*

In health care, bismuth-based drugs with ingredients such as Bi subsalicylate (BSS, Pepto-Bismol), colloidal Bi subcitrate (CBS, De-Nol), ranitidine Bi citrate

(RBC, Pylorid, Tritec), (Fig. **19**), Bi iodoform as well as radioactive ($^{212}Bi/^{213}Bi$) complexes have been obtained and applied in clinical practice to treat numerous illnesses. Ranitidine bismuth citrate has an anti-ulcer effect. It is mediated by two active ingredients. Ranitidine, a blocker of H_2-histamine receptors, suppresses gastric acid secretion. Bismuth citrate shas a bactericidal effect on *Helicobacter pylori* and a protective effect on the gastric mucosa [123 - 125].

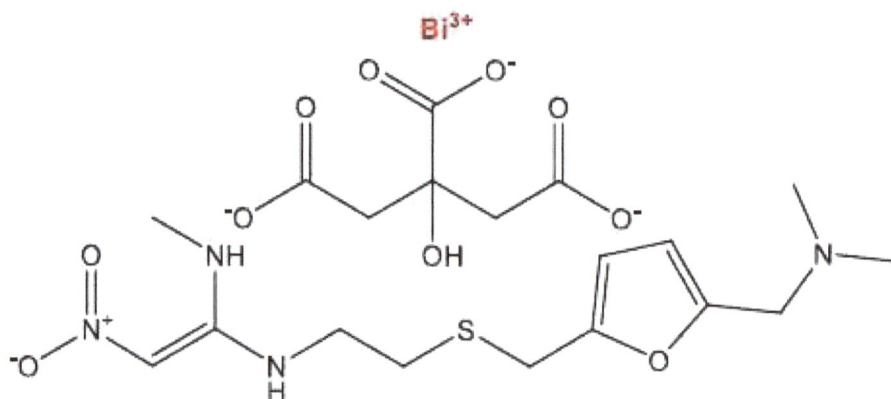

Fig. (19). Ranitidine bismuth citrate (RBC, Pylorid, Tritec).

Bi(III) citrate [Bi(Hcit)] is not soluble in water, but can dissolve in the presence of bases (ammonia and amines like ranitidine, which is a known antiulcer medication). Citric acid exists in three-deprotonated form at neutral pH. Additionally, metal ions, such as Al(III), Fe(III), and Ga(III), like Bi(III), can replace the proton of the central hydroxyl group. Bi(III) complex compounds with citrate have a complex structure, which is based on a dimeric unit [(cit)BiBi(cit)]$^{2-}$, (cit - tetradeprotonated citric acid) containing a tridentate ligand citrate, wherein the terminal carboxylate anion is bound to the neighboring Bi^{3+} cation. The bond of Bi^{3+} with O atom of the alkoxy group is very short, strong, and is part of the five-membered chelate cycle. Bi^{3+}-citrate dimers can be associated with the formation of chain or layered structures through the further formation of bridges and hydrogen bonds. These polymers can be placed on the surface of ulcers [124]. At pH< 3.5 in dilute HCl, BiOCl is precipitated.

Bismuth(III) citrates react easily with thiol-based biomolecules, in particular with the tripeptide GSH, to form [Bi(SG)$_3$], in which Bi^{3+} is bonded to an S atom of the thiol group [124]. The [Bi(SG)$_3$] complex is relatively stable, however, thiol-based ligands are kinetically unstable, and exchange with free thiols takes place within milliseconds. So, Bi(III) is a highly mobile ion in the cell. *H. pylori* bacteria live in acidic conditions in the stomach and use Ni-dependent enzyme urease to produce NH_3 to neutralize the acidic reaction:

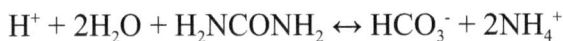

$$H^+ + 2H_2O + H_2NCONH_2 \leftrightarrow HCO_3^- + 2NH_4^+$$

Inhibition of the enzyme urease by Bi(III)- thiolate complexes plays a significant role in the mechanism of Bi(III) antibacterial activity [124, 428]. The acquired resistance of the bacterium to the antibiotic Clarithromycin can be partially overcome by the administration of clarithromycin in combination with CBS or RBC.

Bismuth subsalicylate (BSS) preparations are over-the-counter antimicrobial products for gastrointestinal complaints [124]. In spite of the fact that BSS is very popular and has been used safely by many patients for the last 100 years, its molecular structure and functional mechanisms are still not completely clarified. In the medical practice, bismuth subsalicylate and calcium carbonate are the most commonly used compounds to treat indigestion because of their acid-reducing effects. Bismuth subsalicylate belongs to the class of medicines named antidiarrheal agents, used to manage and treat gastrointestinal discomfort and traveler's diarrhea. It acts by reducing the flow of fluids and electrolytes in the bowel. It reduces intestinal inflammation and kills the microorganisms that cause diarrhea. Bismuth subsalicylate is the main ingredient in the brand names Pepto-Bismol and BisBacter which are used to treat temporary disorders of the stomach and digestive tract, protecting the gastrointestinal tract from stomach acid. These medicines are used for indigestion and acid reflux, diarrhea, and nausea. Bismuth subsalicylate is also an anti-inflammatory agent because of the salicylate component which exerts intestinal anti-inflammatory and antisecretory actions. Bismuth subsalicylate shows aspirin-like activity having an aspirin equivalency conversion factor of 0.479 (about half the aspirin strength). The mechanism of action of bismuth subsalicylate shows that following BSS ingestion other bismuth salts can be formed throughout the digestive tract, for instance, bismuth oxychloride (BiOCl) that also acts upon enteric pathogenic microorganisms. As a salicylate, bismuth subsalicylate can cause serious bleeding problems when used alone in patients with ulcers [429]. The common adverse effects of BSS can be abdominal pain, anxiety, anal discomfort, black tongue (due to the contact with sulfur, which is naturally present in human saliva), lay-colored or gray-black stools, cold symptoms (stuffy nose, sneezing, sore throat), confusion, chronic constipation, *etc.* In the Bi-based triple therapy, bismuth subcitrate potassium (Pylera) or bismuth subsalicylate is included in combination with metronidazole and tetracycline hydrochloride [430 - 432]. It is an effective, safe, and well-tolerated therapy for the treatment of *H. pylori* in clinical practice.

Bismuth colloids are known with their bactericidal action, which corresponds to the treatment of infectious diarrhea and peptic ulcers (*Helicobacter pylori*). To survive in the severe, acidic environment of the stomach, *Helicobacter pylori* bacterium secretes the enzyme urease, which transforms urea to NH_3. The formation of NH_3 around the bacterium neutralizes the acidic stomach reaction, making it more hospitable for the bacterium. Colloidal bismuth subcitrate (DeNol) and bismuth subsalicylate (Pepto-Bismol) are applicable for prevention and treating gastrointestinal and duodenal ulcers [430, 431].

In addition to the well-known gastroprotective effects of bismuth, it also has broad anti microbial, anti fungal, anti leishmanial, and anti cancer properties [433]. Bi(III) complexes containing one or two phenyl groups and a tetrazole/triazolethiolate ligand have been shown to possess high cytotoxic activity, with poor selectivity indices, which is probably a result of their non-specific mechanism of action [434]. The compound tribromophenatebismuth(III), (Fig. **20**), was described at the end of the 19th century. Its external application shows strong antimicrobial properties. The widely studied Bi-thiol compounds are presently advertised for the treatment of chronic wounds, including diabetic foot ulcers.

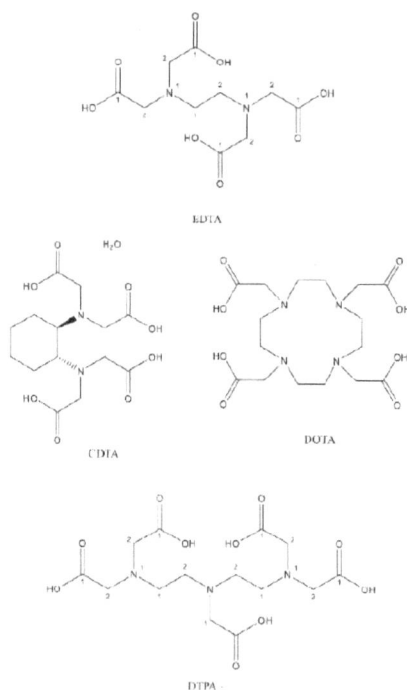

Fig. (20). The structure of tribromophenatebismuth(III).

The highly acidic Bi^{3+} cation forms polymeric complexes with OH-, O-bridges or citrate bridges as in the case of Bi subcitrate. Interest in Bi complexes as anticancer agents is rising as a result of the observation that bismuth administration before chemotherapy reduces poisonous adverse effects related to cisplatin [435]. Normally, bismuth compounds are comparatively non-toxic. Cellular structures are possibly protected from bismuth by thiol-enriched MT protein. Bismuth(III) induces MT synthesis, so pretreatment with bismuth is an efficient mechanism for reducing the noxiousness of Pt preparations.

The antifungal effect of Bi_2O_3 nanoparticles has been proven against *Candida albicans, Candida tropicalis, Candida auris* growth [436 - 438]. Nanostructures enhance the efficiency, solubility, penetration, and drug release to the targeted site of the antifungal agents.

Bismuth, the heaviest stable post-transition metal, has weak radioactivity. The chemical properties of this pnictogen are similar to that of its lighter analogs of VA group As and Sb. Bi(V) compounds are known, but they are strong oxidizing agents. Bismuth-213 (half-life 45.6 min) is an α-emitter for clinical use. Clinical trials of [213]Bi-lintuzumab have established that administration of this radiopharmaceutical agent against relapsed and refractory (R/R) AML was safe and gave rise to remissions in patients [439]. Targeted α-particle radiotherapy produces more efficient tumor killing and spares healthy cells [440]. [213]Bi-lintuzumab showed quick targeting of disease locations without substantial extramedullary toxic effects. The compound bismuth trioxide is lightweight, effective in protecting against ionizing radiations such as gamma rays, and can be produced quickly - making it a promising material for use in medical imaging and radiation therapy [441].

Oxygen

Oxygen therapy is extensively used in the treatment of numerous chronic and acute health indications such as emphysema, pneumonia, some heart disorders, and another kind of diseases. Oxygen in medicine is useful for inhalation in diseases accompanied by oxygen deficiency [129], in case of poisoning with carbon(II) monoxide, hydrocyanic acid, *etc.* A mixture of 95% oxygen and 5% carbon dioxide (carbogen) is often used for this purpose. In anesthesiologic practice, oxygen is widely used in a mixture of inhaled drugs. For therapeutic purposes, oxygen under the skin can be injected, as well as in the form of an oxygen cocktail into the stomach (enteral oxygen therapy).

In recent years, a new field of medicine called hyperbaric medicine has emerged, which is based on the treatment of various diseases at elevated pressure. The healing use of O_2 under pressure is called hyperbaric oxygen therapy (HBOT).

This therapy is recommended for treating burns, carbon monoxide poisoning, radiation injury, and coronavirus [442].

Radioactive oxygen with a half-life of 123 s is used to measure the oxygen content in organs, to determine the change in its concentration. With the help of oxygen-15, it is possible to determine the pharmacological effect of vasodilating drugs, to clarify their dosage, and to register signs of addiction to them with prolonged use.

Hydrogen Peroxide

Hydrogen peroxide shows broad-spectrum of activity against bacteria, viruses, yeasts, and bacterial spores. Diluted solution of H_2O_2 (3%) is applied in medicine for removing dead tissue, cleaning wounds, or as an orally applied debriding agent [22]. Hydrogen peroxide is popular in surgery as a highly useful irrigation solution by virtue of both its hemostatic and antimicrobial effects. Because of its possible harmful effect on wound healing and its cytotoxic effect in higher amounts, there are concerns about the safety of its use.

Ozone

Ozone, an allotropic form of oxygen, possesses unique properties that have been defined and applied to biological systems as well as to clinical practice. The bulk of the ozone produced is used to disinfect drinking water. The disinfecting action of ozone is very effective, although this method is significantly more expensive than conventional chlorination. The sterilizing effect of ozone is connected with the generation of free radicals, which destroy the cell membranes of the microorganisms [132]. In medicine, ozone is used in very small concentrations - for deodorization and disinfection of air in medical premises. Low ozone doses are helpful in the treatment of wound healing, epithelization, and surface caries. Ozonated olive oil provides long-term, low-dose exposure of O_3 and lipid peroxides to tissues. Decubitus ulcers, diabetic ulcers, and mycoses are the main indications for its use.

When inhaling a mixture of air with ozone (ozone therapy), metabolism, and kidney function are improved, the protective functions of the body are enhanced, and appetite, sleep, and general well-being are improved. Therefore, ozone therapy is used in many diseases of the heart, kidneys, food canal, and skin, in the treatment of tuberculosis, coronavirus, *etc.* [443, 444].

Sulfur

In medicine, both sulfur itself and its compounds are used and display a broad spectrum of beneficial chemical and biological properties [154, 155]. Purified sulfur has an antimicrobial and anthelminthic effect. Elemental sulfur is used in dermatology for the treatment of skin diseases (psoriasis, seborrheic dermatitis, scabies) because of its antifungal and anti-seborrheic effects. Sulfur is usually deposited externally in the form of sulfur cream, lotion, ointment, powders, and bar soap used to treat acne and other dermatological complications. In medical practice, purified sulfur is used as a mild laxative.

Sulfur when ingested with organic substances forms sulfides and pentathionic acid $H_2O_6S_5$, which have antimicrobial and antiparasitic effects [155]. It is used in dermatology. Sulfur dioxide is used as an antifungal agent in viniculture. Sulfur(IV) oxide serves as a disinfectant that kills many microorganisms. It is fumigated in order to destroy mold fungi.

Sodium sulfite Na_2SO_3 and sodium bisulfite $Na_2S_2O_5$ act as stabilizing antioxidants of easily oxidizable substances in solutions [154, 155]. Concentrations lower than 100mg/kg can be used for the production of wine, fruit juices, dried fruits, and vegetables for preventing fermentation and changes of color. Sulfates of sodium ($Na_2SO_4.10H_2O$ - laxative), calcium ($CaSO_4.1/2H_2O$- medical gypsum), magnesium ($MgSO_4$ - hypotensive, sedative, laxative, choleretic), and barium ($BaSO_4$ - radiopaque for X-ray inspection of the digestive tract) are widely used in medical practice. Sodium sulfate Na_2SO_4 and magnesium sulfate $MgSO_4$ are constituents of some mineral waters. $CuSO_4·5H_2O$ and $ZnSO_4·7H_2O$ are used as antiseptics.

Sodium thiosulfate and a 30% solution of $Na_2S_2O_3$ for injection are used as detoxifying, anti-inflammatory, anti-allergic, and antiparasitic agents [445]. Its antiparasitic properties are based on the fact that when it interacts with hydrochloric acid, sulfur(IV) oxide, and free sulfur are released. Sodium thiosulfate $Na_2S_2O_3$, applied intravenously, is prescribed as an antidote for the treatment of hydrocyanic acid, cyanides, halogens, arsenic, mercury, lead, bismuth, thallium intoxication and for the control of the toxic indications of cisplatin, forming harmless or less toxic compounds excreted from the body. Sodium thiosulfate is also used for burns with liquid bromine.

Sulfur commonly exists in different oxidation states, enabling it to possess a diversity of forms. Many functional sulfur-containing moieties are included in the acyclic and cyclic structures of familiar sulfur drugs, such as sulfates, sulfoxides, S=C and S=P structures, sulfones, sulfonamides, thioethers, thiazoles, thiophenes, β-lactams, phenothiazines, thionucleotides, macrocyclic disulfides, *etc.* [445].

Derivatives of sulfanilamide streptocide, norsulfazol, etazol, sulfazine are used as antimicrobial agents. Many antibiotics also contain sulfur in their composition. Antibiotics like cephalosporin, penicillin, and sulfanilamides are S-containing compounds. Thiamin, which constitutes vitamin B1, contains sulfur in its ring structure.

The so-called sulfa drugs (active substance - sulfanilamide) have been discovered in the last century. The long life of sulfonamides in drug discovery is attributed to their favorable solubility, high stability, ease of preparation, and the presence of multiple hydrogen bonding donor and acceptor sites [446]. Sulfa drugs are systematically used to effectively treat and prevent bacterial infections in humans. After the detection of penicillin, which is very effective and less toxic, the application of sulfa drugs has decreased significantly.

Despite the success of established sulfur pharmacophores, a large number of sulfur functional groups remain neglected in drug discovery, for instance, sulfoximines, sulfondiimines, sulfonimidamides, sulfur-fluorine compounds, *etc.* Recently, increasing attempts have been made to elucidate the biological effects of these underexplored pharmacophores [447, 448].

Selenium

Inorganic compounds of selenium are used in medicine as part of various mineral-vitamin complexes due to their vital antioxidant functions. Deficiency of nutrient Se frequently results in the incidence of various disorders, such as Keshan disease, thyroid dysfunction, diabetes, arthrophyma, and cognitive limitation. Long-term selenium deficiency or insufficient Se intake can be compensated by the treatment with Na_2SeO_3 or organic Se compounds, the most appropriate is selenomethionine. Se is toxic, but at the same time it can counteract the effects of other toxins like As, Hg, and Cd [162]. Therefore, Se tablets can be healthful for humans. Selenium also impacts skeletal muscle health and mitochondrial function and energetics [449]. Animals in areas with Se-deficient soil are predisposed to develop white muscle disease and have to accept Se additives in fertilizers or in special sprays.

Se sulfide has a fungicidal activity and can be used as a supplement to shampoos to treat dandruff and certain types of dermatitis [450]. Sulfoselen soap (which contains sulfur and selenium) is used in dermatology to treat skin diseases.

It has been found that inorganic (SeO_3^{2-}, SeO_4^{2-}) and many organic Se-based substances, such as methylseleninic acid, diselenides, selenides, selenoesters, selenophene-containing compounds, as well as selenoamino acids (seleno-methionine, selenocysteine, Se-methyl-seleno-L-cysteine, selenocystine) have a great potential for chemoprotective treatment of cancer [451]. The motives for using Se-containing substances as new possible agents or co-adjuvants in anticancer therapy are the greater selectivity and efficiency, less toxicity, and reduced side effects compared to the commonly used antitumor therapeutic agents. Selenium as a pleiotropic agent has attracted considerable attention for biotherapy and drug delivery, in particular, Se-based nanomedicines for cancer and diabetes mellitus.

It needs to be taken into consideration that the interval between the needed intake and the poisonous amount of Se is fairly narrow. Selenium and its compounds (Na_2SeO_3, Na_2SeO_4) are part of the enzymes (in the form of the selenohydryl group SeH^-) and have both activating and inhibitory effects [160, 161].

Tellurium

Recent research on the pharmacology of tellurium and it compounds has revealed some potential applications in medicine [452]. Experimental data show that sodium tellurite is an effective tool in the treatment of acute liver dystrophy. It accelerates the normalization of hepatic secretion, the synthesis of bile acids, and the excretion of cholesterol. Organic tellurium compounds are effective in the treatment of experimental toxicosis of pregnancy, acute pancreatitis, and toxic hepatitis. Tellurium compounds are less poisonous than selenium. Tellurium agar, containing potassium tellurite, is widely used in microbiological and bacteriological practice. Most of the studies have been focused on tellurite, tellurate and a few organic tellurides. Bio-incorporation of telluromethionine offers a new approach to add heavy metal atoms to selected sites in proteins.

The Te(IV) compound ammonium trichloro(dioxoethylene-O,O′)tellurate (AS101), which is not toxic, entered several clinical trials due to its good tolerability for the treatment of external warts, as a supplementation to the standard chemotherapeutic treatment of AML and as a preventive agent of bone marrow poisonousness as a result of chemotherapy [453]. It is a potent Te(IV) immunomodulator prodrug. Experimental studies of the orally and intra-peritoneally administered AS101 have shown that this medication expressively reduces clinical indications of inflammatory bowel diseases. In a dextran Na_2SO_4-induced colitis model, AS101 has exerted its anti-inflammatory and antiapoptotic activity by the blockade of neutrophil and macrophage leucocyte migration into the colon [454]. AS-101 is an effective agent against HIV. Interestingly, an analogous compound of selenium does not have similar properties.

Fluorine

Fluorine is a part of neuroleptic drugs. There are many fluorinated pharmaceutical agents available as anesthetics, antibiotics, antitumor, and anti-inflammatory medications, psychopharmaceuticals, *etc.* [455]. For example, Fluorophenazine is effective in schizophrenia with a prolonged course of the disease. Fluoroacisin has an antidepressant effect; Fluorouracil, Fluorofur, and Fluorobenzotef are used for malignant neoplasms; Fluorotane - is a means for removing inhalation anesthesia; Fluorocort is an ointment used externally for inflammatory and allergic skin diseases. It has been found that fluorine substitution has profound effects on the activity of bioorganic compounds because of the high electronegativity of fluorine, which can modify electron distribution in the biomolecule and affect its absorption, distribution, and metabolism.

Fluoride has long been known to influence the activity of various enzymes *in vitro* and many of the effects associated with fluoride are due to the synergistic action of fluoride and Al. In medicine, NaF in tablet formulations or in toothpastes is applied in small amounts in the treatment of dental caries, mostly in children [169, 170]. Various doses of sodium fluoride are used in the prevention or therapy of osteoporosis. A mixture of calcium chloride and fluoride in a suspension of gelatin can fluoride water. In small amounts, CaF_2 is used as a bactericide and insecticide.

^{18}F-labelled deoxyglucose ($T_{1/2}$ = 110 min), with electron capture, is one of the most extensively used agents in PET imaging for detection of fluctuations in glucose metabolism in pathological processes. The so called ^{18}F-fluoro deoxy glucose-PET (^{18}F-FDG-PET) is mainly used for screening, localization, and monitoring of hypermetabolic processes such as infections, cancers, and autoimmune disorders [456].

Chlorine

Dichlorine (Cl_2) has different oxidation effects, for instance, it oxidizes bromides and iodides to bromine and iodine, and is a disinfectant of water [173, 174]. Chlorine participates as a component of some narcotic and anesthetic drugs. It is part of a number of drugs of the aliphatic series with hypnotic activity. In negligible concentrations, it can serve as an antidote. Chlorine lime is used in hydrogen sulfide intoxication. In this case, hydrogen sulfide oxidizes to sulfur.

In cases of insufficient acidity of gastric juice, diluted hydrochloric acid (with a mass fraction of 8%) can be taken orally in drops and mixtures (often together with pepsin).

NaCl is a common constituent of numerous different infusions. Its 154 mM solution is isotonic with the blood plasma (0.9%) [28]. Administration of large amounts of chlorides (NaCl, $CaCl_2$ or NH_4Cl) moderately drops the content of buffer bases and provides an acidic reaction in extracellular fluids. At Br^- excess in the body, a "salt diet" with a high content of NaCl is recommended to displace Br^- ions.

KCl is applied orally to compensate for the K^+ deficiency (chronic diarrheas), which is associated with the loss of Cl^- and metabolic alkalosis, and in serious cases K^+ ions are added to infusion solutions [33]. KCl is used in cardiac arrhythmias, at intoxication with cardiac glycosides, when myocardial cells are depleted by potassium ions.

Hypochlorous acid HClO is a bleaching agent that can eradicate bacteria [173]. Sodium hypochlorite NaClO is a common disinfectant. ClO^- ions are produced by phagocytosing cells in a myeloperoxidase reaction:

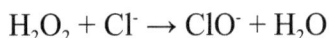

$$H_2O_2 + Cl^- \rightarrow ClO^- + H_2O$$

Ca chloride-hypochlorite $CaOCl_2$ is named chlorine white bleaching lime [173, 174]. It can be prepared by the addition of Cl_2 to $Ca(OH)_2$ and is useful as a basic disinfectant and anti-pollutant. $CaOCl_2$ under the action of CO_2, water and light, releases active O, which destroys the cell membranes of the micro organisms. Calcium decoxide $(Cl\ O_2)_2$ O=O $(Cl\ O_2)_2$ is recognized as a strong agent against aerobic bacteria.

Chlorates $NaClO_3$, $Mg(ClO_3)_2$, $Ca(ClO_3)_2$ are well known herbicides with strong action. In smaller doses, they act as defoliants. Potassium perchlorate $KClO_4$ limits the consumption of I^- ions by the thyroid cells and consequently is useful in the thyroid gland protection throughout the inspection by compounds containing radioactive iodine [457]. Anhydrous magnesium perchlorate $Mg(ClO_4)_2$ readily absorbs water and forms crystalline hydrates. It is one of the most powerful dehumidifiers. Its technical name is anhydron. The use of $Mg(ClO_4)_2$ is convenient because after absorbing the water, it can be dehydrated again when heated.

Among the halogens, Cl_2 is most frequently available in drugs. Currently, a great number of chlorine-containing drugs and many pharmaceutical candidates in clinical trials are available [457]. The organochlorines are characterized by their increased lipophilicity due to the Cl-based substituent, which results to a higher partition of the chlorinated compounds into the lipophilic part of the cellular membrane. This produces a higher local amount of the drug near the biotarget location.

Bromine

In medicine, bromides of ammonium (NH_4Br), potassium (KBr), and sodium (NaBr) are used as depressants, sedatives, and anticonvulsants. Sodium bromide, used as a drug, enhances the activity of the adrenal cortex due to the replacement of I^- in the thyroid gland with Br^-. Especially sensitive to the action of bromine is the central nervous system, which responds to the functions of the Br^- anions by equating the processes of excitation and inhibition, which is manifested in the calming effect of NaBr [175].

Bromine drugs inhibit cerebral functions and are applied for the therapy of epilepsy. However, their adverse effects are serious and the bromine substances are no longer applied. Bromide compounds and organobromines are anyway used in the design of new therapeutic agents [458]. These substances exhibit a varied range of bioactivities: antibacterial, antiparasitic, antifungal, antiviral, antioxidant, antitumor, anti-inflammatory, *etc.* The neutron-deficient isotope bromine-77 (T_{12}= 56 h) has the decay properties required for diagnostic *in vivo* investigations of great potential.

Iodine

This element has diverse medical applications [176 - 179]. Iodine deficiency results in goiter (Derbyshire neck), which can be responded by adding iodide arrangements of, *e.g.,* iodinated water or table salt with iodate [178]. There are many supplementations of iodized salt (NaCl with KI, KIO_3, NaI, and $NaIO_3$) depending on the producer.

Iodine medications are applied externally as antiseptic agents in inflammatory and other diseases of the skin and mucous membranes [176]. The antibacterial iodine tincture (3% I_2 and 2.5% KI in alcohol solution) has long been known. The tincture of iodine is applied as an antiseptic agent for the treatment of wounds externally. Inside it is prescribed for the prevention of atherosclerosis (1-10 drops of a 5% solution). The water solution of KI (Lugol's solution) is applied to lubricate the pharynx and larynx mucous membranes. Povidone-iodine (PVP-I), also known as iodopovidone, is an antiseptic agent used for skin disinfection before and after surgery. Some iodine preparations can be used inside with chronic inflammatory processes of the respiratory tract as expectorants. KI is used for the intoxication with mercury and lead salts. Preparations containing iodide ions are used for the prevention of endemic goiter. Organic compounds of iodine (iodoform, iodinol) are used to treat rheumatism, atherosclerosis, and hyper thyroidism. I_2 is used as a substitute for Cl_2 for drinking water disinfection purposes. Even at small amounts around 1 ppm, I_2 is effective without showing the adverse effects, typical for Cl_2.

The Na^+/I^- symporter (NIS) plays a key role in thyroid pathophysiology and allows very effective use of radio iodide for diagnosis and therapy of thyroid cancer and metastases [177, 459]. Notably, over 80% of breast cancer samples in humans express endogenous NIS, providing the possibility for radio iodide usage in diagnostics and therapy.

For the treatment and diagnosis of thyroid illnesses, radioactive isotopes such as ^{131}I, ^{132}I, ^{124}I, and ^{125}I with a short half-life, are used [180, 181]. With the increasing use of positron emission tomography in pharmacokinetics, medical oncology, and drug metabolism, ^{124}I-labeled radiopharmaceuticals are useful tools for PET imaging, and because of the convenient half-life of I-124 (T_{12}= 4.2 d), they can be applied in PET scanners. In endemic goiter, potassium and sodium iodides are prescribed. Usually, tablets called "Antistrumin" containing KI are used for radioactive isotope prevention. As a result of the high iodine location in the body, thyroid tumors can be effectively identified by using radioisotopes ^{131}I and ^{123}I. Radioactive iodine therapy (RAIT) has long been used to treat hyperthyroidism and thyroid cancer [460].

Astatine

Astatine is the rarest of all occurring on Earth chemical elements. While only short-lived isotopes, with $T_{1/2}$ less than 8 h, are recognized, ^{211}At is the object of growing attention due to its emission of high-energy α particles. The radioactive astatine-211 ($T_{1/2}$ = 7.2 h) has numerous possible advantages for targeted α-therapeutic purposes [461, 462]. α-Emitters have unique characteristics for removal of focal locations of tumor cells which are in close proximity to the normal tissues of the central nervous system. For instance, they may be applied for targeted treatment lacking any risk of toxic effects which occasionally occurs with β-emitters. This specific feature is ideal for delicate areas such as the CNS. The life of astatine-211 is sufficiently long to allow the complex synthetic processes and it is well-matched with the pharmacokinetic characteristics of many other specific target candidates. Consequently, numerous ^{211}At-labeled type systems have been prepared and assessed as targeted radiotherapeutic agents like colloids, DNA precursors, peptides, organic compounds like *meta*-[^{211}At] astatobenzyl guanidine, anti bodies, *etc.* [463]. The practicability, safekeeping, and effectiveness of the chimeric anti-tenascin mAb 81C6 labelled with astatine-211 has been estimated in patients with malignant brain tumors. The radiopharmaceutical ^{211}At-MX35 F(ab')$_2$ has been studied in women in remission of ovarian cancer. By radiolabeling enzyme poly(ADP-ribose) polymerase 1 (PARP1) with astatine-211, the first α-emitting drug targeting cancer nuclei *via* PARP1, [^{211}At]parthanatine ([^{211}At]PTT) was developed [464]. The data of the duality of astatine, which exhibits the characteristics both of a halogen and of a metal, have an impact on the development of radiolabeling strategies to turn ^{211}At into radiopharmaceuticals.

Helium

Helium has been involved in adjunct therapy in some respirational system illnesses like croup, asthma, laryngotracheobronchitis, and bronchiolitis [465]. Helium gas is non-toxic at normal temperature and pressure and is practically physiologically inert. It is non-irritant to the respiratory tract. Mixtures of He and O_2 have been applied as breathing gases for deep-sea diving as well as in the treatment of chronic obstructive pulmonary disease (COPD). Because of its small density, this light gas mixture streams more readily to and from the pulmonary airways than atmospheric air in the lung. Different from N_2, He is not dissolved in the blood, and thus the decompression sickness Caisson disease can be circumvented on climbing, for example.

Helium does not cause myocardial depression or peritoneal acidosis, and, therefore, offer advantages in patients with borderline cardiorespiratory function and those for who prolonged laparoscopy could be likely. Helium has been used efficiency in defense of the myocardium from ischemia, although the protection mechanism is not clear. The use of the safer agent helium in the operating room for replacement of CO_2 for insufflation of the abdominal cavity of patients undertaking laparoscopic operations has been estimated [466]. The first element of the noble gases is a better alternative owing to its superiority in preventing respirational acidosis in comorbid situations that lead to retaining CO_2. Scanning helium-ion microscopy (HIM) is a well-established tool for organs' imaging in the smallest detail [467]. Hyperpolarized He (HP ^3He) for respiratory MRI may be applied for imaging of normal and unhealthy lung tissues.

Argon

Recently, for the study of the impact of argon treatment *in vivo* or *in vitro* models have been used primarily for ischemic pathologies, including cerebral ischemia, traumatic brain injury, and hypoxic ischemic encephalopathy [468, 469]. It has been demonstrated that argon at normobaric and hyperbaric conditions had more potent narcotic effects than nitrogen.

Argon is used in electrosurgery, in the so-called argon plasma coagulation [470]. Illustrations of its use include the restoration of hemorrhages occurring in surgical procedures of ulcers, varices, blood vessels, and tumors, as well as the reduction of tumor tissues.

Krypton

Krypton in the form of quadrupolar isotope ^{83}Kr with an abundance of 11.5% is useful in MRI of respiratory track predominantly for the distinction of hydrophobic and hydrophilic surfaces [471]. Ion laser filled with an argon-krypton mixture is used as a photocoagulator in micropulse coagulation.

Xenon

The effects of xenon as a general anesthetic agent are well known, however, its uses extend beyond this and current studies show that there is much potential for its application in nuclear imaging. Xenon-133 ($T_{1/2}$ = 5 d) with β−decay is useful in lung radio imaging by SPECT, as well as in measuring blood flow [472]. Hyperpolarized ^{129}Xe with 26% abundance is a typical MRI agent applied for imaging of the lung gas flow [473].

Radon

Radon has been found to have positive therapeutic action in physiobalneotherapy for the relief of pain caused by chronic degenerative and inflammatory diseases as a result of the influence of the small radiation doses of radon on the nervous, vascular, and immune systems [474]. Radon therapy is generally recognized and widely applied for the combined treatment of various diseases of the musculoskeletal system, neurological, cardiological, and gastrointestinal disorders, gynecological problems, *etc.*

The biological role, medicinal applications, and toxic effects of p-elements are collected in Table **17**.

Table 17. The biological role and toxic effects of p-elements.

Element	Location and Functions in the Body	Drugs	The Toxic Effect, Antidotes
B	Carbohydrate-phosphorus and fat metabolism; ^{10}B - shield in nuclear radiation (more effective than lead)	H_3BO_3 - disinfectant properties (eye and ear drops); $Na_2B_4O_7$ - antiseptic [61 - 65, 358-363].	Inhibition of amylase, proteinase, and adrenaline [64].
Al	Blood, nerve cells in the brain; epithelial and connective tissues; deposition in the brain	$Al(OH)_3$ - absorbent and antacid activity; $Al_2O_3.2SiO_2.2H_2O$ - kaolin, adsorbing action; $Al_2(SO4)_3$ -antimicrobial agent and in H_2O purification [71, 364, 365] $KAl(SO4)_2.12H_2O$ (alum) - hemostatic, antimicrobial action.	Affects mineral metabolism, and inhibits the synthesis of hemoglobin [68, 69]; antidote - Desferrioxamine.

(Table 17) cont.....

Element	Location and Functions in the Body	Drugs	The Toxic Effect, Antidotes
Ga	Stimulates metabolism; anticancer, antibacterial, anti-inflammatory action; mimicry of the ferric ion	Gallium nitrate - used to treat hypercalcemia, Gallium-based compounds - potential in cancer and infection diseases; ^{68}Ga-labelled radiopharmaceuticals - tumor imaging agents; ^{67}Ga scintigraphy for detection of malignant tumors - Hodgkin's and non-Hodgkin's lymphoma [72, 366-382].	Not particularly toxic [72].
In	Stimulates metabolism; Radioactive [111]In - a radiotracer in nuclear medicine for labeling white blood cells and proteins	[111]In is a readily available γ-emitting radionuclide, used in diagnostic imaging for red cells, platelets, and leukocytes; In(III) ion chelated with DTPA and DOTA -utilized in a number of radiopharmaceuticals for prostate cancer and neuroendocrine tumors [383 - 385].	Damages kidneys; low abundance, its influence is insignificant [73, 74].
Tl	Mitochondrial damage and impairs energy production; interfere with K^+ pathways; peripheral nervous system is the most sensitive	The isotope [205]Tl is used for NMR detection. [201]Tl - extensively used in radio-diagnostic imaging (SPECT) for perfusion tests of the myocardium. Thallous ^{201}Tl chloride injection - used in diagnostics of coronary artery disease and heart attack [386 - 388].	Tl - toxic [75]; Antidotes - dialysis and high supplementation with K^+ with $KFe[Fe(CN)_6]$ (Prussian Blue in colloidal form)
C	Organogen, 21,15%	C (carbol) adsorbs gases and toxic compounds; CO_2 - stimulating effect on lungs, for inhalations and baths; $NaHCO_3$ -antacid agent, solutions of $NaHCO_3$ are used for rinses and lotions [78 - 80].	Coal dust - anthracosis; CO_2, CO [78 - 80]; antidote - O_2
Si	Lens of the eye, hair; gives strength, elastic fabric.	Si carbide and Si oxide - in dental medicine, $Al_2(SiO_3)_3$ - white clay - is used as an adsorbing agent in the form of powders, pastes, ointments; Si-containing phthalocyanine - second-generation photosensitizer [82 - 86, 389-393]	SiO_2 dust produces silicosis [83]
Ge	Increases immunity, eliminates harmful toxins, controls pain, shows antitumor activity	Contains in some medicinal plants, Ge supplements - for treating arthritis, and allergies, reducing cholesterol levels, in preventing high blood pressure, and tumors; Bis-2-carboxyethylgermanium sesquioxide (Ge-132) - in the treatment of cancer, burns, hepatitis, and cardiovascular diseases [394 - 399].	Ge compounds have small solubility, low amounts in nature; not toxic to human cells [86].

(Table 17) cont.....

Element	Location and Functions in the Body	Drugs	The Toxic Effect, Antidotes
Sn	Stimulating effect on animals' growth; enters the bloodstream	Photodynamic therapy agent Purlytin for cutaneous basal cell cancer, *Kaposi's sarcoma* in AIDS, and breast metastases in the chest wall [400 - 404].	Tin contents are very low, non-toxic metal; organotin compounds - toxic [89, 90].
Pb	Collects in erythrocytes and dispersed from blood to soft tissues of other organs; contributes to the toxicity of other metals; disturbs the nervous system	Exclusively for external use; $(CH_3COO)(OH)Pb$ - astringent, anti-inflammatory, and germicide activity; PbO- part of lead patch used in inflammatory skin diseases, furunculosis; ^{212}Pb in radioimmunotherapy, radiolabeled compound ^{212}Pb-TCMC-trastuzumab - antitumor activity [405 - 408].	Saturnism [91 - 96]; Pb^{2+} bind SH-groups of proteins, enzymes; Antidote - cysteine, $CaNa_2EDTA$ with dimercaprol.
N	Organogen; 3,1% in proteins, nucleic acids, *etc.* biomolecules.	NH_4OH - 9.5-10.5% solution, irritating action on CNS; NH_4Cl - diuretic agent; $NaNO_2$ - vasodilator; N_2O in inhaled anesthetics, nitroglycerin, and other nitro-vasodilators; ^{13}N - radioisotope used in PET imaging [80, 99, 101, 334, 335, 409-412].	Toxic nitrites cause oxygen deficiency, Methemoglobinemia antidote - methylene blue or ascorbic acid [97, 98].
P	Organogen; 0,95% in ATP, nucleic acids, bone, and dental tissues in the form of $Ca_5(OH)(PO_4)_3$ or $CaCO_3$. $3Ca_3(PO_4)_2.H_2O$	Calcium glycerophosphate - a means of strengthening; ATP -energy production; Zinc phosphate cement - in dental practice for the cementation of inlays, crowns; ^{32}P in therapeutic and diagnostic oncology for detection of malignant tumors, Phosphocol (^{32}P-radiolabelled preparation) for treatment of malignancies and for therapy of cancer-associated effects like fluid build-up in pleura or peritoneum [107, 109, 413].	White P - poisonous; Hyperphosphatemia, connected to chronic kidney disease [110]; antidote - 0,5% solution $CuSO_4$.
As	Brain tissues, muscles, participates in the synthesis of hemoglobin.	As metalorganic compounds - for therapy of sexually transmitted diseases (Salvarsan in combination with Hg and Bi to treat syphilis); As_2O_3 - necrotizing tissue (used in dentistry); Fowler's solution, containing KH_2AsO_3 - restorative agent; AsI_3 - against leprosy; K_3AsO_3 and Na_2HAsO_4 - for anemia, exhaustion, neurasthenia; As_2O_3 - for promyelocytic leukemia [111, 112, 414-420].	As - poisonous, arsenolysis [112 - 115]; As_2O_3 - white arsenic; powerful poison antidotes - Na_2S, MgS, $Na_2S_2O_3$, dimercaprol, DMPS, DMSA.

(Table 17) cont.....

Element	Location and Functions in the Body	Drugs	The Toxic Effect, Antidotes
Sb	As^{3+} and Sb^{3+} ions are synergistic; accumulates in the thyroid gland	Sb compounds earlier played some role in medicine as antiseptics and emetics. Now Sb is considered toxic. Sb sulfide - for the preparation of ointments; organoantimonial compounds - for the treatment of leishmaniases [421 - 425].	Inhibits the function of the thyroid gland, and causes goiter [120, 121].
Bi	Maximum concentration of Bi is found in kidneys; inhibits enzymes amino- and carboxypolipeptidaze	Bi - in products for the face, eyes, lips, and nails; Pepto-Bismol and BisBacter - used to treat temporary discomfort of the stomach and digestive tract, Bi colloids have an antibacterial action; ^{213}Bi - safe radiopharmaceutical in patients with relapsed or refractory AML; Bi_2O_3 - effective at shielding against ionizing radiation such as γ-rays [123 - 125, 426-441].	Nontoxic, no health risk [122], Bi toxicity is reversible; antidotes - compounds with sulfhydryl groups, aromatic OH-groups or phosphonate; D-penicillamine - most effective antidote.
O	Organogen; 62,4%	O_2 and CO_2 - stimulate the respiratory center; hyperbaric oxygenotherapy [22, 129, 132, 442-444].	Hyperoxia, ROS production [128].
S	Organogen; 0,16% in proteins, amino acids such as cysteine, methionine	S - (cleaned) - antimicrobial action ; SO_2 - disinfectant; Na_2SO_4 - weak purgative; S - organic compounds - sulfa drugs (sulfonamides) treat and prevent bacterial infections in humans; H_3C-S--CH_3; well penetrates through biomembranes, anti-inflammatory effect; $Na_2S_2O_3$ -an antidote to cyanide poisoning; Na_2SO_3 and $Na_2S_2O_5$ - stabilizing antioxidants; [154, 155, 445-448].	Asthma-like allergy [154, 155]; SO_2 - irritates mucous membranes of the pulmonary tract and eyes; H_2S is a highly toxic gas.
Se	Essential in small amounts for normal development, growth, and metabolism; found in selenoproteins; cancer-preventing	Selenium compounds protect against poisoning with As, Hg and Cd [162]; part of mineral-vitamin complexes; Selenomethionine and Se-methyl-sele-o-L-cysteine - for chemoprotective treatment of prostate cancer [449 - 451].	Selenosis [164]; toxic effect of selenites and selenates.
Te	Tellurium is constantly found in the human body; its biological role is not clear	Tellurium compounds (AS101) - in chemotherapy of AML, anti-inflammatory, anti-apoptotic, anti-HIV, ROS-related applications [168, 452-454].	Te and its volatile compounds - toxic for glutathione metabolism [167, 168].

(Table 17) cont.....

Element	Location and Functions in the Body	Drugs	The Toxic Effect, Antidotes
F	Bone and dental tissue $Ca_5(PO_4)_3F$	NaF, KF - sedatives; NaF - to treat increased caries, in toothpastes; ^{18}F labelled deoxyglucose - tracer for PET imaging in glucose metabolism; ^{18}F-fluorodeoxyglucose-PET (^{18}F-FDG-PET) - for screening, localization, and monitoring of malignancies, infections, autoimmune processes [169, 170, 455, 456].	Excess fluoride causes fluorosis or speckled enamel [170].
Cl	In the gastric juice, extracellular anion	HCl - 8,2-8,3% - in cases of low gastric juice acidity; NaCl - 0,9% solution for blood substitution; $CaCl_2$ + $Ca(OCl)_2$, chloramine - disinfectants; HClO - bleaching agent; $KClO_4$ - protection of the thyroid gland at functional inspection by radioiodine-based compounds [28, 33, 173, 174, 457].	Cl_2 - gas, irritating to the mucous; irritates the respiratory system, skin, and eyes [174, 175].
Br	Pituitary gland, kidney, supports the functions of inhibition of CNS; the sedative effect	NaBr, KBr, NH_4Br - sedatives and anticonvulsants, for the treatment of epilepsy [175, 458].	Br_2 vapors - toxic; accumulation of Br^- leads to chronic poisoning "bromism" [175].
I	Thyroid gland (a hormone thyroxine); ^{131}I radionuclide - risk of cancer of the thyroid; iodine tablets block the acceptance of radioactive iodine	I_2 - 5%, 10% alcohol solutions - disinfectant; I_2 + aqueous solution of KI - Lugol's solution - lubricates the mucous membrane of the pharynx and larynx; radioactive isotopes ^{131}I, ^{132}I, ^{125}I - for treatment and diagnosis of thyroid diseases, Na^+/I^- symporter (NIS) - role in I_2 metabolism and thyroid control [176 - 181, 459, 460].	Iodine overload is less common than its deficiency; it is rapidly excreted with urine; I_2 is poisonous; Goiter and thyrotoxicosis [176].
At	Astatine consists only of short-lived radioactive isotopes; accumulates in the thyroid gland, spleen, and lungs	^{221}At, ^{222}At, ^{223}At are α-emitters; Astatine-211 for targeted α-particle therapy in oncology [182, 183, 461-464].	Effects similar to iodine [182, 183].

where: dimercaprol - 2,3-dimercapto-1-propanol, DMPS - 2,3-dimercapto-1-propanesulfonic acid), DMSA - 2,3-dimercaptosuccinic acid

CHAPTER 5

Application of d- and f- Block Elements and Their Compounds in Medicine

THE USE OF D-ELEMENTS AND THEIR COMPOUNDS IN MEDICINE

The Medical and Biological Significance of d-elements of the IB Group

Copper

The therapeutic use of copper, silver, and gold was discovered in the earliest in the field of medicine to treat syphilis and other disease conditions. Copper is an important trace element necessary for the normal functioning of organisms [195]. Complex compounds of copper(II) with bioligands are involved in many metabolic processes, especially in redox reactions.

Compounds of copper are extensively used in medical practice as medicines. Of the copper compounds in medicine, copper(II) sulfate pentahydrate $CuSO_4 \cdot 5H_2O$ has an antimicrobial effect. It is used as an astringent and antiseptic externally in the form of solutions (dilute solution for lubricating the burning surface of the skin, eye drops). The 5% solution of $CuSO_4$ is used to treat white phosphorus burns. Copper sulfate is included in vitamin-mineral complexes as a source of trace element copper [195 - 199]. $CuSO_4.5H_2O$ is used as a fungicide and for the extermination of certain algae. The diluted solution of copper(II) sulfate (2% solution) may be used internally as an antidote for rare white P intoxication or burns because it transforms P into insoluble Cu(II) phosphide Cu_3P_2. Cu(II) sulfate is used for the preparation of the Benedict reagent containing Cu^{2+}-chelate and used for the analysis of compounds, which reduce the Cu(II) chelate to insoluble Cu(I) oxide Cu_2O or copper(I) hydroxide CuOH. Copper is an integral component of the filling material "Hallodent M" and a liquid (an alloy of gallium and tin) for the manufacture of metal fillings. Cu(I) and Cu(II) oxides are parts of microbicidal phosphate cement used as filling materials. Glass ionomeric cement is a "powder-liquid" system. Glass ionomeric cement are used for dental restoration.

Copper coordination compounds are currently found to exhibit antineoplastic activity with a different mechanism of action compared to that of Pt(II) complexes

[475]. Additionally, there are many reports on the SOD-mimic, anti-Alzheimer's, antioxidant, anti-inflammatory, antifungal, *etc.* properties of copper(II) complexes [476].

Silver

The biological role of silver has not been completely established. It is classified as a potentially toxic element with a suspected carcinogenicity. Excessive amounts of silver that enter the human body are deposited in the subepithelial layers of the skin, causing the appearance of gray and brown spots (argyrosis). It has been proven that both Ag and its compounds have antibacterial effects that havee been used for water disinfection and wound management [477 - 480].

All medications of silver used in medical practice are preparations for external use, based on its binding, cauterizing, and antibacterial properties. Between its inorganic compounds, silver nitrate $AgNO_3$ is extensively used for these purposes. In small concentrations, silver nitrate has an astringent, antiseptic, and anti-inflammatory effect, and in concentrated solutions, it cauterizes tissues. It was employed in the treatment of ulcers and Ag(I) cations were recognized as antimicrobic agents [477 - 479]. For preventive purposes, $AgNO_3$ (lapis) can be dropped into the eyes of newborns to prevent inflammation caused by gonococci. Ag(I) nitrate has an astringent and anti-inflammatory effect. Externally, it is used in the form of 1-10% of solutions or ointments, and internally as 0.05% solution to treat stomach ulcers and gastritis. Silver nitrate is used in pediatric dentistry for conservative treatment of caries in children. An ammonia solution of silver oxide, obtained from silver nitrate, and a 10% formalin interact. The chemistry of this process can be expressed as follows:

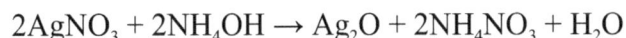

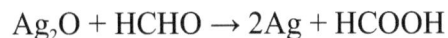

$$2AgNO_3 + 2NH_4OH \rightarrow Ag_2O + 2NH_4NO_3 + H_2O$$

$$Ag_2O + HCHO \rightarrow 2Ag + HCOOH$$

The resulting silver film has a bactericidal effect. Solutions of $AgNO_3$ and $AgCl$ are used to impregnate the dressing materials - paper, cotton wool, and gauze.

In medical practice, along with silver nitrate, colloidal silver preparations are used - collargol and protargol, in which the metal is in solution in the form of the smallest solid particles. Collargol and protargol in the form of aqueous solutions and ointments are used to lubricate the inflamed mucous membranes of the upper respiratory tract, to wash purulent wounds, in eye drops, in erysipelas, *etc.* Silver nitrate in combination with a sulfonamide antibiotic, produces silver sulfadiazine, a local antimicrobial agent for burn treatment [477].

Nowadays many silver-containing medical products are available, as dressings for burn wounds, catheters, wound-care products, and as dental implants. [478]. Silver wound dressings are applied rather than antibiotics due to the development and increase of antibiotic-resistant microorganisms [479]. Ag-based nanoparticles have been assessed as antiviral agents [200, 480]. Alloys of Au, Ag, and Cu in small amounts are widely used in dental practice for prosthetics. Silver is a part of silver-palladium alloys and of powder (an alloy of silver, tin, and copper) used for the manufacture of silver amalgam (AC-2) used in metal fillings. It has to be mentioned that confusion exists over the benefits and hazards associated with silver compounds and alloys.

Gold

For many centuries, it was supposed that gold has medicinal and strong therapeutic value [201, 481-491]. Metallic gold as foil or sand was used as medicine for different diseases in older times. Such elementary Au is relatively ineffective. Alchemists identified that metal Au dissolves in royal water and can be reduced back to Au^0 as a stable colloid (Au ash), the color of which is dependent on the particle sizes and varies from blue to purple. Neutralized solutions "aurum potabile" were extensively used in the Middle Ages, although their actual value is questionable. During the XIX century, gold was called a panacea, a cure for all diseases. The rational use of Au compounds in medical practice dates back to the early XXth century, when microbiologist Robert Koch revealed that $K[Au(CN)_2]$ killed tuberculosis bacteria. Like various other Au(I) complex compounds, $[Au(CN)_2]^-$ contains linear fragments of two-coordinated gold bound to carbon atoms of cyanide ions $[NC-Au-CN]^-$. Complexes of three-coordinated Au(I) and tetrahedral complexes of four-coordinated Au(I) are identified but less studied. Gold(I) belongs to class "b", *i.e.,* to the "soft" ions, thus the most stable compounds should contain heavier bioligands. Thus, P and S are preferable than N and O. Aqua-cation of Au(I) $[Au(H_2O)_x]^+$ is unidentified. Gold(I) stabilizes by π-acceptor ligands. In biosystems, the most favored ligand for gold(I) is the S-atom of thiol (Cys in protein molecules). The attraction of gold(I) to DNA is very small.

Weak gold(I)- gold(I) interactions are often found in the molecules of the gold(I) complexes, which are perpendicular to the axis of linear coordination. The Au-Au bonds are much shorter than the sum of the van der Waals radii. This attraction of Au cations to each other is called "aurophilicity", which may be due to the strong impact of the relativistic effect in Au chemistry (the inner shell electrons, moving at close to the speed of light, cause the shell to contract). Unlike copper, also found in the IB group, Au^{+2}, is not stable. Square planar complexes of Au^{+3} can be easily obtained, but are predisposed to reduction in biosystems (up to Au^+ or Au^0).

Gold compounds can be absorbed by the body and are poisonous in too high amounts. In precise concentrations, they are used for the treatment of tuberculosis and rheumatoid arthritis [201]. In the early XX century in tuberculosis therapy with gold instead of $K[Au(CN)_2]$, the use of less toxic thiolate complexes of Au(I) began. The thiolate ligands RS^- stabilize +1 oxidation state of gold [481]. During the gold decade in 1925−1935 Au compounds, primarily Au(I) cyanide and thiosulfates, were used in the therapy of respiratory tuberculosis. During that time, arthritis has been also thought to be a microbial infection associated with tuberculosis. Numerous Au compounds still in use nowadays have been included into medicine during the early XX century, such as sodium aurothiopropanol sulfonate (Allochrysine, **1**), sodium thiopropanol sulfonate-S-aurate(I) **2**, sodium aurothiosulfate (Sanochrysin, **3**), Myocrisin (sodium thiopropanol sulfonate S-aurate (I)) sodium auro thiomalate (Myochrysine) **4**, aurothio glucose (Aureotan, Solganal **6**), and Auranofin (tetraacetyl-P-D-thioglucoseAu(I) triethylphosphine), **7**, represented in Fig. (**21**). The composition of gold(I) antiarthritic thiolate complexes is defined in the ratio of Au:thiolate of about 1:1, although their structures in solutions are more complicated. Most of thiolate complexes are polymeric. The Au(I) ion should be as a minimum two-coordinated, and the thiolate S-atoms should be bridged to Au(I) cations like -S-Au-S-Au-S-, (**5**), (Fig. **21**). Different linear and ring structures could be produced.

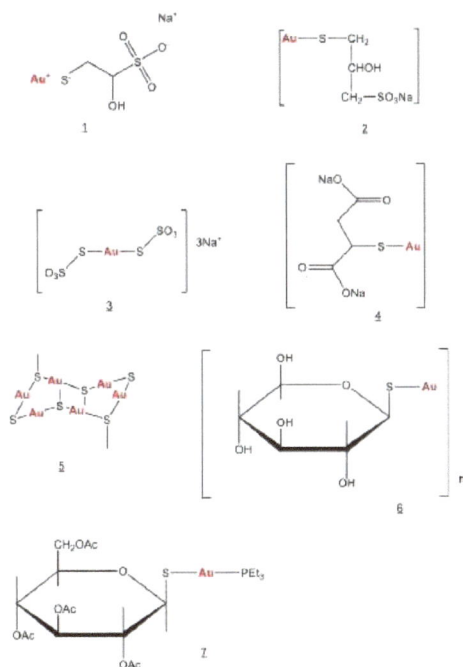

Fig. (21). Gold compounds for the rheumatoid arthritis treatment.

Gold preparations are used in medicine in the form of water-soluble drugs including thiolates like sodium salts of bis(thiosulfo)aurate(I) $Na_3[Au(S_2O_3)_2]$ (Sanocryzine), thiopropanolsulfonate-S-aurate(I) and aurothioglucose (Solganol) for injection in the treatment of chronic arthritis; in the form of suspension in oil aurothiomalate (Myocrizine) or oral Au(I) drugs with phosphine [201, 481]. Sodium salts such as sodium thiopropanol sulfonate-S-aurate(I) and bis(thiosulfate)-sodium aurate(I) are water-soluble drugs administered by injection for the therapy of complicated cases of rheumatoid arthritis. Sodium aurothiomalate (sodium thiopropanol sulfonate-S-aurate(I), Myocrisin), used for its immunosuppressive anti-rheumatic effect, contains intertwined helices. The structure of the compound $[CsNa_2HAu_2\{SCH(CO_2)CH_2(CO_2)\}_2]$ is close to the formula of the drug Myocrysin. The right spirals contain mainly (R)-thiomalate, and the left - (S)-thiomalate.

The first Au substances applied in the therapy of rheumatoid arthritis, are complex compounds with thioglucose-containing ligands, such as aurothioglucose (Solganol, Aureotan). Aurotioglucose contains Au in the oxidation state of +1, like other Au thiolates. It has water solubility with nonionic species having a polymer structure. This drug for rheumatoid arthritis treatment had been in use for more than 70 years, but it was later discontinued along with other gold complexes [201, 481]. A drawback of these Au medications is that they have to be applied through intramuscular injection and thus Au accumulates in organs, mainly in kidneys, causing nephrotoxicity, which results in leakage of proteins and blood in the urine.

All of the mentioned Au(I) complexes are charged, with polymeric structures, and administered as water solution injections into the muscle. A relatively new Au-containing drug that has found extensive usage is auranofin, tetraacetyl-β-D-thioglucose-gold(I)-thioethylphosphine (Crisinor, Crisofin, RidauraTM), which may be administered orally, thus the gold amount in the kidney is significantly less [201, 481]. Its precise mechanism of action is unclear, but it is supposed to work through immuno-mechanisms and by altering the lysosomal enzymatic activity. This drug has received approval from FDA in 1985. It represents a monomeric, neutral coordination complex, containing linear structure with two coordinate Au(I) ions. It is lipophilic and can be applied orally in capsulate forms. Auranofin is a stable complex with a crystalline structure, sparingly soluble in H_2O but with good solubility in organic solutions. Auranofin improves arthritis-associated symptoms including painful swollen joints and typical stiffness. Auranofin finds wide use because at its administration, the gold content in the kidney is significantly fewer.

In spite of the good healing responses of Au drugs in medical therapy, chrysotherapy remains controversial over the years. Gold-containing preparations are "prodrugs" because ligand substitution reactions are easily carried out in Au(I) complexes [201, 481]. These reactions have low activation energies and involve the formation of intermediates of the three-coordinated Au ion. The ligand exchange of thiols is important within the living body. The initial ligands in the gold preparation molecule are cleaved (thiol substitution, displacement, and oxidation of PEt_3 to $OPEt_3$). In blood, most of Au(I) ions are carried with the participation of the thiol group Cys34 of albumin. The gold concentration in the blood can increase to ~ 20-40 μmol/L after injection of the Au drug. The half-life of Au is ≈ 5-31 days, but Au can persist in the human body for years. The main site of gold deposition is lysosomes (aurosomes) associated with the membrane intracellular compartments that contain destructive enzymes. Inhibition of the enzyme that destroys connective tissue may be the cause of the anti-arthritic activity of Au, although the cause of rheumatoid arthritis is not completely clear. Smoking patients who are prescribed treatment with gold-containing drugs achieve a higher concentration of Au in red blood cells than non-smokers. Inhaled tobacco smoke contains HCN, and Au has a high affinity to the cyanide ion. The cyanide ion interacts with the injected Au-containing medication to form particles $[Au(CN)_2]^-$ that easily pass through the cell membranes. Trace amounts of CN^- seem to be always present in the human body (produced from SCN^-), thus $[Au(CN)_2]^-$ is a metabolite of Au-containing drugs even in non-smoking patients, reaching a level of 5-560 nmol/L in the urine. Some of the toxic and adverse effects of Au-containing medicines may be due to the formation of Au(III) [481]. Most Au *in vivo* is present as Au(I). However, strong oxidizing agents, such as HOCl, which oxidizes Au(I) to Au(III), are formed in areas of the inflammatory process. As a result, the leukocytes of the blood of people treated with Au-containing drugs develop sensitivity to Au(III). Additional studies of oxidation-reduction cycles involving Au may lead to clarification of the mechanisms of these adverse effects.

There is also attention given to the possible use of Au compounds to treat asthma, the autoimmune disease pemphigus (a chronic disease, sometimes fatal), cancer, malaria, and AIDS [482 - 491]. Gold cyanide $[Au(CN)_2]^-$, a natural metabolite of Au anti-arthritic medications, inhibits the spread of HIV in white blood cell cultures at small concentrations (20 nmol/L) and can be used to treat AIDS, combined with other medications. The detected concentration of $[Au(CN)_2]^-$ is equal to that found in the blood of patients treated with Au-containing anti-arthritic drugs.

Chrysotherapy studies in the field of oncology have been continuing for the last few decades. Nowadays, this is a likely treatment option and a good alternative to

Pt-based therapy and its frequent disadvantages in regard to the severe adverse effects and cell resistance [482 - 491]. Au(I) and Au(III) complexes, the last isostructural and isoelectronic with Pt(II) complexes, are hypothetically attractive as anti neoplastic agents. Au (III) cation typically produces square- planar complexes in solution due to its similarity with the isoelectronic Pt(II)-d^8 system. Square-planar geometry, less typical in biological systems, is found for d^8 transition metals, specifically for Au(III), Ir(I), Pd(II), Pt(II), and Ni(II) ions in strong ligand fields. Since the square-planar geometry of Pt(II) is significant for its activity as an antitumor drug, Au(III) complexes can definitely be used for the same purposes with the supplementary advantage of their reduced toxicity. However, gold(III) complexes are strong oxidizing agents, being easily reduced to gold(I) or even to gold(0). Gold(III) cation is also more polarizing than Pt(II) ion. Studies of the gold(III) complexes interactions with DNA, the usual target for Pt(II) complexes, indicated that the binding of Au(III) compounds to nucleic acids is not as tight as the binding of Pt(II) drugs, signifying the existence of a dissimilar mechanism for the detected bioeffects, however, the reported data remain very scarce, perhaps as a result of the high chemical activity of Au(III) complexes. It is known that compared to Pt-based medications, complexes with Au tend to be less poisonous. Au complexes as anticancer agents tend to target proteins and enzymes bearing thiol groups, particularly thioredoxin reductase (TrxR). Similarly with Ru and Ga, investigations of new Au coordination complexes with cytotoxic properties are driven by the different deficiencies of modern Pt therapies.

Gold(I) and gold(III) antitumor agents are represented in Fig. (**22**). Tetrahedral bis(diphosphine) complexes of gold(I), such as [Au(dppe)$_2$]$^+$, **1**, (dppe - 1,2-diphenylphosphinoethane), are active against numerous tumor cell lines and kill the cells by damaging mitochondrial function. The ligand bis (di phenyl phosphine) ethane (DPPE) and its Au (III) coordination compounds have shown anti cancer action in transplantable cancer models, as well. Their usage in clinics is not presently allowed because of their cardiotoxicity. Nevertheless, this difficulty can be resolved by a selection of phosphine substituents and by regulating the cation lipophilicity. A gold(I) complex which has monophosphine and diphosphine ligands, **2**, showed high cytotoxicity against several cancer cell lines with IC$_{50}$ values within the micromolar ranges. Gold(I) complexes possessing cytotoxic activity have been widely studied during the last years [485 - 491].

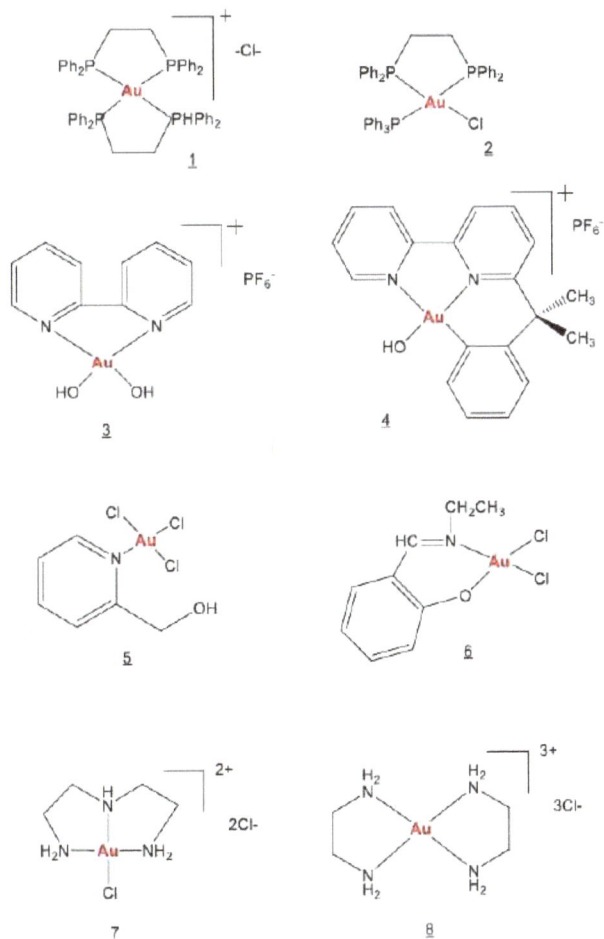

Fig. (22). Gold compounds for the treatment of cancer.

Gold(III) complex compounds have commonly exhibited attractive cytotoxic and anticancer effects, but up to now, their progress has been seriously disadvantaged by their low stability under biological conditions because of their higher ligand exchange rates and higher reduction potential values [483]. However, some Au(III) complexes with organic ligands are stable in relation to reducing agents and show anti tumor activity. Gold (III) complex compounds with multi dentate biologically active ligands, for instance, en (ethylene diamine), dien (di ethylene diamine), and damp (N- benzyl-N, N- dimethylamine) have been identified to be effective against different tumor cells. Numerous Au(III) complexes with bis-pyridyls have been indicated to be hypothetically useful in anticancer therapy, creating new interest in the research of Au(III) interaction with DNA or its components, with regard to the binding sites, the structures, and the stability of studied complexes. The *in vitro* study of their cytotoxicity has demonstrated activity of gold(III) complexes with [Au(bipy)(OH)$_2$]PF$_6$, **3**, and [Au(bipy-H)(OH)]PF$_6$ (bipy = 6-(1,1-dimethylbenzyl)-2,2'-bipyridine), **4**. The cytotoxicity of the representative square-planar Au(III) complexes trichloro(2-pyridylmethanol) gold(III) [AuCl$_3$(Hpm)], **5**; dichloro(*N*-ethylsalicylaldiminato) gold(III) [AuCl$_2$(esal)], **6**; trichlorodiethylendiamine gold(III) [AuCl(dien)]Cl$_2$, **7**, and trichlorobisethylendiamine gold(III) [Au(en)$_2$]Cl$_3$, **8**, (Fig. 2), has been estimated *in vitro* against A2780 human ovarian tumor cells. Notably, all these Au(III) complexes displayed substantial cytotoxic activity, [AuCl$_2$(esal)] demonstrating effectiveness comparable to cisplatin. These Au(III) complexes were able to overcome the resistance to cisplatin to a large degree [481 - 484].

Many Au cytotoxic complexes, such as halo- and pseudohalo- Au(I) complexes with 4,5-diarylimidazoles, gold(I)-N-heterocyclic carbene complexes, NHC-gold(I)-thione complexes, alkynyl-gold complexes, phenanthrene-ethynyl gold(I)-phosphine complexes, *etc.,* (Fig. **23**) have been studied in last decades for their antineoplastic activity [485 - 487].

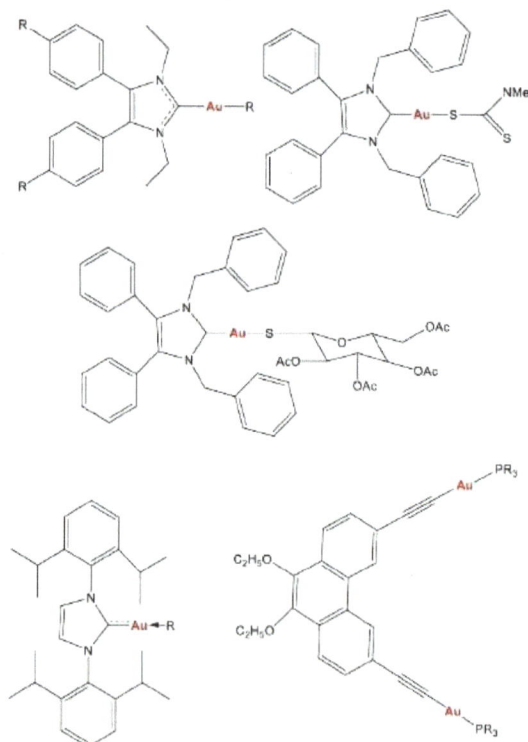

Fig. (23). Recently synthesized gold compounds.

It may be determined that there are numerous results demonstrating that Au(I) and Au(III) coordination complexes may be developed into upcoming medications, but it should be a long time before their pharmacological potential could be explored and applied. It would take longer to find suitable candidates to turn into clinically acceptable drugs [481 - 491].

Some gold alloys with copper and silver are used in dental prosthetics. An alloy, containing 91.6% Au, 4.2% Cu, and 4.2% Ag, is used for the manufacture of bridges, crowns, inlays, half-crowns, and facets. Radioactive gold [198]Au is used to treat malignant tumors. The short half-life of radioactive gold (2.69 days) allows the drug to be injected into the body without its subsequent extraction [489].

Biomedical Significance of d-elements of the IIB Group

Zinc

Zinc, a unique trace element, is a part of the active centers of enzymes that catalyze hydrolysis reactions, oxidation reduction reactions, group transfer reactions, condensation, and isomerization reactions [202 - 206]. The property of zinc to participate in the processes of forming complexes with bioorganic molecules explains why it is widely available in different biological systems. In addition to the catalytic function, zinc also performs a structural function (stabilizes the tertiary structure of the proteins) and a regulatory function. Zinc plays a significant role in the work of the genetic apparatus of the cell, as it is part of the DNA and RNA polymerases, and stabilizes the structure of DNA and RNA. Therefore, zinc deficiency states are a serious problem for the body, including an increased frequency of apoptosis events in tissues [205, 492]. Zinc preparations are used for the prevention and therapy of such conditions. For the prevention and treatment of zinc deficiency states, zinc sulfate, zinc gluconate, and zinc aspartate are used for oral administration. Zinc sulfate is included in the composition of mineral-vitamin complexes as a source of zinc.

In medical practice, ZnO oxide with moderate anti-inflammatory effect and zinc sulfate $ZnSO_4 \cdot 7H_2O$ are used topically as antiseptic, astringent, and drying agents for external use. Zinc sulfate $ZnSO_4 \cdot 7H_2O$ is prescribed in the form of solutions and eye drops with mild antiseptic and astringent effects (0.1 - 0.25%) in ophthalmology. Zinc oxide is used in the composition of various powders, ointments, pastes for skin diseases, liniments, and suppositories.

Anhydrous zinc sulfate is used as a temporary filling material in cement (Vynoxol, Dentin). In dental practice, the mixture of H_3PO_4 with ZnO is used as zinc phosphate cement for filling. $ZnCl_2$ is added into infusions in parenteral nutrition. A suspension of zinc insulin, consisting of zinc chloride and insulin, is used for injections in diabetes mellitus and other complications [203, 205].

Mercury

Although mercury and its compounds are extremely toxic, many of them have been used in medicine [493]. Mercury was applied for centuries both as a medication and a toxin and is still used for many profitable purposes. In the past, mercury was used to treat syphilis (the use of mercury therapy continued into the early 20th century), as an antibiotic and was the active constituent in many therapeutics like antiseptics, diuretics, analgesics, and laxatives. Nowadays, the use of Hg and its compounds in therapy is decreasing. Mercury(II) oxide is used in the form of an ointment for the treatment of skin diseases. Mercury(II) chloride $HgCl_2$ (Sublimate) is highly toxic and a lot of care should be taken when working with it. It is still used as an antiseptic for wounds in some countries. It was used in large amounts during the World Wars. Sublimate was also used for preserving wood. Solutions of $HgCl_2$ in a dilution of 1: 1000 are used to disinfect linen, patient care items, premises, and medical instruments. Due to their high toxicity, the use of mercury, its compounds, pharmaceutical formulations, and products (Hg-based skin lightening soap, cream, powder) in medicine has been severely limited and forbidden, or limited in technologically advanced and many other countries so as to reduce anthropological exposures.

In medicine, not only compounds are used, but also mercury itself and its vapors (mercury thermometers, and mercury manometers in devices for measuring blood pressure) [493]. Thermometers contain the less toxic metal form of mercury and have almost never been a safety problem. In hospitals and physiotherapy rooms of polyclinics, ultraviolet rays obtained from mercury-quartz lamps deeply warm tissues, have a detrimental effect on many microorganisms.

The greatest danger is actually posed by organomercury compounds [494]. Inorganic compounds of mercury under the action of enzymes of microorganisms turn into the ion methylmercury CH_3Hg^+. Methylmercury compounds are soluble in fats (lipids) and, therefore, easily penetrate cell membranes, accumulate in the body, and ultimately cause irreversible destruction in the body and death. Organomercury compounds, like methylmercury (CH_3-Hg^+ X^-) and di methyl mercury (CH_3 -Hg- CH_3), are reserved by the body much more powerfully than the simple Hg substances. Inorganic mercury compounds can be also easily converted by marine bacteria to organomercury compounds. Such substances, predominantly CH_3HgSCH_3, can be absorbed by the fatty tissue of fish, and then pass to humans at consummation. Another major danger is organomercury fungicides.

Certain Hg compounds are active germicide agents such as aryl complexes of Hg(II). Bacteriological resistance to Hg(II) compounds is well clarified. In bacteria, with the participation of lyase enzymes, organomercury compounds are desarylated, and the resulting Hg(II) ion is reduced to Hg^0 by the enzyme mercury reductase. Resistant microorganisms produce these enzymes and a number of other proteins, that capture Hg on their cell membranes, and transport it to reductase. DNA-binding Hg-sensory proteins switch from a repressor to a transcription activator when bound to Hg(II). The organomercury compound ethylmercury thiosalicylate (Thimerosal, Thiomersal), (Fig. **24**), possesses antiseptic and antifungal properties. In the mid-twentieth century this compound was generally used as an antimicrobic vaccine preservative to prevent side effects such as *Staphylococcus* infections without reducing the potency of the vaccines. Research studies comparing ethylmercury and methylmercury have suggested that they are processed in a different way in the human body [494]. Ethylmercury is excreted more quickly than methylmercury. Hence, ethylmercury is significantly less probable than methylmercury to be accumulated in the human body and to cause damage. Thiomersal, used for vaccine preserving, should be refrained from the administration of children.

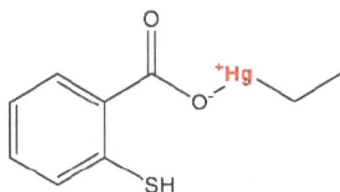

Fig. (24). Ethylmercury thiosalicylate (Thimerosal, Thiomersal).

The ethylmercuri-thio ion of Thiomersal can bind easily to thiol-groups in proteins blocking their enzyme action [494]. The numerous applications of Hg and its strong neurotoxicity have been controversial for decades and debate on the use of Hg for medical purposes continues.

In dental practice, amalgams (Hg, Cu, Ag, Cd, *etc.*) are utilized as filling materials [493]. These amalgams soften readily when heated, and at physiological temperature, they become solid to form a solid filling. The predisposition of Hg to form amalgams has long been used in dentistry. Dental amalgam fillings are about 40% Hg by weight. Typically, amalgams for dental fillings can be composed of 52% Hg, 35% Ag, and 13% Sn. It can be prepared by stirring an Ag-Sn alloy into Hg. The health problems caused by dental amalgams have been widely discussed. Hg in solid state vaporizes at a slow rate, but this can be increased with increasing the temperature, for instance, with the consumption of hot drinks and food. Filling of teeth with amalgams is unacceptable if there are gold crowns in the oral cavity nearby. The fact is that gold is easier to form an amalgam, and therefore the presence of an amalgam filling can quickly lead to the destruction of the golden crown.

Medical and Biological Significance of d-elements of IIIB Group

Scandium

Scandium has attracted the attention of researchers and nuclear physicians, due to the existence of matched radionuclides for the possibility of theranostic applications. Radioisotopes of scandium have potential in PET and SPECT imaging, and in radiotherapy, especially ^{44}Sc and ^{47}Sc, which display suitable characteristics for diagnostic or therapeutic purposes [218, 495]. When combined ^{44}Sc and ^{47}Sc can be used for theragnostic applications. The radioisotope ^{44}Sc is an applicant for PET imaging with radio-metallated peptides or some small targeting biologically active molecules, like DOTA-functionalized biomolecules. The isotope ^{44}Sc can be a beneficial radioactive isotope for medical nuclear imaging and preclinical therapeutic dosimetry before treatment with the healing ^{177}Lu labelled DOTA derivatives. The radioisotope ^{47}Sc is a beta-emitter having the potential as a therapeutic radioactive nuclide and in combination with ^{44}Sc could permit the use of matching radio-drugs with the same pharmacokinetic characteristics. The application of ^{43}Sc and ^{44}Sc ($T_{1/2}$ = 3.9 h and 4.0 h, respectively) for PET is beneficial with regard to several aspects over longer periods when comparing it to the commonly employed ^{68}Ga ($T_{1/2}$ = 68 min).

Yttrium

In medical practice, Y-based substances are used in therapeutic lasers and medical implants. This is extended by the arrangement of accessible Y radioisotopes to allow roles for ^{90}Y complex compounds as radiopharmaceutical drugs and ^{86}Y tracers for PET imaging [496]. Yttrium is not among the essential elements, but is used clinically in anticancer therapy as the radionuclide ^{90}Y, which is a pure beta-emitter lacking gamma photons. ^{90}Y can be produced by the nuclear decay of ^{90}Sr ($T_{1/2}$ = 29 y) which is a fission product of U. Yttrium-90 decays because of the emission of beta-particles ($T_{1/2}$ = 2.67 d), making it susceptible to various targeted radiotherapy applications including ^{90}Y-labeled colloid, tumor-targeting antibodies, somatostatin-receptor targeting peptides, and resin/glass microspheres for catheter-directed embolization of hepatic malignancy and metastases. It is useful for metabolic radiotherapy, for instance, non-Hodgkin B-cell lymphoma radiotherapy and immunotherapy. It can be delivered to cells as strongly chelated complexes. In the form of microspheres, it is suitable for selective arterial injection. The radioactive isotope ^{90}Y is inserted into tiny particles and used to deliver a high dose of radiation directly to tumors *via* long, thin catheters.

Yttrium-90 radiotherapy is harmless and well-tolerated. It is also helpful in preserving healthy tissue, as the radiation releases close to the tumor. The radionuclide [86]Y, which decays by electron capture, plays a corresponding role to ^{90}Y for PET imaging of the *in vivo* biological distribution and dosimetry of ^{90}Y pharmacotherapeutics. The isotope yttrium-89 is naturally occurring and is quite stable. Yttrium-76 through 88 and yttrium-90 through 107 are artificially produced and are radioactive.

Medical and Biological Significance of d-elements of IVB and VB Groups

Titanium

Titanium is used in prosthetics because it doesn't react with the body tissues. It is recognized in medicine as a light and strong metal, suitable for implants [230, 497]. Ti compounds, patented as fodder supplements, are claimed to expand weight gain in domestic animals.

Titanium is used for the synthesis of anticancer complexes and nanomaterials, some of which have been approved by clinical trials [15, 498]. Titanium(IV) complexes were one of the first classes of metal complexes to enter clinical trials after Pt anticancer complexes. Budotitane (Fig. **25**) and titanocene dichloride exhibit antitumor activity with small toxicity in many tumor cells.

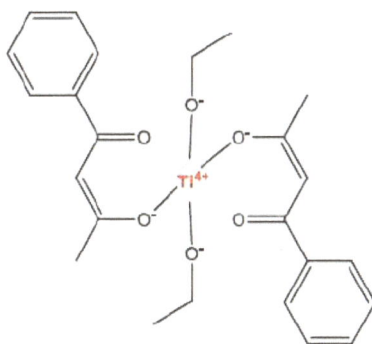

Fig. (25). The structure of Budotitane.

The clinical trials of these complexes started in the 1980s have been finally abandoned because of their low stability in water solutions. Thereafter, new Ti(IV) compounds have been designed with the purpose of overcoming this low stability. Between these, titanocene derivatives and titanium salan compounds have shown potential [498, 499]. The Ti complexes Ti-Salan and titanocene-Y exhibit contrasting behavior concerning their interactions with DNA and albumin, cellular uptake, and intracellular circulation. Ti-Salan demonstrates comparatively low binding to biological molecules but increased serum-dependent cellular uptake while titanocene-Y displays lower cellular accumulation and high binding to albumin and DNA. Biodistribution data have indicated that for titanocene-Y the transport into nuclei and DNA reactions are critical whereas mitochondrial targeting is significant for Ti-Salan.

The success of cisplatin has encouraged scientists to search for similar metal complexes containing reactive Cl⁻ ions as ligands in the cis-position. The metallocene dihalides (Fig. **26**) are a class of small, hydrophobic antineoplastic agents that exhibit activity against many tumor cells such as leukemias P388 and L1210, B16 melanoma, colon 38, and Lewis lung carcinomas, solid and fluid Ehrlich ascites tumors, and several human colon and lung carcinomas [15].

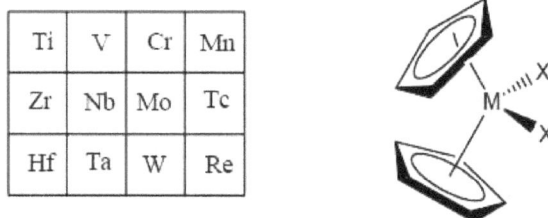

Ti	V	Cr	Mn
Zr	Nb	Mo	Tc
Hf	Ta	W	Re

Fig. (26). Structures of antitumor metallocene dihalides.

The antitumor activity of metallocene complexes $[MCp_2Cl_2]$ depends on the nature of the metal: complexes with M = Ti, V, Nb, Mo are active, but complexes with M = Ta and W show insignificant activity, and with M = Zr and Hf are not active. Variations of the halide ligands have been widely studied for titanocene dichloride. The halides do not appear to affect expressively the antitumor activity, and in the series, Cp_2TiX_2 correspondingly strong tumor inhibition was shown for various halide and diacido ligands. Partial studies have been performed on the substitution of Cp ligands, and all the studies up to now have been restricted to titanocene [498].

Titanocene and vanadocene dichlorides have exhibited the best action against lung, breast, and gastrointestinal cancers *in vivo*, but these findings have not yet been confirmed by clinical trials. Complexes $[MCp_2Cl_2]$ in water undergo rapid hydrolysis [499]. These compounds have distorted tetrahedral structures where two Cp ligands and two halide- or acido- ligands (X) are coordinated to the metal in +4 oxidation state. The two Cp rings with delocalized negative charges are bonded to the metal center in a bent sandwich configuration.

The titanium complex titanocene dichloride (MTK4) is the most extensively studied between metallocenes. It has shown antineoplastic activity and was the first non-Pt complex to undergo clinical trials as a chemotherapeutics. Clinical trials have been conducted for the tetrahedral organometallic complex Ti(IV)-titanocene dichloride $[TiCp_2Cl_2]$ (Cp - cyclopentadienyl). However, the detected hepatotoxicity and gastrointestinal toxicity did not allow the use of the required doses. The dissociation reaction of the first ligand Cl^- from $[TiCp_2Cl_2]$ is too fast to measure its rate, and the half-life of the intermediate containing the second ligand Cl^- is around 45 min. The ion $[TiCp_2(H_2O)_2]^{2+}$ is an acid. It remains unclear whether DNA is the main target for Ti(IV). The binding of Ti to N atoms in DNA bases seems to be weak at neutral pH, though the stability of such complexes increases at low pH values. Phosphate groups may be preferred ligands for Ti. Binding proteins may also play a significant role. It is assumed that the Ti(IV) ion binds to Fe(III)-transport protein transferrin and thus is involved in the biochemical processes of iron transport [498, 499]. In addition to antineoplastic activity, titanocene dichloride exhibits anti-inflammatory, antiviral, and insecticidal actions.

Titanocenes and vanadocenes inhibit DNA and RNA synthesis and Ti and V accumulate in nucleic acid-rich parts of cancer cells. Nevertheless, in contrast to the known Pt-based antineoplastic drugs, their active species responsible for antitumor action *in vivo* has not been determined and the mechanism remains not clear. Moreover, the studies of the hydrolysis processes, stability at different pH and the interactions with nucleic acids have established that each of the metallocene representatives has its own mechanism of functions depending on the respective metal center. Most studies have focused on $[TiCp_2Cl_2]$ and a few studies have discussed the other complexes of this series [498, 499].

The titanocene derivative of tamoxifen (Fig. **27**) with anticancer activity, revealed an unpredicted proliferative action on the estrogen-dependent tumor cells MCF7, derived from a breast cancer line holding ER+ [498]. Similar effects were detected with Cp_2TiCl_2 alone. Resistance to tamoxifen treatment, encountered in many breast cancers, remains the most important problem.

Zirconium

Use of Zr for biological and medical purposes is progressively rising, especially in dental implants, whole knee and hip replacements, and surgery reconstructing middle-ear ossicular chains. Similar to aluminum(III), zirconium(IV) can form O-bridged complexes with polymeric structures (Zr-O(H)-Zr bridges) and is broadly used in antiperspirants. An illustration is a chloride-, glycine-, hydroxide-substance called aluminum zirconium tetrachlorohydrex gly, used in many deodorant products [500]. It contains a mixture of monomeric and polymeric Al(III) and Zr(IV) complexes with the above ligands. The radionuclide zirconium-89 ($[^{89}Zr]Zr^{4+}$) has found extensive use for positron emission tomography imaging when it is coupled with proteins, antibodies, and nanoparticles.

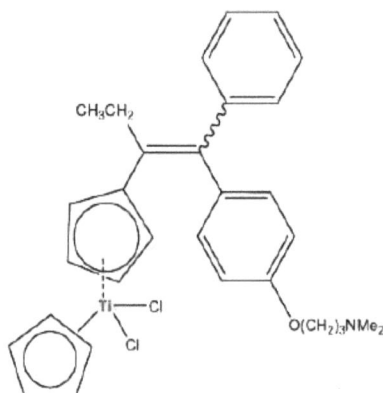

Fig. (27). The structure of titanocene derivative of the anticancer drug tamoxifen.

Hafnium

Hafnium (Hf) is a reactive metal, closely related to titanium (Ti) and zirconium (Zr), used as an implant material for biomedical applications in bone and soft tissue. There is information about the use of functionalized hafnium oxide nanoparticles with negatively charged surfaces (for example NBTXR3). NBTXR3 nano species are taken up by tumor cells and amplify the effects of radiotherapy [501]. NBTXR3 could be used to effectively treat any type of solid tumors, in the cases of sarcomas, and head and neck cancers [502]. Hafnium also is used as a scavenger metal, especially against oxygen and nitrogen.

Vanadium

Though the biological role of vanadium in the human body has not been established up to now, certain interest was given to the research of the healing usages of V complexes. It was revealed that they are involved in the inhibition of cancerous tumor growth or can be applied as insulin-mimetics drugs. Many investigations have demonstrated that V reduces tumor growth and provides anti-cancer protection [225, 228,503]. Different structures of metallocenes and vanadocene complexes are presented in Fig. (8). It is supposed that the vanadium mechanism of anticancer activity includes DNA binding, OS, cellular cycle regulation, and programmed cellular death. More information is obviously needed to fix its specific functions in the human body. Vanadium is a biologically vital element, found in anions and cations, with different oxidation states from +1 to +5. This flexibility provides V complexes with unique characteristics. Particularly, the cation form of V complexes with oxidation state +IV exerts functions in various biosystems by catalyzing ROS generation. In addition to the capability of V metal to adopt several oxidation states, its coordination chemical behavior also plays a crucial role in its reactions with many biological molecules. Principally, organometallic V(IV) complexes with bis(cycopentadienyl) fractions or vanadocenes (Fig. **28**) display *in vitro* and *in vivo* anticancer properties, mainly through oxidative damage. It is likely that the mechanisms of vanadocene-mediated cytotoxic effects are dissimilar from that of titanocenes or other metallocenes. Although the wide investigations on titanocene dichloride have shown certain insights into the mechanism of antitumor action, simultaneously, there is unsatisfactory structure-action information on the other metallocene dihalides, including vanadium complexes, to propose their molecular mechanisms of activity.

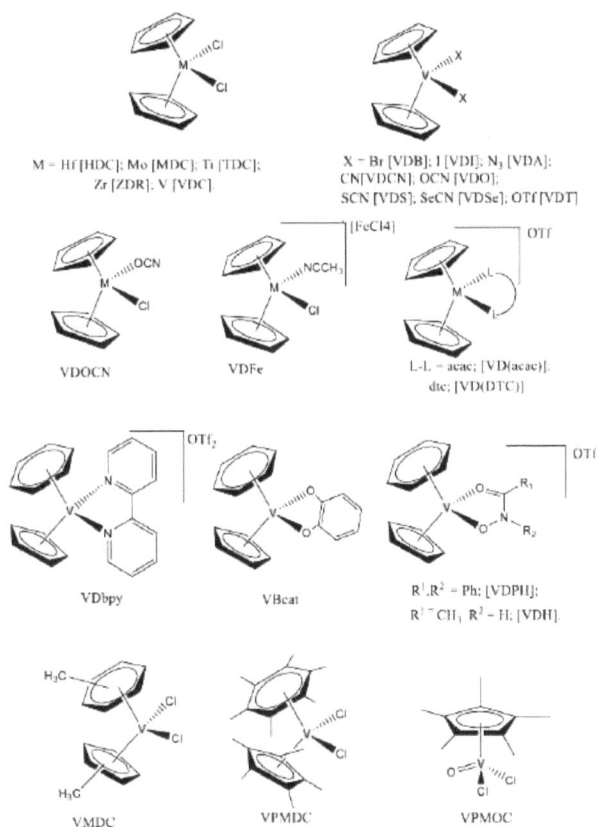

Fig. (28). Vanadocene and other metallocene complexes.

The physiological role of V compounds as insulin-mimetic or insulin-enhancer agents has been widely discussed in the literature [225, 226, 504]. Insulin-like activity incorporates the capability to lower the higher blood glucose amounts *in vivo*. Vanadium arouses the glucose acceptance and the consequent oxidation in glucose-metabolizing cell structures along with the synthesis of glycogen *in vitro*. Additionally, it helps the inhibition of glycolysis and gluconeogenesis, and prevents lipolysis (stimulates lipogenesis). V complex compounds may be used to improve the conditions associated with the deficient insulin response in diabetics. They cannot fully compensate the lack of insulin (type 1 diabetes), but can decrease the dependence on exogenous insulin, or substitute the other oral hypoglycemic agents (type 2 diabetes).

Some V complexes have been posted on clinical trials as antidiabetic candidates [225 - 228, 50, 5]. Much investigations have been described about the complex compound produced by maltol and vanadyl sulfate, bis (maltolato) oxovanadium (IV) (BMOV). BMOV has been reported as a gold standard reference compound. The complex BMOV is easily oxidized *in vivo* to form particles of di-oxovanadium(V). Ligand maltol itself belongs to approved food additives, so that BMOV is currently a common component of dietary supplements. The ethyl-substituted version of maltol, eatol, is used as a ligand for interaction with vanadyl sulfate to form bis(ethyl-maltolato) oxovanadium(IV) (BEOV). BMOV and the ethylmaltol analogue BEOV, depicted in Fig. (**29**), have experienced wide pre-clinical testing for safety and efficiency.

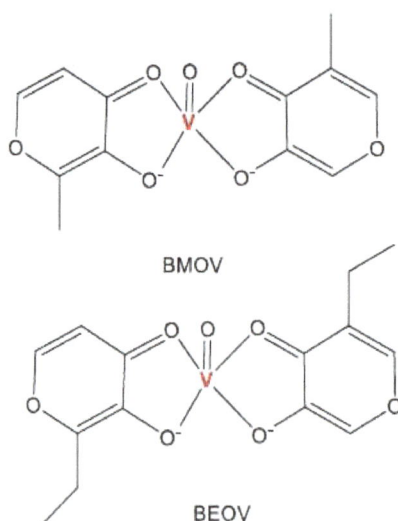

BMOV

BEOV

Fig. (29). Vanadium complexes BMOV and BEOV.

BMOV and BEOV appeared as lead complex compounds, demonstrating improved bioavailability relating to VOSO$_4$ in vivo [225 - 228, 504, 50, 5]. Vanadyl in the form of VOSO$_4$ is not suitable, since due to low oral absorption it must be used in high doses. The insulin-enhancing action of BMOV and BEOV is supposed to originate from the stimulation of the insulin receptors through the inhibition of insulin receptor tyrosine kinase IRTK-associated phosphatases. It is unclear what degree of oxidation of vanadium, V(IV) or V(V) is responsible for the activity of insulin mimetics. Vanadates act as phosphate analogues, and there is reason to believe that they inhibit phosphotyrosine phosphatase. Insulin receptors are single membrane-penetrating tyrosine specific protein kinases triggered by insulin from the outside of the cell for catalysis of intracellular phosphorylation of tyrosine residues. Vanadium is collected in bone and kidney tissues. Vanadium, accumulated in the bones, is then slowly released and transferred to other tissues through the bloodstream, which can provide prolonged activity, and therefore a rare intake of the drug. Challenges with first generation V complexes BMOV and BEOV have been the high doses required to reach the therapeutic effects [225, 231, 504, 505]. Further generation bioligand systems like these in bis((5-hydroxy-4-oxo-4H-pyran-2-yl)methylbenzoatato)oxovanadium (IV) (BBOV) show half the acute oral toxic effects as compared to BMOV. The important developments in VO^{2+} insulin mimetics have encouraged further investigations into the biochemical significance of V complexes predominantly for pharmacological control of malignances and diseases activated by viruses, microorganisms, amebae, and parasites.

Niobium

Niobium and tantalum are transition metals that are almost always found together in nature because they have very similar physical and chemical properties. There have been no reports which suggest their harm to a living body. Niobium is applied in therapeutic practice as implantable medical devices with excellent biocompatibility, pacemakers, since niobium is biologically very inactive and consequently hypoallergenic and safe [229, 506]. There is information about some polyoxometalates comprising Nb(V) which possess potential antiviral activity.

Tantalum

The extremely biologically inert tantalum (both *in vivo* and *in vitro*) has been effectively used in medical practice and has found a wide range of diagnostic and implant applications, with apparently overall excellent results in pacemaker electrodes, cranioplasty plates, and as radiopaque markers. Pure metal and its oxide possess low solubility and toxicity; however, halide compounds are more biologically active. Since the metal is strongly radiopaque because of its atomic number, this characteristic is extensively employed for bone marking in orthopedics and in endovascular medical devices [230, 507]. Additional significant development is the formation of tantalum-based nanoparticles, which are perfect for iodinated contrast agents for blood pool imaging. These properties of tantalum nanoparticles are similar to gold nanoparticles, even though replace gold in x-ray-based imaging.

Medical and Biological Significance of d-elements of VIB and VIIB Groups

Chromium

There is interest in the conceivable therapeutic activity of chromium and its compounds, but their positive effects still remain uncertain [232 - 235]. Chromium is widely used in medical and dental implants, appliances and tools, where sufficient content s of this chemical element can provide a protective corrosion-resistant oxide on the alloy surface. Metallic chromium is a part of cobalt-chromium alloys. In addition to cobalt and chromium (major components), the alloy contains molybdenum and nickel. Chromium and nickel stainless steel is widely used in orthopedic practice. At low concentrations, chromium is used for medical purposes, and it is also involved in natural human lipid and protein metabolism. However, at sufficiently high concentrations particularly hexavalent chromium is toxic and carcinogenic. Chromium(III) tris(picolinate) is used in the treatment of carbohydrate and fat metabolism disorders and is widely used as a constituent in mineral supplements for bodybuilding, although the possible damage to DNA is a great concern [508]. Chromium(III) oxide Cr_2O_3 is a component of dental pastes. Chromium(VI) (in the form of chromate) is known to be a genotoxic carcinogen. The toxicity appears probably to arise from cellular oxidation-reduction interactions which generate Cr(V) 1,2-diolato species, such as carbohydrates, glycoproteins, and sialic acid derivatives, which may lead to oxidative damage to DNA. The chromium(V) complex compounds with several monosaccharides and the ligand cis-1,2-cyclopentanediol provided a suggestion of possible nuclease action [509]. The chromium(V) complexes cause oxidative DNA damage without the occurrence of reducing or oxidizing agents, supporting the contribution of Cr(V) 1,2-diolato compounds in the bioactivity of Cr(VI) and Cr(III) ions.

Molybdenum

Molybdenum is one of the ten essential biogenic metals [236 - 243]. Metal alloys, particularly stainless steel, Co, Mo, Cr alloys, and Ti-based alloys find wide applications in orthopedics for making joint replacement prostheses, systems for external or internal fixation of bone fractures, surgical correction of degenerative conditions, or in the composition of staples, screws, and wires. Apart from the use of molybdenum as alloys and steels, other uses include the application of molybdenum sulfide as a lubricant. Medical applications of low-toxic molybdenum are numerous including avoidance of dental caries, cure of anemia, enhancement of immunological reactions, as antibacterial, antifungal, antiulcer, anticancer, and antidiabetic agents. Molybdenum has an antagonistic action against copper; that is, high concentrations of molybdenum can decrease copper absorption and afterward cause copper deficiency. In medical literature, molybdate anion (MoO_4^{2-}) is described to prevent lipid oxidation and defend antioxidant biosystems *in vivo*, consequently it may be useful for diabetic mellitus therapy. Tetra-thiomolybdate MoS_4^{2-} is a relevant Cu chelator not only for its capability to decrease Cu amounts but also for breast cancer and esophageal carcinoma therapy being in clinical trials [510]. The clinically approved copper chelator ammonium tetra-thiomolybdate, useful in treating Wilson's disease (Cu overload) and Menkes disease (Cu deficiency) has been redeveloped as an anti-cancer agent.

$(NH_4)_2MoO_4$ and Na_2MoO_4, in micro-amounts, can be added to vitamin-based supplements, since Mo(VI) improves the blood phagocytic function [236 - 245]. In therapeutic practice, molybdenum radioactive isotopes are utilized for diagnostic determinations for liver scanning and examination of blood circulation in muscles. The key molybdenum isotopes are ^{95}Mo, ^{96}Mo, ^{98}Mo, and ^{99}Mo, the last being the most commonly used diagnostic medical isotope.

Tungsten

The inorganic salt sodium tungstate (Na_2WO_4) possesses antidiabetic properties [244, 246, 511]. Tungstate ion WO_4^{2-} normalizes glycemia at oral administration without causing hypoglycemic episodes. In primary cultured hepatocytes, Na_2WO_4 behaves in an analogous way to insulin, raising the glycogen synthesis and accumulation. The exact mechanisms of activity of Na_2WO_4 are not clear. In addition, along with its positive effect, Na_2WO_4 has been reported to be toxic and carcinogenic. Therefore, the possible balance between long-term treatment and a higher risk of renal carcinogenesis in diabetics should be considered. Tungsten disulfide (WS_2) nanotubes and nanoparticles are among the most extensively studied, and are used for, *e.g.*, polymer reinforcement, lubrication and electronic devices. Their biocompatibility and low toxicity make them suitable for biomedical applications. One potential application is photothermal therapy (PTT), a method for the targeted treatment of cancer, in which a light-responsive material is irradiated with a laser in the near-IR range.

Polyoxometalates, a type of O-cluster anions formed by transition metals such as V, Nb, Ta, Mo, W in their highest oxidation states, can implement a variety of sizes, shapes, and compositions. This adaptive nature allows their application in many medical fields [512]. Polyoxotungstates in medicine have been studied for their application as antiviral, antimicrobial, and antitumor agents, and for a range of other medicinal applications [513]. Nevertheless, they are not close to a clinical trial or a final application in the treatment of infectious or malignant diseases.

Manganese

Manganese is one of the most important trace elements [247 - 251]. It is part of many enzymes that catalyze redox reactions, reactions involving ATP, *etc.* Manganese enhances the immune response of the body to the action of foreign proteins, accelerating the synthesis of antibodies. That is why, manganese is available in a wide variety of forms, involving manganese salts ($MnSO_4$, $MnCl_2$, gluconate) and manganese chelates such as aspartate, picolinate, fumarate, malate, succinate, citrate, and amino acid chelates. Manganese additives can be taken in the form of tablets or capsules, commonly in combination with other vitamins and minerals such as multivitamins. Manganese has an effect on many metabolic processes, but not all mechanisms of this influence are well understood. In medical practice, potassium permanganate $KMnO_4$ is used in the form of diluted aqueous solutions as an antiseptic for washing wounds, gargling, *etc.* In analytical practice, potassium permanganate is used as an important reagent. A method of quantitative analysis based on titration with a standard solution of potassium permanganate is called permanganatometry.

Mn salts and complexes are investigational ambiguous cancerogenic agents. Manganese(II) ion has numerous characteristics that are valuable for MR, PET, and PET/MR imaging, such as long relaxation time, kinetic lability, high spin number, and fast water exchange. Mn(II) cation is one of the most promising options for gadolinium(III) ion because of its lower thermodynamical stability and kinetic inertness than that of gadolinium(III) or other transition metal ions. This is as a result of the smaller charge of the manganese(II) cation and the minimum ligand-field stabilization energy (d^5 electron configuration) [514].

Several radionuclides of manganese are known for their beneficial properties, for instance, manganese-51, manganese-52m, and manganese-52g, are positron emitters for application in MR, PET, and PET/MR imaging [252, 515]. ^{51}Mn ($T_{1/2}$= 46 min) has a favorable β^+ branching fraction comparable with that of ^{68}Ga ($T_{1/2}$= 68 min), which is suitable for the imaging of fast biological processes. The β^+ energy of ^{52m}Mn is higher than that of ^{51}Mn. In contrast to the manganese-51 and manganese-52m isotopes, the most promising ^{52g}Mn has a convenient long half-life ($T_{1/2}$= 5.6 d), which is advantageous for target separations and chemical handling of the radionuclide. In addition, its half-life is well suited for the investigation of slow biological processes, *e.g.,* the pharmacokinetics of antibodies. For medicinal imaging, the attention is on the long-living manganese-52g and its potent use for radiolabeling of molecules, the imaging of manganese-dependent bioprocesses, and the development of PET/MRI probes in combination with paramagnetic [nat]Mn as a contrast agent. Since [nat]Mn(II) is paramagnetic and PET isotopes of the metal are available, isotopically radiolabeled Mn-based PET/magnetic resonance imaging contrast agents could be interesting candidates with high potential to become new emerging radiometals for applications in nuclear medicine. The chief challenge is the possibility to find appropriate chelators, which could provide Mn(II) complexes of adequate stability and relaxivity. Various approaches towards the progress of these Mn(II) complexes have been widely described [252, 515].

As a hard Lewis acid, the most stable Mn(II) complexes have been obtained with ligands coordinating with Mn(II) through O and N donors. Mn(II) cations form stable complex compounds with EDTA, CDTA, DOTA, their derivatives and other chelators for the coordination of Mn(II). Mn(II) ions in their octahedral high spin complexes own five unpaired electrons, which results in a high paramagnetic moments. That is why Mn(II) complexes obtained with EDTA, CDTA, DOTA, DTPA have been studied as possible magnetic resonance imaging (MRI) contrast agents [516-518] (the molecular structures of EDTA, CDTA, DOTA, DTPA ligands, mentioned in the text, are represented in Fig. (**30**).

Technetium

As members of group VIIB of the periodic table, the elements technetium and rhenium possess a rich coordination chemistry. Technetium is a radioactive element, with no stable isotopes. Technetium-99m is the most extensively used radioisotope in nuclear diagnostic imaging. Its short half-life ($T_{1/2}$= 6 h), easy assimilation into a variety of carrier molecules, low energy γ-emission, and fast excretion make it perfect for obtaining images of the most important internal organs and skeleton of the human body. Technetium-99m is easily generated at the bedside from the long-lived radioisotope molybdenum-99. Many ^{99m}Tc radiopharmaceutical drugs, mainly coordination complexes, are currently in use for imaging of different body organs, including bones, brain, lungs, thyroid gland, myocardium, liver, *etc.* [253, 519]. Modern trends in the radiopharmaceutical chemistry of technetium focus on the 'labeling' of biologically active molecules such as peptides, steroids or other receptor-seeking units. The bioligands play a central role in the targeting functions of the complexes, for instance, phosphate and phosphonate complexes for bones. Bone scanning by means of ^{99m}Tc methylene diphosphonate (^{99m}Tc-MDP) is used to estimate renal osteodystrophy. Methylene diphosphonate adsorbs bones and shows a better affinity to locations of new bone formation [253, 520]. SPECT with ^{99m}Tc-glucoheptonate (^{99m}Tc-GHA) has shown promising results in brain scans for differentiation of recurrent brain tumors from radiation necrosis. Cardiolite (^{99m}Tc-sestamibi) and Neurite (^{99m}Tc-disicate) have been used for folate receptor-positive tumor tissues. ^{99m}Tc-MIP-1404 is used for prostate cancer imaging [253, 521].

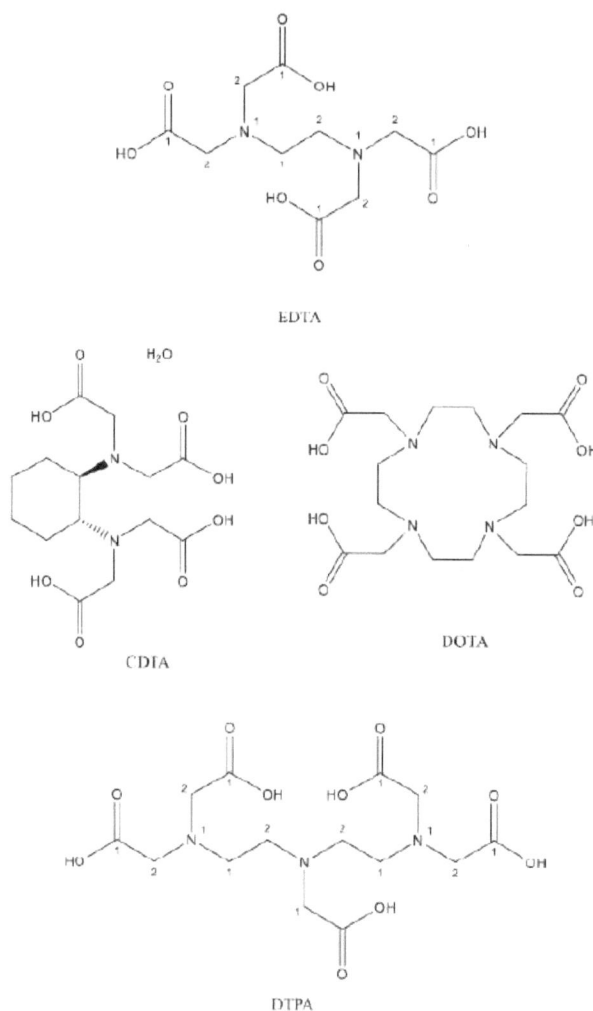

Fig. (30). Structures of the EDTA, CDTA, DOTA, DTPA ligands.

Rhenium

There is a great interest for the application of rhenium in medical diagnostics for imaging determinations based on its radioactive beta-emitter isotopes [186]Re ($T_{1/2}=$ 16.9 h) and [188]Re ($T_{1/2}=$ 89.2 h) that combine diagnosis by radio imaging with conventional γ-cameras with therapeutic actions, allowing an effective energy transfer to cancer tissue. Radioisotopes of rhenium, [188]Re ($\beta-$ emitter) and [186]Re with decay by electron capture and beta−emission, are used in the treatment of malignant cancers, bone metastases, rheumatoid arthritis, *etc.* diseases. Colloidal S-particles labelled with rhenium-186 are used in radiosynovectomy in rheumatoid arthritis therapy and [188]Re-1,1-hydroxyethylidenediphosphonate ([188]Re-HEDP) for bone pain palliation in the cases of prostate cancer [255, 522]. Rhenium radioisotopes have both particle emissions with characteristics appropriate for targeted treatment and photon emissions, that may be used for diagnostic investigation purposes by SPECT. The best studied coordination complexes of technetium and rhenium are those with carbonyl and nitrosyl ligands such as $[M(CO)_3]^+$, $[M(CO)_2(NO)]^{2+}$, which is isoelectronic to $[M(CO)_3]^+$, as well as $[ReCl_2(CO)_2(NO)]_2$ and $[M(CO)_3X_3]^{2-}$ anions (M = Re, Tc; X = Cl, Br). It is clear from the structures that for both metals, substitution of more than one CO ligand was not observed. Further studies with biologically relevant organic ligand systems and chelators (*viz.*, cyclic thioethers, diimines, aminocarboxylic acids, N-heterocyclic carbenes, phenylimido, *etc.*), which are promising for the bifunctional approach, are currently in progress and it is to be expected that this new class of technetium and rhenium compounds will play a role in future radiopharmaceutical research.

Medical and Biological Significance of d-elements of VIIIB Group

Iron

For the prevention and treatment of iron deficiency anemia, as well as with weakness and exhaustion of the body, mainly iron(II) compounds are used, as they are better absorbed by the body [265 - 267]. Both inorganic iron salts and salts of organic acids are used as medicines. The following iron preparations are used in medical practice: ferrous(II) sulfate heptahydrate $FeSO_4 \cdot 7H_2O$ (included in different complex preparations), Fe(II) gluconate, Fe(II) fumarate, Fe(II) chloride, Fe lactate trihydrate $(CH_3CH(OH)COO)_2Fe \cdot 3H_2O$. These preparations may also include other salts of Fe(II) and Fe(III) such as ascorbate, glycerophosphate, citrate, sorbate, and saccharate. Only exceptionally, iron stores in the body can be supplemented by delivering a calculated basic dose of iron parenterally (in the form of Fe(III) compounds).

In medicine, the iron(II)-based compound ferroquine (an organometallic chloroquine-ferrocene conjugate), is utilized for the treatment of malaria [523]. It is supposed to apply its anti-plasmodial activity by reaction with free heme and by the generation of ROS. Complexes, comprising ferrocene and tamoxifen components (ferrocifen and its derivatives), show capacity as potential drugs for breast cancer treatment. Currently, ferrocifen is in pre-clinical trial against cancers [524].

Superparamagnetic Fe oxides composed of nanosized crystals are used as MRI contrast agents with substantial applications in the diagnostics of many diseases like vascular pathological deviations and inflammation conditions apart from malignancies [525].

Sodium nitroprusside, sodium pentacyanonitrosylferrate(III) $Na_2[Fe(CN)_5NO]$, (Fig. **11**), which slowly releases NO, can be prescribed as a hypertensive agent. Sodium nitroprusside is used in infusions acting as a vasodilator agent and as a reagent for detecting the ketone bodies (acetone and acetoacetic acid) in urine used in medical laboratories [334, 335, 526].

Fe excess, as in the genetic disorder thalassemia, can be treated with Fe-chelating agents, for instance, the injectable deferoxamine or deferasirox for oral applications [527].

Cobalt

Preparations containing cobalt are effective anti-anemic agents, such as vitamin B_{12} (cyanocobalamin), hydroxocobalamin, and cobamamide. Vitamin B_{12} is used to treat megaloblastic anemia, dystrophy, and liver disease [268 - 270]. Cobalt is known to mimic hypoxia on the cellular level by stabilizing the α subunit of hypoxia-inducing factor (HIF), when chemically applied as cobalt chloride $CoCl_2$. It has been shown to promote angiogenesis, erythropoiesis and anaerobic metabolism through the transcriptional activation of genes such as vascular endothelial growth factor (VEGF) and erythropoietin (EPO), contributing significantly to the pathophysiology of major categories of disease, such as myocardial, renal and cerebral ischemia, high altitude related maladies and bone defects.

The main application of cobalt is in its metal form in cobalt-based alloys and superalloys in orthopedic implants [528].

Some radioisotopes of cobalt, such as ^{57}Co or ^{60}Co, are used in nuclear medicine applications and in scientific investigations [529]. The radioactive isotope Co-60 is used in radiotherapy as a trace and tumor fighter. Additionally, it is used in studying defects in the absorption of vitamin B_{12}. By the injectable vitamin B_{12}, labeled with radiocobalt, the path of the vitamin through the organism and possible anomalies can be detected. The radioactive isotope of cobalt ^{60}Co is used to diagnose and treat malignant tumors. It is also used for sterilization of medical equipment.

Perhaps unexpectedly, there are some known cobalt-based drugs that provoke bioeffects by protein inhibition, alteration of drug activity, and bio-reductive activation. Cobalt, like other transition metals, can adopt a wide range of coordination numbers, oxidation states, geometries, and ligand binding affinities, that can be used in the design of advanced therapeutics [530]. Up to the present time, the only Co-containing therapeutic agent that has got clinical trials is Doxovir. It is a Co(III) Schiff base complex Co(III) bis(2-methylimidazole), which is effective against drug-resistant herpes simplex virus 1, though its mechanism of action is not quite clear [531].

Currently, the research is concentrated on the potential of cobalt-containing nanoparticles for a theragnostic such as multifaceted imaging signal probes, improved thermo/radiation therapy, microrobots, and drug release [532]. Cobalt ferrite nanoparticles with high coercivity and moderate saturation magnetization are one of the most important materials for nanomedicine. They are a good candidate for hyperthermia and magnetic resonance imaging because of their high relaxivity, anisotropy energy and initial susceptibility.

Biomedical Significance of Platinum Metals

Ruthenium

Among the presently examined metal-containing chemotherapeutics for various cancers, Ru and its complexes have shown promising results because of their different oxidation states and minor toxic effects in comparison with other metal complexes [285, 287, 288, 291 - 293]. Ruthenium complexes are more effective, less noxious, and target-specific non-covalent DNA-binding antineoplastic agents. Ru compounds have the capability to mimic Fe binding to some macromolecules such as serum transferrin and albumin, which makes them perfect applicants for medical purposes. The best benefit of Ru-containing antitumor agents is their efficiency against metastatic processes and their activity against a wide variety of tumor cells. This is a result of their two essential characteristics: Ru agents are activated by the reduction of the Ru(III) core and selectively transported through the transferrin pathway. In fact, the precise mechanism of their action is still indefinable in spite of many research suggestions.

The coordination chemistry of Ru complexes, with consideration of their electron-transfer effects, has received constant attention for the last few years. Ru has various oxidation states ranging from -2 in $[Ru(CO)_4]^{2-}$ to +8 in RuO_4. Consequently, Ru complexes are redox-active giving rise to different chemical applications which makes them attractive objects of study [285, 287, 291-293].

A wide range of Ru-based agents have been obtained and established for their anticancer activity in the past decades, [292] (Fig. **31**). Most of these Ru complexes, regardless of the ligands coordinated to Ru cation, have exposed comparatively low cytotoxic activity and lesser toxicity than cis-platin, respectively requiring higher therapeutic doses. Extensive binding to numerous cellular and extracellular constituents may explain this fact.

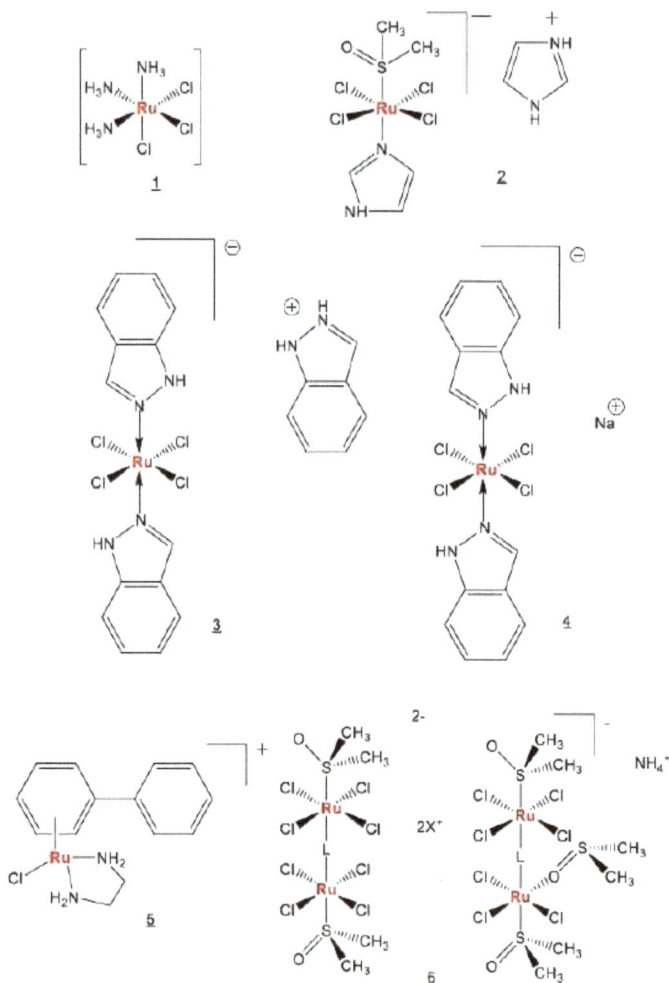

Fig. (31). Structures of ruthenium complexes.

The octahedral Ru(III) complexes like fac-[RuCl$_3$(NH$_3$)$_3$], **1**, have been revealed to possess high anticancer activity, but they have very low solubility for pharmacological use [285 - 288, 291]. Solubility can be improved by increasing the amount of Cl$^-$ ligands. Clinical trials have been conducted for Ru(III) octahedral complex of imidazole (Im) and dmso trans-$[Ru^{+3}Cl_4((CH_3)_2SO)$ (Im)](ImH) (NAMI-A), **2**, with antimetastatic properties. The anticancer agent NAMI-A, imidazolium trans-tetrachloro-(dimethylsulfoxide)imidazole-ruthenate(III) has low toxic effects to primary cancer cells and is capable of stopping the distribution of cancerous cells, meaning metastasis. Some NAMI-A-type mono- and dimeric ruthenium(III) complexes have been found to possess antimetastatic action comparable to that of NAMI-A. In such complexes, the coordination sphere of each ruthenium(III) nucleus is analogous to that of NAMI-A. Particularly, the biochemical features of the next classes of complexes were presented: NAMI-A-type complexes, derived from NAMI-A by changing the N-ligands; dinuclear NAMI-A-type complexes comprising heterocyclic bridge N-N ligands; and Ru-DMSO nitrosyls derived from NAMI-A-type coordination compounds.

The Ru(III) complex, indazolinium-[tetrachloro(bisindazole)ruthenate(III)] (KP1019), **3**, is the second Ru(III) compound in clinical trials. This complex has activity against colon carcinoma and its metastases. The 35-fold better soluble Na^+ salt NKP1339, **4**, is used for the synthesis of KP1019. While NAMI-A shows activity against lung metastasizes *in vivo* and tumor cell invasion *in vitro*, KP1019 is useful for metastatic cancers and cisplatin-resistant tumor cells. It exhibits strong cytotoxic activity against primary tumor cells, predominantly in colorectal malignancy. Though a great number of ruthenium complexes have demonstrated excessive promise as possible anticancer agents, only three of them, NAMI-A, KP1019, and NKP1339, have passed clinical trials with minimal side effects [292, 533]. The indazole complex KP1019, trans -$[RuCl_4 (In)_2]$ InH (its sodium salt is NKP1339) is more toxic to the primary tumor cells than trans -$[RuCl_4 (Im)$ (DMSO)] ImH, NAMI -A, a better antitumor metastasis inhibitor. KP1019 induces apoptosis *via* the intrinsic mitochondrial pathway. Ru(III) ion in the mentioned complexes can be transported to tumor cells by iron(III) transport protein serum transferrin, receptors for which are over-expressed on cancers. When in cells Ru(III) can be activated by the reduction to Ru^{2+}, though Ru^{4+} is also available under physiological conditions.

As with cisplatin, hydrolysis is believed to be the significant mechanism for activating Ru(III) complexes. It is supposed that the second important mechanism of activation of Ru(III) is its reduction to Ru^{2+} [285 - 292]. Tumor cells are often characterized by hypoxia (low concentration of oxygen) and contain reduction agents such as thiols (GSH). Reduction of Ru^{3+} to Ru^{2+} weakens the bonds with π-donor ligands and rises the rate of ligands substitution. For instance, π-acceptors, such as DMSO, can increase the redox potentials (trans-$[Ru(III)Cl_3(dmso)(Im)_2]^-$ instead of trans-$[Ru(III)Cl_4(Im)_2]^-$). Ru(III) and Ru(II) ions bind strongly to DNA bases, preferably to G-N7. Binding to proteins additionally plays a significant role in the mechanism of Ru complexes' action. The acceptance of Ru(III) by cells appears to be mediated by transferrin, a plasma glycoprotein with two Fe(III)-binding centers. Ruthenium(III) can reversibly bind to these active centers, and Ru complexes with transferrin themselves exhibit antitumor activity. Malignant tumor cells have a high content of transferrin receptors on their surface, and rapid cell division requires a high rate of iron uptake. Ru, an analogue of Fe, can thus exhibit a similar type of activity and participate in biochemical processes typical for iron. Targets for Ru can also be the enzymes topoisomerase and matrix metalloproteinases.

Organometallic Ru(II)-arene complexes have attracted rising attention as antitumor compounds with the potential to overcome the disadvantages of known drugs like *cis*-platin with regard to resistance, selectivity, and toxic effects [292]. The stable Ru^{2+} complexes with arenes [(η^6 -arene)Ru(en)Cl]PF_6, **5**, (en= ethylenediamine), have a specific piano-stool geometry exhibiting strong anticancer activity. These complexes contain a reactively capable bond Ru-Cl and in water solutions undergo hydrolysis. They bind to G by coordination with the N7 atom and form hydrogen bonds (en)NH···OC6(G). In addition, arene-purine interactions are observed if the arene molecule is large enough (biphenyl or tetrahydroanthracene). These coordinated arene ligands can thus intercalate into DNA.

An improvement in Pt pharmacological medicine was the multinuclear complexes which highlighted the opportunity to overcome resistance problems, perhaps owing to the improved interchain DNA binding [285]. The search for new anticancer compounds based on ruthenium has brought to the description of a sequence of binuclear ruthenium complexes, **6**. They show the ability to interact with tumor cells *in vitro* quite similar to that of NAMI-A. Homo-binuclear (Pt,Pt) and hetero-dinuclear (Ru,Pt) metal complexes with the general formula $M_aNH_2(CH)_4NH_2M_b$ were identified to produce specific DNA lesions which may capably cross-link proteins to DNA. The homodinuclear case is signified by $M_a = M_b = [cis\text{-}PtCl_2(NH_3)]$ and the heterodinuclear case is represented by $M_a = [cis\text{-}RuCl_2(DMSO)_3]$ and $M_b = [cis\text{-}PtCl_2(NH_3)]$. These binuclear metal complexes could be valuable agents for the study of many protein-DNA interactions.

Ru(II)-arene compounds seem to have different profiles of bioactivity compared to the metal antitumor complexes in medical use [534]. The best known arene-Ru (II) complexes such as RM175, [(η6-biphenyl) (ethylene diamine) ruthenium(II)-chloride], RAPTA-C, [(η6-para-cymene-(1,3,5-triaza-7-phosphaadamantane) ruthenium(II)-dichloride], and NP309, [(η6-cyclopentadiene)-[N,N-(9-hydroxy-pyridol)-(2, 3-a-pyrrolo)-(3,4-c-carbazole)-(5,7-dione)] ruthenium(II) depicted in Fig. (**32**), have displayed optimistic results in numerous *in vitro* and *in* *vivo* screenings and continue to develop new complexes of other transition metals, like Os (II) and Ir (III).

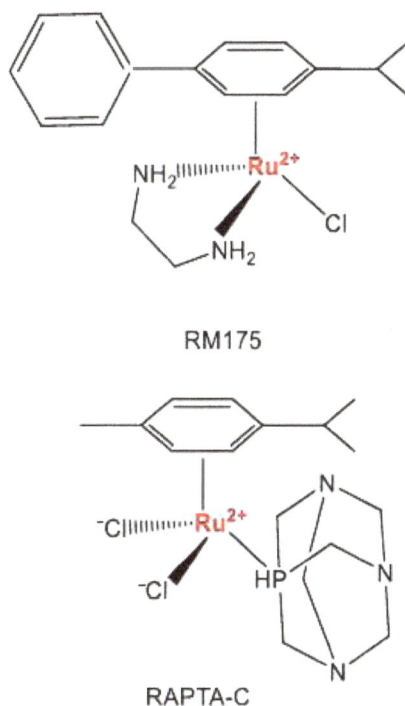

Fig. (32). Structures of RM175 and RAPTA-C.

Some prominent examples of the huge experimental work in the last years into the examination of new anticancer Ru complexes are introduced in Fig. (33), [535-544].

Ruthenium complexes are also used as antimycobacterial and anti-HIV therapeutic agents [289, 290, 300, 545]. Ruthenium coordination compounds with numerous bioligands provide good platform and appropriate building blocks for the design of new antifungal compounds which overcome microbial resistance [546].

Brachytherapy is a form of internal radiation therapy, which treats many cancerous tumors. The radioactive sources used for brachytherapy are radionuclides with relatively short half-lives, such as [106]Ru. Ruthenium-106 brachytherapy is an efficient and sparing therapy that provides tumor control and a good survival rate [293, 547].

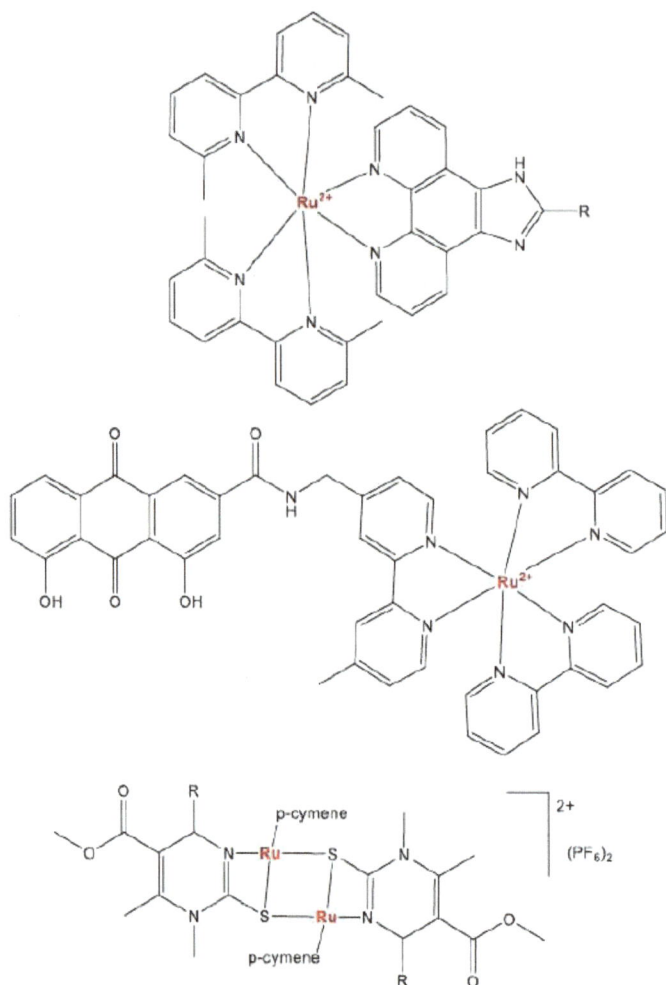

Fig. (33). Recently synthesized Ru-coordination compounds.

Rhodium

As a rare element with no known natural biological function, rhodium has a limited history in biochemistry and chemical biology. Nevertheless, rhodium complexes have unique structure and reactivity attributes, and many scientific groups have increasingly used these attributes to probe and perturb living systems [294 - 296]. Investigations of Rh(I), Rh(II), and Rh(III) complex compounds have attracted lots of consideration due to their tunable chemical and biological properties as well as their specific mechanisms of action. Many indications of their anticancer, antiparasitic, and antiviral activity have been detected [294 - 296]. The rhodium radionuclide [105]Rh (β−emitter) with a half-life of 35.4 h is useful in medicine. The complex of [105]Rh with ethylenediamine tetra(methylene phosphonic acid ([105]Rh-EDTMP) is a capable pharmaceutical for the therapy of pain due to bone metastases, exhibiting fast blood clearance and selective uptake into the bones [548].

Palladium

Up to now, Pd has found only partial use in treatment. Nowadays, palladium is commonly used in dental appliances [297]. Palladium mono- and polynuclear coordination compounds possess antimicrobial activity [300].

A Pd-bacteriopheophorbide (TOOKAD) can be photoactivated by long-wavelength light. It is a photosensitizer, established for the therapy of bulky tumors, allowing deep penetration into tissues and exhibiting quick release from the bloodstream [549].

Between the non-Pt complexes studied for anticancer activity, Pd(II) derivatives have been readily selected due to their similarity with those containing Pt(II) [298, 299, 301, 302]. Platinum(II) complexes are more stable than those of Pd(II) from a thermodynamical and kinetical point of view. The ligand substitutions in Pd(II) compounds are much quicker than for Pt(II) analogues. It means that Pd(II) compounds tend to engage in adverse interactions before reaching DNA. To overcome this high liability and the formation of very reactive species of Pd(II) compounds, different bulky bioligands with appropriate functional leaving groups were used to afford thermodynamically stable and kinetically inert complexes. Numerous Pd complexes with N- and N,N-containing aromatic ligands such as quinoline, pyridine, pyrazole, and 1,10 phenanthroline derivatives, as well as complexes with N,S-chelating bioligands such as thiosemicarbazone and dithiocarbamate derivatives, have exposed very strong antineoplastic properties.

Palladium is mainly used in radiotherapy for the treatment of prostate cancer and choroidal metastases, among others. [103]Pd needles are used in the clinic for prostate cancer and choroidal melanoma brachytherapy [550]. The radionuclide [103]Pd ($T_{1/2} = 17$ d) decays by electron capture. It has been used in brachytherapy. Application of [103]Pd for plaque radiotherapy of choroidal melanoma improved visualization when compared to the usage of [125]I. The radionuclide [103]Pd has also been used for the treatment of prostate cancer.

Osmium

In medicine, osmium is used in injections of osmic acid solutions (aqueous solutions of OsO_4) for destroying diseased tissues in irritated arthritic joints. Osmium tetroxide acts as a SOD mimic, catalyzing the dismutation of superoxide radicals, the main inflammatory species [551].

Recent investigations have shown that the chemical reactivity of osmium complexes can be finely tuned by the choice of osmium oxidation state, the ligands (including C- and N-bound), and the coordination geometry and stereochemistry, so opening up a wide range of new potential biological and medical applications. Osmium complexes have been reported to inhibit human cancer cell growth and proliferation [303 - 306]. Osmium cancer therapeutics can have diverse modes of action and targets, including DNA interactions, redox modulation, and protein inhibition. Though this area is basically dominated by Ru, certain Os complexes possessed equivalent activity at least *in vitro*. Osmium compounds are usually isostructural and isoelectronic with the respective Ru derivatives. Organoosmium complexes with arenes showed potential as anticancer agents, though up to now there were no Os complexes in clinical trials.

Resent applications of Os include photodynamic therapy, a less aggressive approach that uses the photo-physicochemical characteristics of Os complexes and cellular imaging [552]. Polypyridyl Os(II) compounds have potential advantages for luminescent cell imaging and photodynamic therapy due to their favorable photophysical and photochemical properties, such as long-wavelength metal-ligand charge transfer (MLCT) absorptions, high photostability and useful near-infrared (NIR) emission [303 - 306, 552]. The best advantage of osmium complexes with novel mechanisms of action over Ru is the coordination sphere stability with regard to ligand exchange, hydrolysis, and following deactivation of the complex.

Iridium

Ir and Ru are used in minor quantities in dental alloy materials with improved uniformity within the alloys. This field has been recently developed [307, 553].

The oxidation states of Ir in its coordination compounds are +1 and +3, though complexes of all possible oxidation states (ranging from −1 to +6) have been produced. Ir species with low oxidation states usually contain CO or P donor ligands, while those with high oxidation numbers contain predominantly hexahalide ligands [554]. The electronic configuration of Ir(III) ion d^6, the most common coordination number six with octahedral geometries is typical for iridium(III) complexes. Donor atoms to Ir(III) are various, with nitrogen being the most common.

Ir(III) complexes are inhibitors of protein kinase and protein-protein interactions [555]. Phosphorescent iridium(III) complexes and nanomaterials have gained increasing attention in biological applications owing to their excellent photophysical properties and efficient transportation into live cells [556-557]. Photoactive Ir(III) complexes with polypyridyls are promising candidates for photodynamic therapy [556]. Organoiridium(III) cyclopentadienyl complex compounds have shown potential as anticancer agents [557]. Certain seem to catalyze the cellular conversion of NADH to NAD^+ by transferring of hydride to iridium(III). The second most frequent oxidation state of iridium is Ir(I) having d^8 electron configuration, observed in square planar arrangements with most of the donor atoms. Iridium coordination compounds in the other oxidation states are commonly rare. The most frequent use of iridium complexes persists in the catalytic reactions, though interest is emerging in the luminescent activities of Ir coordination compounds.

Iridium is used clinically as β–emitter radionuclide ^{192}Ir with a half-life of 73.8 days [312, 558] in cancer brachytherapy. This method is a high-precision, hypo-fractionated, minimally invasive technique in the field of modern radiation oncological therapy for liver, prostate, endometrium, and intrathoracic malignancies.

Platinum

Platinum is extensively used in clinical practice because of its high biocompatibility. Pt materials (pacemakers and hearing aids), being resistant to corrosion, do not have any adverse toxic actions on human tissues in the body. Pt metal is widely not only in the design of drugs but also in the development of therapeutic apparatuses and devices such as urinary catheters, cardiovascular catheters, cardiac pacemakers and defibrillators, neuromodulation devices, and more [314 - 316, 559]. Catheters are used to remove body fluids, to deliver certain medications to a patient, to keep patients fed and hydrated. Pacemakers and defibrillators are developed to observe heart rate and help prevent cardiac arrests. Neuromodulation devices (brain pacemakers) are projected to send electric signals to CNS, a process helping control and treatment of many chronic conditions.

Platinum compounds are important chemotherapeutic drugs used to treat cancers. Breast, ovarian, lung, testicular, and other cancers are usually treated with platinum-based agents [313, 560]. The initial drug cisplatin, cis-dichlorodiammi-neplatin $[Pt(NH_3)_2Cl_2]$ (**1**), originated in the middle of XXth century, is combined by its correspondent equivalents carboplatincis-[Pt(1,1-dicarboxycyclobutane)$(NH_3)_2$] (**2**), oxaliplatin [Pt(1R,2R-1,2-diaminocyclohexane)(oxalate)] (**3**), nedaplatin (**4**), lobaplatin (**5**), heptaphane (**6**), satraplatin (**7**), and BBR3464 (**8**), which have been approved worldwide, (Fig. **34**), [561].

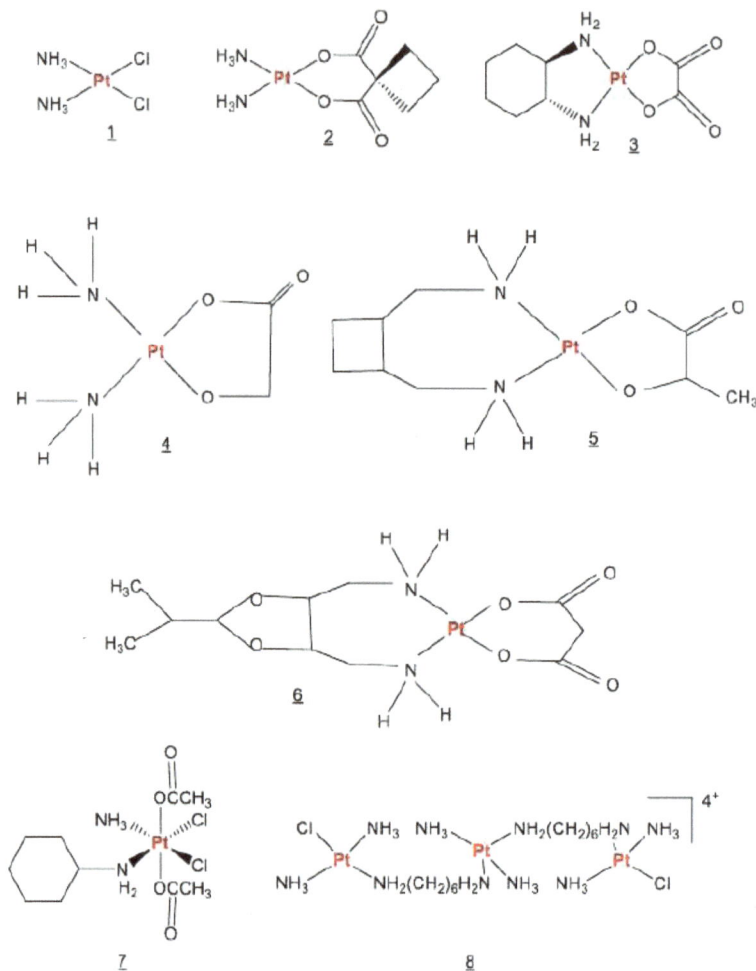

Fig. (34). Platinum chemotherapeutic drugs.

The complex *cis*-[PtCl$_2$(NH$_3$)$_2$], denoted as cisplatin, is applied for treatment of germ-cell, epithelial ovarian, and small cell lung cancers, as well as for palliation of cervical, esophageal, nasopharyngeal, and head or neck cancers [274, 561]. *cis*-[PtCl$_2$(NH$_3$)$_2$] interacts with DNA in the cell nucleus, where the amount of Cl$^-$ is lower than in the extracellular environment. In the intracellular fluids comprising low quantities of Cl$^-$ ions, the drug loses its Cl$^-$ ligands forming mono- and di-aqua cationic complex ions: [Pt(NH$_3$)$_2$(OH$_2$)Cl]$^+$ and [Pt(NH$_3$)$_2$(OH$_2$)$_2$]$^{+2}$ when H$_2$O attacks the Pt coordination center. After losing the chloride anions, hydrolyzed drug interacts with DNA and forms bonds with N-atoms of nucleobases. The active species inside the cell is therefore [Pt(NH$_3$)$_2$]$^{2+}$, not cisplatin. H$_2$O molecules are substituted by nucleobases (N7-atom of guanine) from DNA strands and cross-link adducts are formed. These adducts lead to noticeable conformational modifications in DNA inhibiting DNA and RNA synthesis, and inducing cell death. Therefore, the crucial basics in the activity of cisplatin and the corresponding Pt compounds on DNA are the controlled hydrolysis, cellular transport, and specific binding to DNA through the adjacent guanine bases, followed by DNA distortion and alteration of protein interactions, which leads to repair of the damage or apoptotic cell killing.

Nevertheless, some cancer cells have shown resistance to cisplatin and some side effects associated with its application [561]. Most often the adverse effects of cisplatin treatment include kidney and digestive complications due to enzyme inhibition through Pt coordination with the -SH protein groups. That is why, more research is carried out to design the second-generation Pt drugs with improved toxicology and the third-generation drugs which overcome the resistance.

The best-known similar Pt-based anticancer drugs in clinical practice are carboplatin and oxaliplatin which have a broader spectrum of activity or improved toxicological protection [313]. Carboplatin (diamine[1,1-cyclobutane dicarboxylato(2-)]-O,O'-platinum(II)) shows some what lower toxicity but its therapeutic efficiency to malignancies is not higher than that of cisplatin. The chelate effects of the 6-membered ring reduce its reactivity and probable adverse effects and damages (ototoxicity and nephrotoxicity). Further efforts to decrease the toxic effects and drug resistance have led to the development of oxaliplatin, (1R,2R)-(N,N'-1,2-diamminocyclohexane)-(O−O')-ethanedioato) platinum(II), which has been approved for the therapy of colorectal cancer in combination with 5-fluorouracil.

Drugs of a similar design are nedaplatin (cis-diamine-glycolate-O^1,O^2)Pt(II),254-S), lobaplatin (1.2-diaminomethyl-cyclobutane-Pt (II) lactate; D-19466), and heptaplatin (cis-[(4R,5R)-4,5-bis (aminomethyl)-2-isopropyl-1,3-dioxolane] malonate Pt (II)), which are in clinical usage in Japan, China, and South Korea, correspondingly. Nanoparticle formulations of Pt agents are also of interest [315, 562]. New liposome nanoparticles of cis-platin (Lipoplatin) and oxaliplatin (Lipoxal), which reduce the side effects, are presently under clinical trials. Lipoplatin, produced by cis platin and liposomes of dipalmitoyl phosphatidyl, soy phosphatidyl choline (SPC-3), cholesterol and methoxy polyethylene glycol-distearoyl phosphatidylethanolamine (mPEG2000-DSPE) has already accomplished clinical trials.

Platinum(IV) anticancer agents are also under continuous investigation. Pt(IV) complexes (for instance, cis-tetrachlorodiammineplatin [$Pt(NH_3)_2Cl_4$]) with the low-spin d^6 electronic configuration are interesting as pro-drugs which may be reduced to active Pt(II) species *in vivo* by light irradiation or chemically (through thiols or ascorbates) [314]. Polymer nanoparticles containing covalently bonded Pt(IV) polymer conjugates are quite stable. They enter cells by endocytosis and the rapid intracellular release is triggered by acidic surroundings [315]. The Pt(IV) complexes show potentials as a result of their larger stability and bioactivation, thus permitting a better amount of drugs to reach the target cells. The platinum(IV) complex JM216 (Satraplatin), *cis,trans,cis*-[PtCl$_2$(Ac)$_2$(NH$_3$) (C$_6$H$_5$NH$_2$)], shows activity by oral application in therapy of advanced prostate cancer. Satraplatin is an analog of cisplatin. On the whole, Pt(IV) octahedral low-spin complexes with d^6 configuration show higher kinetical inertness than square-planar Pt(II) complexes. Platinum(IV) complexes can be easily reduced *in vivo* to Pt(II) by reducing agents, for instance, ascorbate or thiols in cysteine and glutathione. Satraplatin undergoes rapid biotransformation in red blood cells in spite of the presumed inertness of Pt(IV) complexes.

Another group of Pt complexes that bind to DNA in a dissimilar way from that of cisplatin are the multinuclear complex compounds. The highly positively charged multinuclear Pt complexes form a new class of potent chemotherapeutics [563]. These compounds contain between two and four Pt centers with *cis* or *trans* configuration. An illustrative trinuclear complex, BBR3464, triplatin tetranitrate, showed activity against lung, pancreatic, and melanoma malignancies.

Studies have shown that the variety of Pt complexes with advantageous cytotoxic effects and anticancer activity is not firmly limited to cisplatin analogous structures. It has been supposed earlier that *cis*-configuration is required for the anticancer action of Pt compounds. Nevertheless, it has been found that some *trans*-Pt complexes possess *in vitro* and *in vivo* antineoplastic activity.

Both binuclear *bis*-Pt and *trans*-Pt complex compounds possess their own specific model which is different from that of cisplatin. Further on, the newest Pt(II) and Pt(IV) coordination compounds released in the literature in recent years have been introduced, (Figs. **35-36**), [314, 315, 564-573]. The variety of platinum complexes with antibacterial and anticancer activity includes complexes with modified pyriplatin, with triphenylphosphonium moiety, Pt(II)-terpyridine complexes, folate-containing Pt(II) complexes, pyridine-based Pt(II) complexes (Fig. **35**), complexes with pyrrole-substituted Schiff bases, phenanthriplatin complexes, pyridine co-ligand functionalized cationic compounds, diazido-Pt(IV) complexes (Fig. **36**), *etc.*

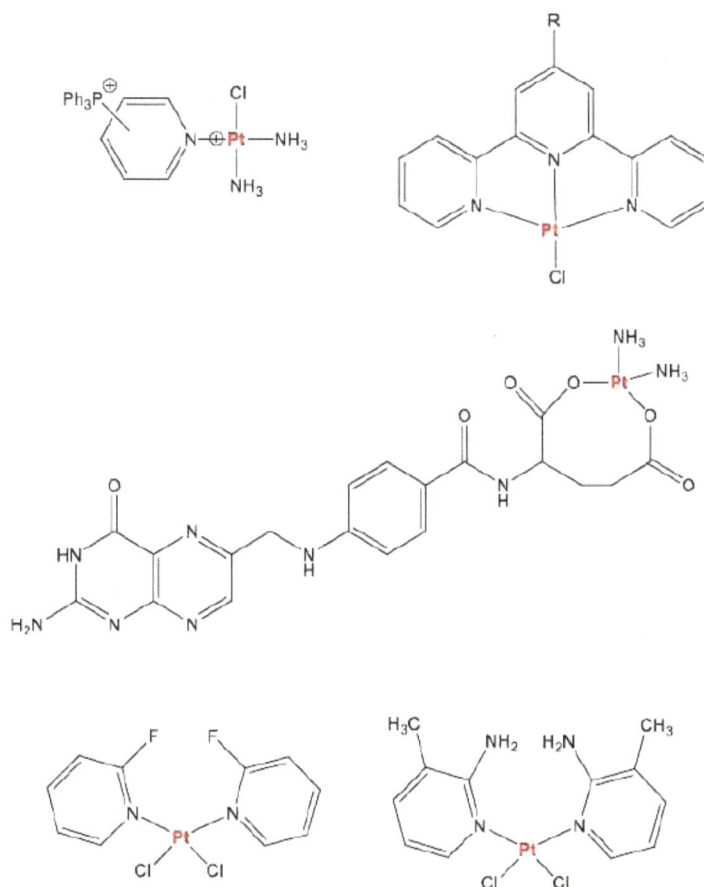

Fig. (35). Recently synthesized Ru-coordination complexes according to [564-573].

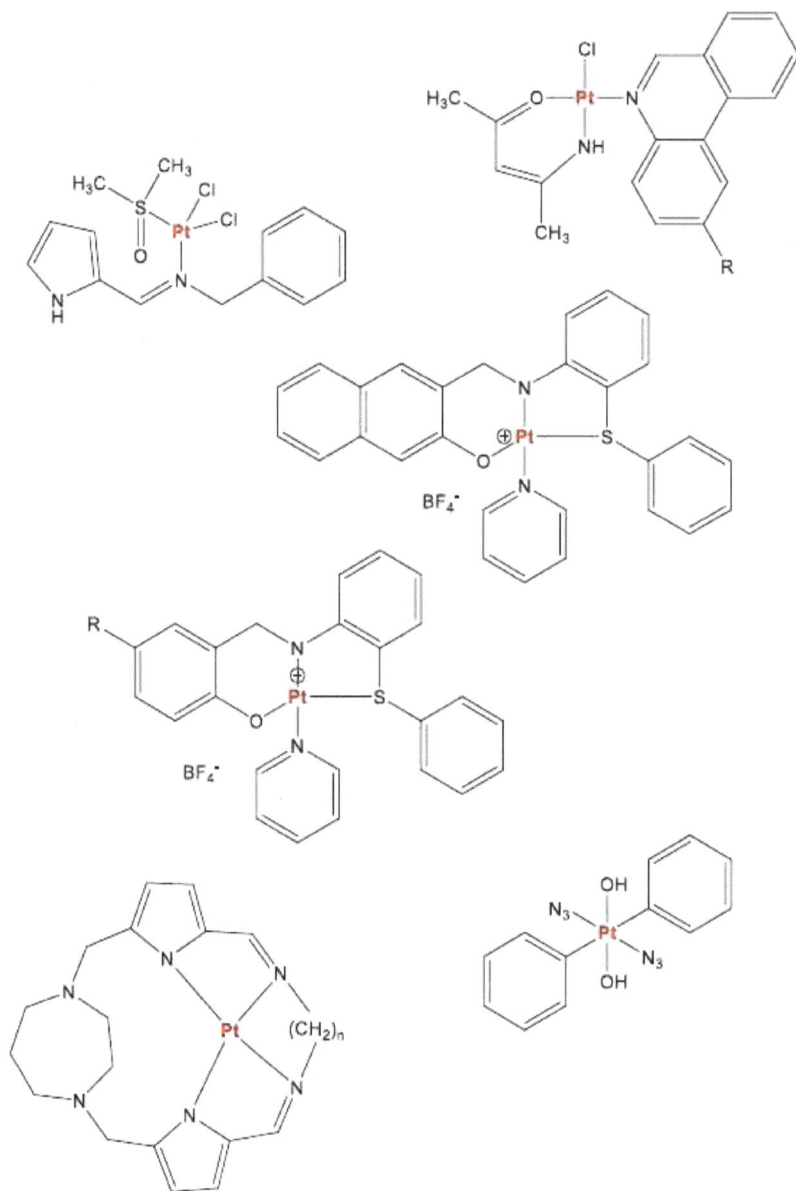

Fig. (36). Recently synthesized Ru-coordination compounds according to [564-573].

The biological role, medicinal applications, and toxic effects of d - elements are listed in Table **18**.

Table 18. The biological role and toxic effects of d elements.

Element	Location and Role in the Body	Drugs	Toxic Effect, Antidotes
Cu	Concentrates mostly in the liver, kidney, and brain; processes of respiration, hematopoiesis, angiogenesis, and neuromodulation; Cu-based proteins and enzymes (around 1% of total proteome) .	$CuSO_4 \cdot 5H_2O$ - antimicrobial effect, astringent, and antiseptic; 5% solution of $CuSO_4$ treats white phosphorus burns; $CuSO_4$ and CuO - part of vitamin-mineral complexes; alloys of Au, Ag, and Cu - in dental practice for prosthetics; Cu(II) complexes - SOD-mimic, anti-Alzheimer, antioxidant, anti-inflammatory, antifungal [475, 476].	Excess of Cu — Wilson's disease [196, 199]; $CuSO_4$ — an antidote for poisoning by white phosphorus; antidote - cysteine, D-penicillamine.
Ag	Found in the liver, kidney, endocrine glands, erythrocytes; bactericidal action.	Protargol (protein complex of silver) and colloid silver (colloidal Argentum) $AgNO_3$ (lapis) — bactericidal, astringent, and anti-inflammatory; Ag nanoparticles - antiviral agents [477 - 480].	Interacting with proteins containing S, deactivates enzymes, and deconstructs proteins [200].
Au	Gold forms stable complexes with sulphur and phosphorus, particularly with thiol (-SH) groups of blood proteins; inhibits ROS	Ag(I) and Au(III) complexes in chrysotherapy or aurotherapy, effective in the therapy of rheumatoid arthritis, reduce inflammation [201]; anticancer candidates [481 - 491]	Cytotoxic potency [481 - 491]
Zn	In the enzyme carbonic anhydrase, endocrine glands, reproduction processes.	$ZnSO_4$ (0,1-0,25%) — astringent, anti-inflammatory activity (eye drops); ZnO — antibacterial and astringent (in dermatology) [202 - 206, 492].	Severe vomiting [206]; antidote - D-penicillamine
Hg	Hg vapor absorbs in the lungs, dissolves in the blood, and then to the brain, which leads to irreversible damage to the CNS; accumulates mainly in the liver, kidney, and brain	$HgCl_2$ (sulema)) (1:1000) — antiseptic; Hg_2Cl_2 ((calomel) - laxative; HgO (ointment) — in dermatology [493]; Hg — in thermometers; amalgams in dentistry, composed of 52% mercury; Thimerosal (ethylmercury thiosalicylate) - for preserving vaccines [494]	A pair of Hg and $HgCl_2$ affect the CNS; spilled mercury binds $FeCl_3$, S, $KMnO_4$; antidotes - dimercaprol, DMPS, DMSA, D-penicillamine [214 - 217].
Sc	Scandium is not a biogenic element; its radioactive isotopes are potential PET and SPECT imaging agents.	^{43}Sc and ^{44}Sc - in PET imaging, while ^{47}Sc is used in radiotherapy [218, 495].	Elemental Sc is non-toxic, some Sc compounds -cancerogenic [219].
Y	Yttrium is not a vital element, but yttrium-based materials (^{90}Y, ^{86}Y) are used in medical lasers and biomedical implants.	Y - used in anticancer treatment as ^{90}Y radionuclide (β-emitter): non-Hodgkin B-cell lymphoma radiotherapy and immunotherapy; ^{86}Y -tracer for PET imaging [496].	Hazardous, causes lung embolisms, chances of lung cancer [220].

(Table 18) cont.....

Element	Location and Role in the Body	Drugs	Toxic Effect, Antidotes
Ti	Known to act as a stimulant; one of the most biocompatible metals.	Ti - in prosthetics, and implants [497]; Ti compounds - fodder additives, for animals' weight gain; Ti(IV) complexes - for treatment of cancer [498, 499].	Ti is not harmful or toxic; TiO_2 - a carcinogen [221].
V	Stabilizes blood sugar levels; helps bones and teeth form properly; antidiabetic agent.	Vanadium compounds - in inhibition of cancerous tumor growth or as insulin-mimetic drugs [225 - 228, 503-505].	Not a serious hazard [226, 227]; V_2O_5 is more toxic.
Ta	Compatible and non-reactive with body tissues.	Used for long-term surgical implants and bone defects repair [230, 507].	Moderately toxic; Ta compounds are nonpoisonous - low solubility [230].
Cr	Enzymes pepsin, trypsin, exchange of glucose.	Chromium picolinate - for treatment of carbohydrate and fat metabolic conditions, for diabetes; Cr_2O_3 is a component of dental pastes [234, 508, 509].	Heart rhythm disturbance; Cr^{+6} causes skin and mucous membrane disorders [232, 233, 235].
Mo	Enzyme xanthine oxidase, purine metabolism	MoO_4^{2-} prevents oxidation of lipids and protects antioxidant systems, for the treatment of diabetic mellitus. MoS_4^{2-} - copper chelator, for treatment of breast cancer and esophageal carcinoma; $(NH_4)_2MoO_4$ or Na_2MoO_4, - used in many vitamin complexes [237 - 245, 510].	Excess disturbs purine metabolism — endemic gout [236, 243].
W	Essential for certain anaerobic bacteria	Polyoxotungstates - antiviral, antibacterial, anticancer agents, and for the treatment of Alzheimer's disease. Na_2WO_4 - anti-diabetic effects [244, 511-513].	The concentration of W in nature is very low and W is considered nontoxic [246].
Mn	Bone, liver, lungs, muscles, pancreas, and kidney typically have higher manganese concentration, an activator of enzymes-glutamine synthetase; Mn superoxide dismutase in mitochondria.	$KMnO_4$ — antiseptic; $MnSO_4$, $MnCl_2$, and Mn gluconate, aspartate, picolinate, fumarate, malate, succinate, citrate, and amino acid chelates - Mn supplements in the form of multivitamins; beneficial for MR, PET, and PET/MR imaging [252, 514-518].	Excessive Mn, manganism, a neurodegenerative disorder; ROS production [247, 248, 250].
Tc	Used in medical radiation imaging as a tracer; ^{99m}Tc concentrates in the thyroid gland and gastrointestinal tract; the short half-life and its rapid excretion minimize the toxic effects.	[99m]Tc, a γ-emitter - used in SPECT and allowing rapid and safe diagnosis; non-invasive diagnosis on the brain, heart, kidneys, and thyroid; radiation treatment of cancers with minimal side effects [253, 519-521].	Unstable isotopes and never presents a risk; radiological toxicity [519-521].

(Table 18) cont.....

Element	Location and Role in the Body	Drugs	Toxic Effect, Antidotes
Re	Re(I) coordination complexes display potential anticancer properties and reduce ROS production	^{186}Re and ^{188}Re combine diagnosis by radio imaging with therapeutic properties on malignant tumors, bone metastases, and rheumatoid arthritis [255, 522].	No reports on the metal or its compounds toxicity [254]
Fe	Hemoglobin (Fe^{2+}); catalase and peroxidase ($Fe^{2+} \rightarrow Fe^{3+}$); cytochrome c ($Fe^{2+} \rightarrow Fe^{3+}$) hematopoietic processes and electron transfer.	$FeCl_3.6H_2O$ — hemostatic; iron supplements to treat iron deficiency anemia; Fe(II) containing ferroquine - utilized for treatment of malaria, cancer; $Na_2[Fe(CN)_5NO]$ -hypertensive agent; Fe oxides - MRI contrast agents [334, 335, 523-527].	Hemochromatosis, cirrhosis of the liver, blockage of blood vessels [257, 265]; antidote - Desferrioxamine [527].
Co	Stored in the plasma, liver, spleen, kidney, and pancreas; Processes of hematopoiesis; Radiation of ^{60}Co many applications	Vitamin B_{12} (cyanocobalamin); ^{60}Co anticancer agent in cobalt therapy, radiotherapy for the treatment of malignant tumors; for sterilizing medical supplies and waste [268 - 270, 528-532]	Hypothyroidism; overproduction of erythrocytes, fibrosis in lungs, and asthma [271, 272]
Ni	Pancreas; effect on carbohydrate metabolism	Nickel and its compounds are almost not used in medicine	Carcinogen; Ni allergy [283, 284].
Ru	Retained strongly in bones; Ru complexes - antineoplastic agents with antimetastatic properties, selectivity and low total toxicity; Ru mimics the binding of Fe.	Ru immunosuppressant (Ru(III) complex of Cyclosporin A), antimicrobial agent (Ru(III) complex of Chloroquine) [289], antibiotic agent (Ru(III) complex of Thiosemicarbazone), an inhibitor of nitric oxides (ruthenium polyamine carboxylates); NAMI-A possess anti-metastasis activity; photodynamic agent [285, 287, 288, 291-293, 533-547].	Carcinogenic, RuO_4, is highly toxic and volatile [286].
Rh	Rh(II) complexes - anticancer, antiparasitic, and antiviral agents or enzyme inhibitors.	Rh(I), Rh(II), and Rh(III) complexes - antitumor and antimicrobial agents [294 - 296]; ^{105}Rh-EDTMP - potential therapeutic agent for pain treatment in bone metastatic cases [548].	Rh compounds - toxic and carcinogenic [294 - 296].
Pd	Pd - component of dental alloys; Pd complexes with lower toxicity are closely related to Pt antitumor analogs; ^{103}Pd used in radiotherapy.	Pd in dental appliances [297] and ^{103}Pd needles - for prostate cancer and choroidal melanoma brachytherapy; Pd chloride - treatment of tuberculosis; Pd complexes - against prostate and lung cancer; in radiotherapy ^{103}Pd - in brachytherapy, for choroidal melanoma, prostate cancer [298, 299, 301, 302, 549, 550].	Non-toxic; Pd compounds are relatively rare, but highly toxic and carcinogenic [298, 299, 301, 302, 550].

(Table 18) cont.....

Element	Location and Role in the Body	Drugs	Toxic Effect, Antidotes
Os	The chemistry of Ru and Os is typically comparable.	Osmium-containing sensors to check the blood glucose levels continuously; Os complexes - anticancer and antimicrobial agents; used in photodynamic therapy [303 - 306, 551, 552].	Os is not toxic and unreactive, but all Os compounds are highly toxic [303 - 306].
Ir	Ir(III) organometallic complexes - anticancer and antimicrobial activities	Ir(III) complexes - inhibitors of protein kinase and protein-protein interactions; photoactive polypyridyl Ir complexes - for photodynamic therapy; organoiridium(III) cyclopentadienyl complexes - anticancer agents; ^{192}Ir - for cancer brachytherapy and prostatic carcinoma; GAMMA-Iridium-192 catheter for coronary artery disease [307 - 312, 553-558].	Metal has low toxicity, but all Ir compounds are highly toxic [308]; ^{192}Ir-acute radiation [312].
Pt	Absorbed Pt accumulates in kidneys, excreted in urine; Pt complexes - the most extensively used medicines in cancer chemotherapy.	Pt - used to build dental crowns and dentistry instruments; Pt materials - pacemakers and hearing aids; Pt complexes - chemotherapeutic drugs used to treat cancers [314 - 316, 559-573].	Pt is biologically inert, almost all Pt compounds are highly toxic [313].

where: dimercaprol - 2,3-dimercapto-1-propanol, DMPS - 2,3- dimercapto-1-propanesulfonic acid, DMSA - 2,3-dimercaptosuccinic acid.

MEDICAL AND BIOLOGICAL SIGNIFICANCE OF LANTHANIDES AND ACTINIDES

In spite of their unnecessary biogenic nature, the lanthanides (Ln) in compounds can participate in and influence the functions of biosystems in a notable variety of ways [317 - 326]. It is expected that this variability may rise, especially in the fields of therapeutic diagnostics and imaging [574-576]. The outstanding magnetic, catalytic, and optic properties of lanthanides endorse them as exceptional biosensors, fluorescent dyes, and contrast agents in medicinal investigations, spectral examinations, and sensor and laser agents, used in biological applications [577]. The approach proved very successful, increasing the sustained interest in the biochemistry of lanthanides. Their luminescence activity and photophysical performance emphasize their use as imaging representatives in visible and NIR regions [578]. As far as radioactive Ln are concerned, most of their applications are therapy related. Positron-emitting radionuclides of lanthanides are used in PET. The growing tendency to use one type of compound for both diagnosis and therapy has resulted in the development of the arena of theranostics [579]. On the other hand, numerous nonradioactive lanthanide(III) complexes have been extensively investigated for their promising antineoplastic and antioxidant activity [319, 323-325, 580, 581]. Non-radioactive Ln have proven their usefulness in the therapy of diseases like osteoporosis, ROS related and cardiac diseases, including the replacement of Ln(III) for vital biogenic metal cations in various proteins, enzymes, *etc.*

Lanthanum

The properties of lanthanides are best suited to their biological and chemical interactions, and special consideration is paid to their resemblances to Ca(II) ions as this forms the foundation of many biochemical studies using Ln. The approach of replacing Ca(II) by lanthanide(III) cations (especially La(III) and Gd(III)) in biosystems has been evidenced valuable for the reason that Ca(II) is one of the most significant metal cations in biology. In view of the fact that La(III) and Ca(II) have similar ionic radii, coordination numbers and donor atom preferences (O>N>S) the Ln metals imitate calcium [322, 581]. This resemblance lets lanthanum(III) ions exchange with calcium(II) cations in bones when the bone remodeling cycle is changed, thus stimulating the proliferation of osteoblasts, cells that redevelop bones. Lanthanum carbonate $La_2(CO_3)_3$ (Fosrenol) was approved as a phosphate-binder for the therapy of hyperphosphatemia, an electrolyte disproportion that leads to higher concentrations of phosphate in the bloodstream. This overload disease usually arises in patients with renal disorders. Fosrenol reacts with phosphate bioligands at low and higher pH values, decreasing phosphate absorption by the complexation formation of low soluble La(III) phosphate $LaPO_4$ which can then cross the digestive tract unabsorbed and can be excreted efficiently. Lanthanum(III), cerium(III), and praseodymium(III) compounds have been widely used as feed additives for growing animal production where small amounts of these supplements can result in greater weight improvement. Lanthanum(III) compounds are also used as biological tracer elements [324].

In recent decades the popularity of La(III) complex compounds in anticancer investigations has been progressively increasing, generally because of lanthanum's capability to mimic biogenic metals and to coordinate with bioligands. La(III) ions have interacted with variety of ligands such as 2,2'-bipyridine, 1,10-phenanthroline, and many others. Very recently La(III) complexes (Fig. **37**) with pyridine-2,6-dicarboxylate were screened against different tumor cell lines and comparted with oxaliplatin. The complexes have been found more active than the ligands [582].

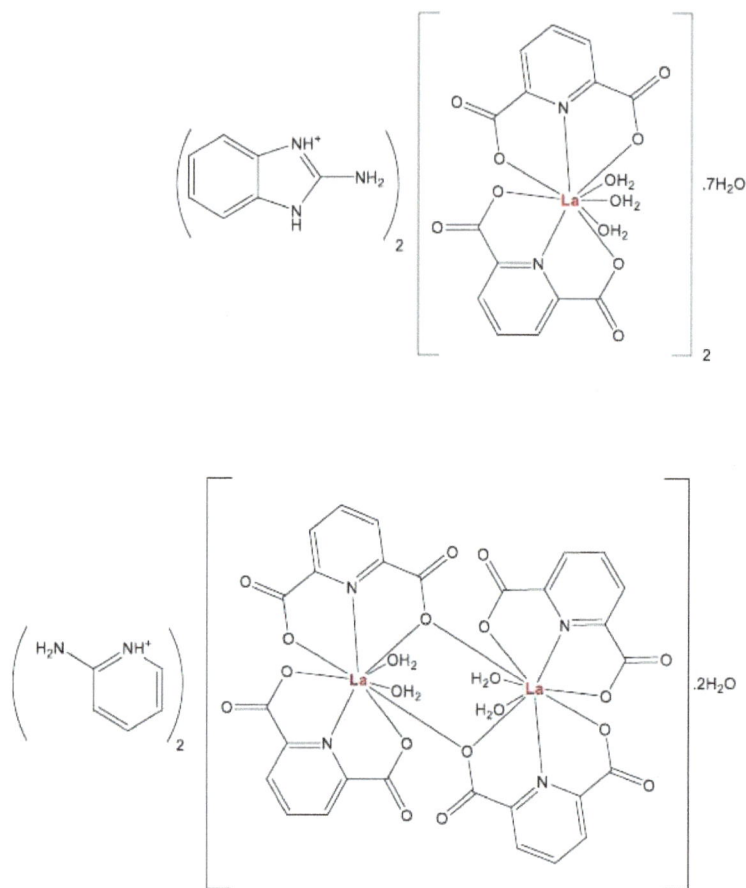

Fig. (37). Recently synthesized La(III) complexes.

Cerium

Unlike other lanthanides, which typically exhibit (+3) oxidation state, cerium can exist in either +3 (reduced) or +4 (oxidized) state. Cerium produces various salts, such as $Ce(NO_3)_3$, which attracts much medicinal attention. Water solutions of Ce^{4+} salts are stable only in highly acidic conditions at pH < 3. Ce(IV) cation is a strong oxidizing agent of no biological significance. In contrast, Ce(III) is unaffected by oxidation and interacts only with very powerful oxidizing agents [325]. $Ce(NO_3)_3$ has attracted most consideration in the therapy of deep burns, connected with its antimicrobic activity. It has effective bacteriostatic properties against a wide variety of microorganisms in a pH-dependent manner [583]. In addition to antimicrobial actions, immunomodulatory activity has been documented as the most important mechanism by which Ce contributes to the prevention of sepsis in burn wounds. $Ce(NO_3)_3$ has been shown to possess antioxidant activity [584]. The complex formulation of Ce(III) nitrate in combination with Ag(I) sulfadiazine (Flammacerium) is currently used in burn wound treatment [585]. $Ce(NO_3)_3$ is supposed to exert protective effects against postburn immunosuppression triggered by lipid-protein complexes with high molecular weights. Nanoparticles of Ce^{3+} oxide are of specific interest as promising therapeutic agents with a strong antioxidant effect which is beneficial for different biological and medical purposes, particularly for ROS-related conditions together with Alzheimer's disease, cardiac diseases, and cancer [586]. Ca(II) ion is analogous to Ce(III) in relation to the size, binding, and affinity to donor functional groups. In biosystems, they are likely to precipitate together, hence the higher preference of cerium(III) to the mineral bone matrix and its induction of calcification due to Ce(III) precipitates with pyrophosphate. Because of the similar ionic radii of Ca^{2+} and Ce^{3+}, Ln(III) substitutes Ca(II) ions in many biologically active molecules, without automatically replacing functionality. This includes the interference in Ca-dependent interactions of the blood clotting cascade and their anticoagulant and antithrombotic properties [587].

Samarium

The samarium isotope ^{153}Sm is a potent theranostic radioactive nuclide and one of the most widely used radiopharmaceuticals for many years [588]. ^{153}Sm (β−decay) has a half-life of 1.93 days. In parallel, ^{153}Sm co-emits gamma-rays that allow SPECT imaging. These properties make ^{153}Sm favorable for targeted radionuclide therapy (TRNT). In relieving severe pain related to bone cancer, targeting of bone by exchange with Ca(II) of ^{153}Sm(III) delivered as complexes with multidentate bioligands is a major therapeutic aspect. In the form of ^{153}Sm-ethylenediamine-tetramethylphosphonic acid (^{153}Sm-EDTMP) it stabilizes pain in patients suffering from osteoblastic metastatic bone lesions. ^{153}Sm-EDTMP can be used for the therapy of bad osteosarcoma and breast cancer with metastasis to bone, multiple myeloma, and bone pain. It is well tolerated by the human body. Its range of emission in bone is very small, consequently limiting exposure of bone marrow and other radiated tissues. In clinics, comparing ^{153}Sm-EDTMP and ^{177}Lu-EDTMP for pain palliation in bones, it has been found that these radiopharmaceuticals are similarly active and can be used interchangeably [589].

Europium

A small number of reports are known about the usage of Eu in medical applications. It has the potential as a paramagnetic chemical exchange saturation transfer (PARACEST) MRI contrast agent [590]. The complex Eu(III)-DOTA-tetraamide was designed as an MRI sensor of $^1O_2$. The metal-chelated 1,4,7,10-tetraazacyclododecan-1,4,7,10-tetraacetic acid-tetraamide (DOTA, (Fig. **30**) framework has been extensively used for the production of contrast agents for diagnostics in PET and MRI. The Eu(III) complex rapidly reacts with $^1O_2$ forming an endoperoxide derivative. This may be useful for the detection of $^1O_2$ in cells throughout photodynamic therapy [591]. Luminescent Eu^{3+}-doped nano-porous silica nanoparticles have received great interest in biomedicine [592].

Gadolinium

The progress of Gd-containing relaxivity enhancement agents to improve tissue contrast in MRI is a key feature of this currently widely utilized imaging technique. The reason for using gadolinium(III) is that this cation has the largest number of unpaired electrons of any metal cation in the periodic table, thus being a basis of prevailing paramagnetic properties. Gd(III) is unique with its 7 unpaired electrons, its long electron-spin relaxation time, and large magnetic moment giving rise to contrast in MR images. During the last decades Gd(III) chelates have become commonplace in medical diagnosis. Nowadays, about 50% of the examinations with MRI are completed after treatment with gadolinium(III) chelated complexes as contrast agents [593]. Related complex compounds of Dy(III) and Tm(III) with shorter electronic relaxation times are very efficient NMR shift reagents. Gadolinium(III) compounds can be considered one of the safest drugs known. Because of the higher thermodynamical and kinetical stability of Gd(III) complex compounds, for instance, $[Gd(DTPA)(H_2O)]^{2-}$ (Magnevist) and $[Gd(DOTA)(H_2O)]^-$ (Dotarem), (Fig. **38**), they can be safely administrated as injections with no serious adverse effects.

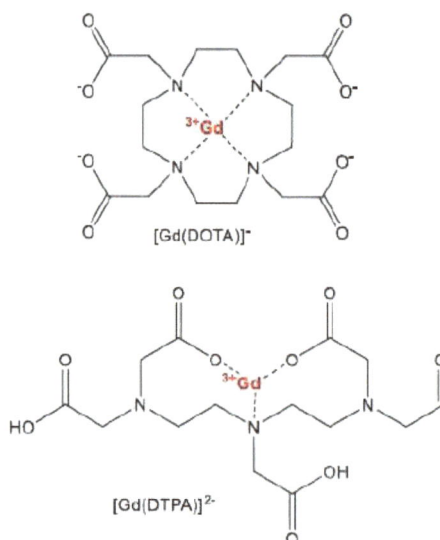

Fig. (38). Gd-based agents Magnevist and Dotarem.

The use of the macrocyclic chelators like DOTA and DTPA see Fig. (10) as SPECT and PET radiopharmaceutical drugs provides perspectives on theranostics for personalized therapy with radioactive analogues. The approved Gd(III) complexes for clinical usage as contrast agents for MRI are as follow: $[Gd(DTPA)(H_2O)]^{2-}$ (Magnevist; $[Gd(DOTA)(H_2O)]^-$ (Dotarem); [Gd(DTPA-BMA)(H_2O)] (Omniscan); $[Gd(HP-DO3A)(H_2O)]$ (ProHance); [Gd(bopta)(H_2O)]^{2-} (MultiHance); $[Gd(DO3A-butrol)(H_2O)]$ (Gadovist), where DOTA-1,4,7,10-Tetraazacyclododecane-1,4,7,10-tetraacetate, DTPA-BMA - (bis) methylamide derivative of DTPA, HP-DO3A-hydroxypropyl derivative of DOTA, bopta-(9R,S)-2,5,8-tris(carboxymethyl)-12-phenyl-11-oxa-2,5,8-triazadodecane-1,9-dicarboxylate (derivative of DTPA), DO3A-butrol-1,4,7,-tris(carboxymethyl)-10-(1-hydroxymethyl-2,3-dihydroxypropyl)-1,4,7,10-tetraaz-acyclododecane (derivative of DOTA). Macrocyclic derivatives provide Gd(III) complexes with more than the required stability for injection application and improved safety. In the past years, problems have arisen regarding the toxicity of clinically used MRI contrast agents [594]. Gd(III) ion is noxious at the amount used in MRI and it could not be injected per se. DTPA is a good ligand since it produces a very stable complex with Gd^{3+} and enables renal excretion. Cyclic polyaminocarboxylates of Gd(III) similar to DOTA are less favored. The large Gd(III) ion can readily hold eight donor atoms from the chelating ligand which exchanges quickly with bulk H_2O. Additionally, Gd(III) ion has an analogous radius to that of Ca(II), allowing them to interfere with Ca-mediated signaling pathways. There are concerns about possible adverse effects (displacement by Ca^{2+}), resulting from any release of Gd^{3+} particularly for contrast agents with low stability. It is expected that the information obtained with the MRI technique can be increased substantially by the use of Ln(III) chelates as shift reagents [595].

The rapid development of MRI and MRS methods generates a growing demand for more effective and more specific contrast and shift reagents and, accordingly, to a large research activity in this important field. Gd-based nanomaterials are another class of contrast agents for MRI [596]. Gadolinium-containing carbon nanomaterials have shown better results than conventional Gd contrast agents [597]. As a result of the enhanced proton relaxivity, they can afford reduced toxicity, excellent cell penetration, contrast selectivity, and good cell, tissue or organ imaging with lesser doses than Gd agents presently used in clinics. Gadolinium(III) texaphyrin (Fig. **39**) is applied as XRT enhance agent and MRI contrast agent. This medication is utilized for the treatment of brain tumors and metastases. Additionally, lutetium(III) texaphyrin finds applications not only in radio oncology. Lu(III) texaphyrin (Lu-tex) is used for locally recurrent breast cancer.

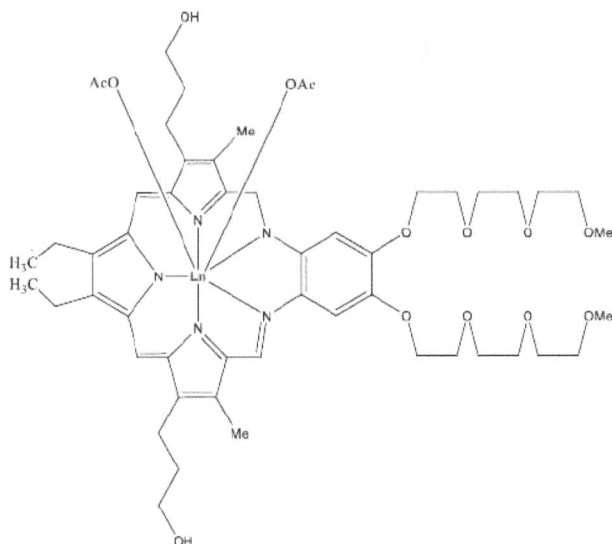

Fig. (39). Ln(III) texaphyrin, where Ln = Lu; Lu(III) Texaphyrin (LUTRIN); Ln = Gd; Gd(III) Texaphyrin (XCYTRIN).

Texaphyrins are a group of porphyrins produced by Schiff base condensation between diformyltripyrrane and aromatic 1,2-diamines. These macrocycles are soluble in H_2O tripyrrolic-pentaaza- expanded porphyrins, which are able to bind large ions such as Ln(III). Their capability to produce stable complex compounds with Ln(III) gives them an exclusive place in the medical fields. Gd(III) complex with the ligand motexaphrin (a derivative of texaphyrin) is also very promising [593-595]. This substance improves the radiation response of cancer by mechanisms that include catalytic oxidation of intracellular reducing metabolites such as GSH and ascorbate. Nonradioactive gadolinium(III) compound of the expanded porphyrin texaphyrin with a long wavelength absorption, appropriate for its excitation by NIR radiation, gives species deactivated by the conversion of the triplet oxygen to its cytotoxic singlet form [598].

Promethium

Promethium is the only lanthanide with no stable isotopes. It is not obtainable in large amounts in the Earth's crust. All promethium isotopes emit radiation, for instance, [145]Pm ($T_{1/2}$ = 17.7 y), [146]Pm ($T_{1/2}$ = 5.4 y), [147]Pm ($T_{1/2}$ = 2.6 y) [599]. It experiences radioactive decays such as electron capture and β-emission. Although promethium has 38 known isotopes, promethium-147 is the most beneficial. Promethium has remarkable number of applications. The radioisotope [147]Pm is commercially existing and has certain uses, *e.g.,* for the production of miniature long-life atomic batteries which have been tested as pacemakers and in radiotherapy. Promethium has substituted radium for health purposes. Improperly stored promethium becomes an environmental hazard. Pm compounds proved to be harmless in terms of radioactivity. In medical practice, Pm β-therapy can cure lumbosacral radiculitis [600]. Promethium-142 has been used in an *in vivo* generator for pre-clinical PET. ^{149}Pm, in turn, as a medium-energy β-emitter, is an appropriate radio-lanthanide for receptor-targeted radiation therapy [601]. A great benefit of promethium-149 is its low-intensity emission of imageable gamma-rays, which offers *in vivo* tracking of the therapeutic doses. Furthermore, Pm can stop hair loss, help hair regrowth, and black hair formation, as well as eliminate or even prevent dandruff [602].

Thulium

The rare metal thulium has approximately no practical uses. The gamma-radiation from the radioisotope ^{170}Tm has been studied for application in materials testing and as a portable X-ray source for therapeutic use. This radioisotope is one of the significant radionuclides which may be applied for metastasis bone pain palliation along with samarium-153 (^{153}Sm), lutetium-177 (^{177}Lu), ytterbium-175 (^{175}Yb), and holmium-166 (^{166}Ho). Apart from emissions of β-particles, ^{170}Tm has some γ-photons which offer track, dose calculations, and imaging studies [603]. One of the most popular chelators for bone-seeking agents with a high affinity for bone minerals is ethylenediamine tetra(methylene phosphonic acid (EDTMP). EDTMP is a phosphonate equivalent of EDTA which has high chelating ability. It also has high affinity for bone tissues and deposition in locations with enlarged bone metabolism. As a result of the advancement of targeted radiotherapy in the treatment of malignancies, ^{170}Tm-EDTMP was established for medical applications. The β−radiation of ^{170}Tm is considerably lower than that of ^{188}Re and ^{89}Sr, so the bone marrow captivates a lower radiation dose [603]. Thulium oxide nanoparticles with multi-modal biological applications have the potential as novel nanoparticles for image-guided radiotherapy of brain cancer.

Holmium

A wide range of applications of the radioisotope ^{166}Ho have been established. The radionuclide holmium-166 is used as a substitute for ^{188}Re by reason of its appropriate features for internal radiotherapy. Holmium-165 is attractive because of its high β-energy emission, used for therapeutic effects, and low γ-energy for nuclear imaging purposes. Certain complexes labelled with ^{166}Ho are now clinically used, such as ^{166}Ho-labelled microspheres for liver cancer, ^{166}Ho-labelled chitosan for hepatocellular carcinoma and ^{166}Ho-DOTMP (1,4,7,10-tetraazacyclododecane-1,4,7,10-tetramethylene-phosphonic acid) for bone metastases [604]. Presently, two types of ^{166}Ho-microspheres for intratumor applications were tested, *i.e.,* [166]Ho-labelled acetylacetonate and [166]Ho-labelled poly(L-lactic acid) microspheres. They are used for intraarterial radioembolization in patients for therapy of liver metastases and unresectable liver malignancies. [166]Ho-labelled poly(L-lactic acid) microspheres have been applied as a palliative administration in the cases of recurrent head-and-neck squamous cell carcinoma showing relatively low therapeutic efficacy and no adverse effects [605]. [166]Ho-labelled chitosan complex, which has been tested in various tumors such as brain, liver, and prostate cancer. Chitosan has a polymeric structure. It is synthesized from the deacetylation of chitin. Holmium-165 medications and therapeutic devices labelled with radioholmium are used for internal radiation therapy. Many other uses have been established, like patches for therapy of skin cancer and Ho-labelled antibodies and peptides. One of the most important applications that is presently clinically used is selective internal radiotherapy (SIRT) for liver malignancies. As the half-life of [166]Ho is 26.8 h, over 90% of the radiation is deposited in less than 4 days. Another type of intratumoral treatment is the use of [166]Ho-labelled ceramic seeds, which were tested in animal brain tissues and in human breast tissues by computational simulation [606]. Ho-containing nanoparticles with different compositions were utilized for various applications [607]. The observed high stability and paramagnetic characteristics make them appropriate for therapy and multimodal imaging with SPECT and MRI.

Ytterbium

The production of radio lanthanides with optimum properties for various uses is attracting great research interest. The radioisotope of ytterbium [175]Yb shows favorable β-decay characteristic features for therapeutic applications. [175]Yb-labelled polyaminophosphonates are promising agents for bone pain palliation in the treatment of bone metastases [608]. They have high bone acceptance with minimal uptake in soft tissues and fast blood clearance. Multidentate polyaminopolyphosphonic acid derivatives can produce stable coordination compounds with numerous heavy metal ions, including Ln(III). Between them, triethylenetetraminehexamethylene phosphonic acid (TTHMP) can be predicted as a perfect carrier moiety, for the production of β-emitter radioactive medications, for bone palliation purposes. The radioisotope ytterbium-169 emits primarily gamma-photons with a much longer half-life of 32 days, and is used as a promising therapeutic for intravascular brachytherapy [609]. The [169]Yb seeds produce more isotropic dose distributions, and for permanent implants, they can deliver it at a greater initial dose rate. However, for temporary implants, ytterbium-169 may prove to be a useful substitute for ^{192}Ir or ^{137}Cs radioactive isotopes because of its relatively lower energy emissions. The non-toxic and inert ytterbium fluoride has been experienced as an additive to composite plastic dental fillings. Traces of fluoride anions are constantly released, providing defense against caries. In addition, ytterbium fluoride is not transparent to X-rays [610].

Lutetium

Lutetium is the last element in the Ln series. Its chemical behavior plays an essential role in the research of a wide range of radiotherapeutics that show considerable *in vivo* stability. The radionuclide of lutetium ^{177}Lu with its beta- and gamma- emissions could be applied for targeted radionuclide therapy (TRT) and SPECT imaging in the treatment of many diseases [611]. It is one of the most significant theranostic radioisotopes utilized for the treatment of numerous oncologic and non-oncologic conditions. Being a hard Lewis acid, Lu^{3+} forms strong complexes with chelators which have high Lewis bases such as carboxylates. Due to lanthanide contraction, Lu^{3+} has the smallest ionic radius among the lanthanides. Consequently, a limited number of ligands can be placed around Lu^{3+} because of its high charge density and narrow coordination field [612]. A wide variety of ^{177}Lu radiopharmaceuticals, comprising small molecules, large biomolecules, and nanoparticles, has been effectively established and evaluated for various therapeutic procedures including peptide receptor radionuclide therapy, bone pain palliation, radiation synovectomy, and radioimmunotherapy. Among the chelators, DOTA and its derivatives are the most extensively used for preparation of ^{177}Lu-based radiopharmaceuticals. Some phosphonate equivalents of aminocarboxylates, like ethylenediaminetetra-(methylene phosphonic acid) (EDTMP) and 1, 4, 7, 10-tetraazacyclododecane- 1, 4, 7, 10-tetramethylene phosphonic acid (DOTMP) have also been used for the production of radiopharmaceuticals for bone pain palliation [613]. ^{177}Lu has numerous advantages in comparison to other intrinsically theranostic radiometals [614]. The nuclear decay properties of ^{177}Lu such as its comparatively long half-life, the energy of β$^-$ particles, and the energy and abundance of the γ-photons make it suitable for use in preparation of theranostic radiopharmaceuticals for targeting small-sized primary tumors and their metastatic sites.

Actinium

The radioactive isotope of actinium ^{225}Ac, which decays by β$^-$, α, and β$^+$ emissions, is a valuable radiopharmaceutical in nuclear medicine for malignant tumors treatment, favorable for usage in targeted alpha therapy (TAT). It can be applied to produce ^{213}Bi, both having favorable decay characteristics and chemical properties combined with the inherent advantages of alpha radiation of high energy and short-range in human tissue. It can be used alone as α- and β− emitter valuable for targeted alpha therapy (TAT). Alpha-emitters are suitable for the administration of minimal diseases, including hematologic cancers, infections, and compartmental tumors like ovarian cancer [615]. ^{225}Ac-Lintuzumab combined with Cytarabine is used for adults with untreated acute myeloid leukemia (AML) [616]. The monoclonal antibody moiety of ^{225}Ac-lintuzumab selectively binds to the cell surface antigen CD33, delivering a cytotoxic dose of α-radioactivity to cells expressing CD33 which is useful for patients with advanced myeloid leukemia malignancies.

Plutonium, Americium and Californium

Three trans-uranium isotopes, of plutonium, americium, and californium (^{238}Pu, ^{241}Am, and ^{252}Cf), have demonstrated considerable practical applications in space exploration to deliver energy [617]. Plutonium has been used for pacemakers to generate the electricity that stimulates the heart. The radioisotope of plutonium ^{238}Pu ($T_{1/2}$ = 87.7 y) seemed an attractive option for powering pacemaker batteries. Later, these devices were taken out of fashion by the introduction of Li-powered batteries, combined with the refinement of pulse generators.

The most common americium isotope ^{241}Am has a major γ-ray energy and a long half-life of 433 years for decay by the emission of α-particles, which make it predominantly useful for a wide range of industrial measuring applications (in radiography and X-ray fluorescence spectroscopy), and for the diagnosis of thyroid syndromes [618]. When mixed with Be, ^{241}Am generates neutrons at a high rate. Gamma rays from ^{241}Am are used to afford passive diagnosis of thyroid function. This application is now outdated. ^{241}Am γ-rays can provide sensible quality radiographs with a 10-minute exposure time. Meanwhile, ^{241}Am radiographs have only been tested empirically because of the possible damage to cells and DNA.

Californium isotope ^{252}Cf is a powerful neutron source. This isotope has been tested for applications in neutron activation analysis and neutron radiography. Although its usage in medicine requires protection precautions, it is attractive for brachytherapy applications where high-LET radiation is beneficial [619].

The chemical elements of the periodic table with therapeutic and diagnostic activity are listed in Table **19**.

Table 19. Chemical elements and their compounds with medical purposes.

Element	Medically-relevant Uses	References
Hydrogen	H_2O_2 -antiseptic; deuterium - labels pharmacokinetics of drugs, tritium is used in radioisotope diagnostics.	[22, 327-329]
Lithium	Li_2CO_3 - treatment of mental illnesses.	[24 - 26, 330-333]

(Table 19) cont.....

Element	Medically-relevant Uses	References
Sodium	$NaHCO_3$: antacid, $Na_2B_4O_7 \cdot 10H_2O$ - antiseptic, NaI for thyroid diseases, NaBr: sedative, $NaNO_2$: coronary dilator for angina pectoris, $Na_2S_2O_3$: antitoxic and desensitizing agent, Na_2-EDTA - anticoagulant.	[28, 334, 335]
Potassium	KI for thyroid diseases, KBr: sedative, KCl - cardiac arrhythmias, KMnO4 - antiseptic, ^{40}K: β− emitter.	[33]
Rubidium	^{82}Rb: radionuclide for PET myocardial perfusion imaging.	[34, 336, 337]
Cesium	^{131}Cs - treatment for prostate cancer, ^{129}Cs (γ-particle emitter) for myocardial imaging.	[34, 338]
Magnesium	MgO - antacid, $MgSO_4 \cdot 7H_2O$ - laxative, choleretic, hypotensive, sedative, and analgesic, $MgCO_3$ - antacid and antiulcer agent, Mg(lactate)$_2$: dietary supplement.	[45, 339-341]
Calcium	$CaCO_3$: antacid, $CaSO_4.1/2H_2O$: plaster ingredient, Ca(lactate)$_2$: dietary supplement, $CaCl_2.6H_2O$: serum sickness, urticaria.	[53, 342]
Strontium	Sr(II) salts - toothpaste additives, ^{89}Sr - β-emitter for the therapy of breast and metastatic prostate cancer.	[343 - 350]
Barium	$BaSO_4$ meals - contrast agent for gastrointestinal tract's X-ray imaging.	[59, 351]
Radium	^{223}Ra - α-emitter for skeletal metastases and prostate. $^{223}Ra^{2+}$ - Ca^{2+}mimetic.	[352 - 357]
Boron	H_3BO_3 - antiseptic, Boromycin - antibiotic, Borinic picolinate (AN0128) - antimicrobial and anti-inflammatory, Kerydin (AN2690) - antifungal.	[61 - 65, 358-363]
Aluminum	$Al(OH)_3$ - adjuvant in vaccines, antacid; $KAl(SO_4)_2 \cdot 12H_2O$ - astringent, $AlPO_4$ - antacid, antiulcer	[71, 364, 365]
Gallium	$Ga(NO_3)_3$: treatment of cancer-related hypercalcemia, ^{68}Ga scintigraphy - detects malignant tumors, including Hodgkin's and non-Hodgkin's lymphomas.	[72, 366-382]
Indium	^{111}In - γ-emitting radionuclide for prostate cancer and neuroendocrine tumors.	[383 - 385]
Thallium	^{205}Tl - for NMR detection, ^{201}Tl - in SPECT for perfusion tests of the myocardium.	[386 - 388]
Carbon	activated carbon, bicarbonate buffer system (HCO_3^-/H_2CO_3), liquid CO_2 for cryotherapy or for local analgesia.	[78 - 80]
Silicon	$Al_2(SiO_3)_3$ - adsorbing agent, $2MgO \cdot 3SiO_2 \cdot nH_2O$ - adsorbent and antacid agent, talc $3MgO \cdot 4SiO_2 \cdot H_2O$ in powders, pastes, and tablets, SiC - for grinding fillings and plastic prostheses, SiO_2 - silicate dental cement.	[82 - 86, 389-393]
Germanium	Ge: dietary supplement, Bis-2-carboxyethylgermanium sesquioxide (Ge-132) - for therapy of cancer, burns, hepatitis, cardiovascular diseases.	[394 - 399]
Tin	Sn in photodynamic therapy, Purlytin for cancers, breast metastases, organotin compounds - anticancer and antiviral agents.	[400 - 404]

(Table 19) cont.....

Element	Medically-relevant Uses	References
Lead	PbO - in inflammatory skin diseases, $Pb(CH_3COO)_2$ - astringent, ^{212}Pb (β−emission) in radio-immunotherapy, ^{212}Pb-TCMC-trastuzumab - antitumor	[405 - 408]
Nitrogen	Nitroglycerin, nitrosorbide - coronary drugs, $NaNO_2$ - vasodilator for angina pectoris, in cyanide poisoning, N_2O for anesthesia, NH_4OH to excite breathing, ^{13}N - in cardiac PET imaging.	[80, 99, 101, 334, 335, 409-412]
Phosphorus	ATP and creatine phosphate - for muscle dystrophy and atrophy, phosphate buffer system ($H_2PO_4^-/HPO_4^{2-}$), zinc phosphate cement - in stomatology, ^{32}P (β-emitting radionuclide) for detection of malignant tumors, Phosphocol - therapeutic for cancer-related effects.	[107, 109, 413]
Arsenic	As_2O_3 - for pulp necrotization, K_3AsO_3 and Na_2HAsO_4 - for anemia, exhaustion, neurasthenia; Salvarsan and Neosalvarsan - antibiotics to treat syphilis; Darinaparsin - cancer therapeutic.	[111, 112, 414-420]
Antimony	Organoantimonial compounds (Glucantime and Pentostam) - treatment of leishmaniases.	[421 - 425]
Bismuth	Bismatrol, Diotame, Kola-Pectin, Pepto Bismol, Kaopectate, Kapectolin, antidiarrheal agents - Bi citrate, Bi subsalicylate, bismuth iodoform, BiOCl, Bismuth colloids - antibacterial, Bi_2O_3 nanoparticles - antifungal, Sulbogin - for wound healing, Bismuth-213 (α-emitter), ^{213}Bi-lintuzumab for alpha-targeted radiotherapy in patients with AML.	[123 - 125, 426-441]
Oxygen	Oxygen therapy, hyperbaric oxygenotherapy, H_2O_2 (3%) for cleaning wounds, removing dead tissue, or as an oral debriding agent, O_3 for disinfection.	[22, 129, 132, 442-444]
Sulfur	S - laxative, antimicrobial, anti-seborrheic, and anthelminthic, for treatment of skin diseases, sulfanilamides - streptocide, norsulfazol, etazol, sulfazine - antimicrobial agents; SO_2 - fungicide agent, Na_2SO_3 and $Na_2S_2O_5$ - stabilizing antioxidants, $Na_2S_2O_3$ - for detoxication of cyanide or Tl poisoning.	[154, 155, 445-448]
Selenium	Se - part of mineral-vitamin complexes, Na_2SeO_3 - for Se deficiency; selenomethionine and Se-methyl-seleno-L-cysteine for chemopreventive treatment of prostate cancer, Se sulfide - an antifungal agent.	[449 - 451]
Tellurium	AS101 (non-toxic Te(IV) compound - for treatment of external genital warts, in chemotherapy - anti-inflammatory and antiapoptotic.	[168, 452-454]
Fluorine	NaF - for prevention of dental caries, and osteoporosis. ^{18}F labelled deoxyglucose - tracer for PET imaging, ^{18}F-fluorodeoxyglucose-PET (18F-FDG-PET) for screening, localization, and monitoring of malignancies, infections, autoimmune processes.	[169, 170, 455, 456]
Chlorine	NaCl in isotonic solutions, HOCl, $CaOCl_2$ - bleaching agents, NaClO - disinfectant. $KClO_4$ for the protection of the thyroid gland at inspection by radioiodine.	[28, 33, 173, 174, 457]
Bromine	NH_4Br, KBr, NaBr - depressants, sedatives, and anticonvulsants.	[175, 458]

(Table 19) cont.....

Element	Medically-relevant Uses	References
Iodine	Supplementing iodide preparations (NaCl with KI, KIO_3, NaI, $NaIO_3$); ^{131}I, ^{132}I, ^{125}I, and ^{123}I - for the therapy and diagnosis of thyroid diseases, alcohol solution of iodine (tincture of iodine) - antiseptic, water solution of KI (Lugol's solution), iodoform, iodinol - treatment of hyperthyroidism, *Povidone-iodine* (PVP-I) - antiseptic for skin.	[176 - 181, 459,460]
Astatine	^{221}At, ^{222}At, ^{223}At (α-emitters) for targeted therapy of central nervous system and malignant brain tumors.	[182, 183, 461-464]
Helium	^3He for pulmonary MRI.	[465 - 467]
Argon	Ar for ischemic pathologies; argon plasma coagulation.	[468 - 470]
Krypton	^{83}Kr in MRI of the respiratory track.	[471]
Xenon	Xenon-133 in lung radio imaging by SPECT, ^{129}Xe - MRI contrast agent for imaging of the gas flow in the lungs.	[472, 473]
Copper	$CuSO_4{\cdot}5H_2O$ - antimicrobial effect, astringent, and antiseptic, Cu(histidine)$_2$: Menke's disease treatment, $CuSO_4$ - antidote of phosphorus poisoning.	[475, 476]
Silver	Colloidal Ag (collargol, protargol) - bactericidal effect, astringent, antiseptic, and anti-inflammatory, $AgNO_3$: cauterizing agent, histology: silver staining, Au, Ag, Cu alloys - in dental practice for fillings and prosthetics.	[200, 477-480]
Gold	Au(I) - treatment of rheumatoid arthritis (Myocrizine, Aureotan, Solganol), anticancer; ^{198}Au - treatment of malignant tumors.	[201, 481-491]
Zinc	Zn(gluconate)$_2$ - dietary supplement, ZnO, $ZnSO_4{\cdot}7H_2O$ - antiseptic, astringent, and drying agents - skin ointments, eye drops, H_3PO_4 with ZnO - stomatology cement, $ZnCl_2$ - infusions in parenteral nutrition, zinc insulin - injections in diabetes mellitus.	[202 - 206, 492]
Mercury	mercury thermometers, amalgams (40% Hg) in dental practice, HgO - treatment of skin diseases, $HgCl_2$ - antiseptic for wounds, Thimerosal (ethylmercury thiosalicylate) - for preserving vaccines, organomercury fungicides.	[493, 494]
Scandium	^{44}Sc and ^{47}Sc - in PET and SPECT imaging and radiotherapy.	[218, 219, 495]
Yttrium	^{90}Y (β-emitter) - for non-Hodgkin B-cell lymphoma radiotherapy and immunotherapy, ^{86}Y tracer for PET imaging.	[220, 496]
Titanium	Ti in prosthetics and implants, Ti(IV) for anticancer treatments (Budotitane, Ti-Salan and titanocene derivatives).	[221, 497-499]
Zirconium	Zr in dental, knee, and hip implants, reconstruction of the middle-ear ossicular chain, Al(III)-Zr(IV) tetrachlorohydrex gly in deodorants.	[222, 500]
Hafnium	Hafnium - scavenger metal against oxygen and nitrogen, hafnium oxide nanoparticles (NBTXR3) in anticancer and radiation therapy.	[223, 501, 502]
Vanadium	Insulin mimetics, V(IV) and V(V) complexes - for diabetes mellitus type 2, vanadocene derivatives - for the treatment of cancer.	[225 - 228, 503-505]

Element	Medically-relevant Uses	References
Niobium	Nb in pacemakers, Nb(V) polyoxometalates - potential antiviral agents.	[229, 506]
Tantalum	Ta radiopaque for marking in orthopedics and in endovascular medicine, Ta nanoparticles - iodinated contrast agents for blood pool imaging applications.	[230, 507]
Chromium	Cr and Ni stainless steel - in orthopedic practice, Cr(III) tris(picolinate) - therapy of carbohydrate and fat metabolism disorders, Cr_2O_3 - in dental pastes.	[234, 508, 509]
Molybdenum	MoO_4^{2-} prevents oxidation of lipids and protects antioxidant systems for treatment of diabetic mellitus, MoS_4^{2-} - copper chelator, for treatment of breast cancer, and esophageal carcinoma; $(NH_4)_2MoO_4$ or Na_2MoO_4, - in vitamin complexes, Mo radioisotopes - for liver and blood circulation diagnostics.	[237 - 245, 510]
Tungsten	Polyoxotungstates - antiviral, antibacterial, anticancer, Na_2WO_4 - antidiabetic.	[244, 511-513]
Manganese	Mn - part of enzymes catalyzing redox reactions, Mn salts ($MnSO_4$, $MnCl_2$, and gluconate), and Mn chelates (aspartate, picolinate, fumarate, malate, succinate, citrate, and amino acid chelate) in Mn supplements with vitamins; $KMnO_4$ - antiseptic, for washing wounds, gargling.	[252, 514-518]
Technetium	^{99m}Tc - in nuclear diagnostic imaging of bone, brain, lungs, thyroid, myocardium, and liver. SPECT ^{99m}Tc-glucoheptonate (^{99m}Tc-GHA) - for brain scans, Cardiolite (^{99m}Tc-sestamibi), Neurite (^{99m}Tc-disicate), ^{99m}Tc-MIP-1404 for cancer imaging.	[253, 519-521]
Rhenium	^{186}Re and ^{188}Re (β-emitters) - for diagnosis and radio imaging in the treatment of malignant tumors, bone metastases, and rheumatoid arthritis; ^{188}Re-HEDP for bone pain palliation in prostate cancer, ^{188}Re-P2045 - for therapy of small cell lung cancer and advanced neuroendocrine carcinomas.	[254, 255, 522]
Iron	$FeSO_4$, complex organic Fe(II) salts (gluconate, succinate, fumarate, lactate, ascorbate, sorbate, saccharate) - for iron deficiency anemia, Ferroquine (ferrocene derivative) - for treatment of malaria; superparamagnetic Fe oxides - MRI contrast agents, $Na_2[Fe(CN)_5NO]$ - hypertensive agent.	[334, 335, 523-527]
Cobalt	vitamin B12 - treatment of pernicious anemia, ^{57}Co and ^{60}Co - in nuclear medicine: ^{60}Co for diagnostics and treatment of malignant tumors, Co(III) complex Doxovir (CTC-96) - against drug-resistant herpes simplex virus.	[268 - 270, 528-532]
Ruthenium	Ru complexes (KP1019, NKP-1339, IT-139, NAMI-A) - anticancer drugs, Ru(III)- EDTA complexes - NO scavengers for therapy of septic shock.	[285, 287, 288, 291-293, 533-547]
Rhodium	Rh complexes - anticancer, antiparasitic, and antiviral, ^{105}Rh (β-emitter), ^{105}Rh-EDTMP - for therapy of pain due to bone metastases.	[294 - 296, 548]
Palladium	Pd - in dental appliances, ^{103}Pd needles - for prostate cancer and choroidal melanoma brachytherapy.	[298, 299, 301, 302, 549, 550]

(Table 19) cont.....

Element	Medically-relevant Uses	References
Osmium	OsO_4 - in chronically inflamed arthritic joints, OsO_4 - SOD mimic, Os complexes - anticancer, redox activation, DNA targeting or inhibition of protein kinase; in photodynamic therapy (PDT).	[303 - 306, 551, 552]
Iridium	Ir and Ru - in dental alloys, Iridium(III) complexes - anticancer, inhibitors of protein kinase and protein-protein interactions, in photodynamic therapy; ^{192}Ir ($\beta-$ emitter) for cancer brachytherapy and prostatic carcinoma; GAMMA-Iridium-192 catheter for coronary artery disease.	[307 - 312, 553-558]
Platinum	Pt materials - pacemakers and hearing aids, urinary catheters, cardiovascular catheters; Pt compounds - chemotherapeutic drugs: carboplatin, oxaliplatin, and cisplatin for the treatment of breast, lung, ovarian, and testicular cancers; nedaplatin, lobaplatin, and heptaphane - potent anticancer agents.	[313 - 316, 559-573]
Lanthanides and actinides	La(III) ions - substitute Ca(II) ions in bones, $La_2(CO_3)_3$ (Fosrenol) - for treatment of hyperphosphatemia; $Ce(NO_3)_3$ - bacteriostatic, Ce-Ag sulfadiazine (Flammacerium) - for treatment of burn wounds; ^{153}Sm ($\beta-$decay) in ^{153}Sm-EDTMP - in osteoblastic metastatic bone lesions for therapy of high-risk osteosarcoma and breast cancer metastatic to bone, multiple myeloma; Eu - MRI contrast agent: Eu(III)-DOTA - MRI sensor of $^1O_2$ during photodynamic therapy; Gd(III) chelates - contrast agents in MR images: $[Gd(DTPA)(H_2O)]^{2-}$ (Magnevist) and $[Gd(DOTA)(H_2O)]^-$ (Dotarem), related Dy(III) and Tm(III) - NMR shift reagents; ^{166}Ho - substitute for ^{188}Re for internal radiation therapy; ^{175}Yb (β-decay) - for bone pain palliation in the therapy of bone metastases, ^{169}Yb - for intravascular brachytherapy; ^{177}Lu (β- and γ-emitter) - for targeted radionuclide therapy (TRT) and SPECT imaging; ^{225}Ac (β^-, α, and β^+ decay) - for malignant tumors, hematologic cancers, infections, and ovarian cancer, acute myeloid leukemia (AML) treatment.	[317 - 326, 574-619]

REFERENCES

CONCLUDING REMARKS

The book titled "BIOLOGICAL AND MEDICAL SIGNIFICANCE OF CHEMICAL ELEMENTS" is devoted to the chemistry and biological role of biogenic essential and trace elements. It deals with issues related to the prevalence of chemical elements in nature, the ratio of the chemical elements and their compounds in living organisms and the environment, the biological role of elements depending on their position in the periodic table of elements, the use of compounds of s-, p-, d- and f-elements in medicine, and environmental aspects of the action of their compounds.

Chemical elements are present in different forms in nature, and these elements are very essential for the body to perform different functions. It is known that the human body contains nearly all the elements of the periodic table, many of which go into the body from the environment and can participate in biochemical processes in health and disease. When considering the chemistry of biogenic elements on the basis of the periodic law, an approach is used to find out which properties and features of the elements are responsible for their different amounts in living organisms, which determines the specific role of elements in biological systems. The study of chemical and biological properties provides information about the patterns of individual properties of chemical elements and their compounds. Here an element-by-element journey through the periodic table is made, starting with the main groups IA-IIA (s-elements: hydrogen, alkali and alkaline earth metals), IIIA-VIIIA (p-block elements, mostly non-metals, metalloids, and noble gases), followed by groups IB-VIIIB, including d- and f-elements such as transition metals, lanthanides, and actinides.

Special attention in the book is paid to the chemistry and biology of the essential biogenic elements and their compounds. However, the periodic table also offers potential for novel therapeutic and diagnostic agents, based on not only essential elements, but also non-essential elements, and on radionuclides, which provide new challenges in biology, bioinorganic chemistry, and medicine. Future advances in the design of inorganic, organic, organometallic, metal-based coordination compounds, and supramolecular drugs require more knowledge of their mechanism of action, including target sites and metabolism.

The most characteristic patterns of modern human beings are the deficiency of essential elements and the excess of toxic trace elements. The accumulation or deficiency of the elements may stimulate an alternate pathway that might cause diseases. Chronic toxicity, acute intoxication, and their effects on the living body have also been considered.

This book highlights the current knowledge of essential biogenic elements, trace elements useful in diagnosis and therapy, and notable features in their chemistry which relate to their biological activity. The book may be of interest to researchers working in the field of bioinorganic and medicinal chemistry, as well as in medicine and biology.

ACKNOWLEDGEMENTS

The author would like to thank the European Union-NextGenerationEU, through the National Recovery and Resilience Plan of the Republic of Bulgaria, project N° BGRRP-2.004-0004-C01 for the administrative support provided.

REFERENCES

[1]   Lindh, U. Biological Functions of the Elements. In: *Essentials of Medical Geology*; Selinus, O., Ed.; Springer: Dordrecht, **2013**.
        [http://dx.doi.org/10.1007/978-94-007-4375-5_7]

[2]   Maret, W.; Blower, P. Teaching the chemical elements in biochemistry: Elemental biology and metallomics. *Biochem. Mol. Biol. Educ.,* **2022**, *50*(3), 283-289.
        [http://dx.doi.org/10.1002/bmb.21614] [PMID: 35218613]

[3]   Kostova, I.; Soni, R.K. Bioinorganic Chemistry. Shree Publishers & Distributors: New Delhi, India, **2011**.

[4]   Goswami, A.K.; Kostova, I. Medicinal and biological inorganic chemistry. Walter de Gruyter GmbH & Co KG, **2022**.
        [http://dx.doi.org/10.1515/9781501516115]

[5]   Anbar, A.D. Elements and evolution. *Science,* **2008**, *322*(5907), 1481-1483.
        [http://dx.doi.org/10.1126/science.1163100] [PMID: 19056967]

[6]   Eggins, B.R. Biological Elements. In: *Biosensors*; An Introduction. Teubner Studienbücher Chemie: Verlag, Wiesbaden, **1996**.
        [http://dx.doi.org/10.1007/978-3-663-05664-5_2]

[7]   Aversa, R.; Petrescu, R.V.; Apicella, A.; Petrescu, F.I. The basic elements of life's. *Am. J. Eng. Appl. Sci.,* **2016**, *9*(4), 1189-1197.
        [http://dx.doi.org/10.3844/ajeassp.2016.1189.1197]

[8]   Fränzle, S.; Markert, B. The biological system of the elements (BSE)—a brief introduction into historical and applied aspects with special reference on "ecotoxicological identity cards" for different element species (e.g. As and Sn). *Environ. Pollut.,* **2002**, *120*(1), 27-45.
        [http://dx.doi.org/10.1016/S0269-7491(02)00126-4] [PMID: 12199465]

[9]   Ghosh, S.; Mugesh, G. The elements of life. *Curr. Sci.,* **2019**, *117*(12), 1971-1985.
        [http://dx.doi.org/10.18520/cs/v117/i12/1971-1985]

[10]   Needham, R.J.; Sadler, P.J. A periodic table for life and medicines *The Periodic Table II,* **2019**, 175-201.
        [http://dx.doi.org/10.1007/430_2019_51]

[11] Fraga, C.G. Relevance, essentiality and toxicity of trace elements in human health. *Mol. Aspects Med.,* **2005**, *26*(4-5), 235-244.
[http://dx.doi.org/10.1016/j.mam.2005.07.013] [PMID: 16125765]

[12] Sigel, H.; Sigel, A. The bio-relevant metals of the periodic table of the elements. *Z. Naturforsch. B. J. Chem. Sci.,* **2019**, *74*(6), 461-471.
[http://dx.doi.org/10.1515/znb-2019-0056]

[13] Maret, W. The metals in the biological periodic system of the elements: Concepts and conjectures. *Int. J. Mol. Sci.,* **2016**, *17*(1), 66.
[http://dx.doi.org/10.3390/ijms17010066] [PMID: 26742035]

[14] Kaim, W.; Schwederski, B.; Klein, A. Bioinorganic Chemistry--Inorganic Elements in the Chemistry of Life: An Introduction and Guide. John Wiley & Sons, **2013**.

[15] Barry, N.P.E.; Sadler, P.J. Exploration of the medical periodic table: Towards new targets. *Chem. Commun.,* **2013**, *49*(45), 5106-5131.
[http://dx.doi.org/10.1039/c3cc41143e] [PMID: 23636600]

[16] Cammack, R. Origins, evolution and the hydrogen biosphere. In: *Hydrogen as a Fuel*; CRC Press, **2001**; pp. 21-28.
[http://dx.doi.org/10.1201/9780203471043-6]

[17] Wike-Hooley, J.L.; Haveman, J.; Reinhold, H.S. The relevance of tumour pH to the treatment of malignant disease. *Radiother. Oncol.,* **1984**, *2*(4), 343-366.
[http://dx.doi.org/10.1016/S0167-8140(84)80077-8] [PMID: 6097949]

[18] Mindell, J.A. Lysosomal acidification mechanisms. *Annu. Rev. Physiol.,* **2012**, *74*(1), 69-86.
[http://dx.doi.org/10.1146/annurev-physiol-012110-142317] [PMID: 22335796]

[19] Mayle, K.M.; Le, A.M.; Kamei, D.T. The intracellular trafficking pathway of transferrin. *Biochim. Biophys. Acta, Gen. Subj.,* **2012**, *1820*(3), 264-281.
[http://dx.doi.org/10.1016/j.bbagen.2011.09.009] [PMID: 21968002]

[20] Jeffrey, G.A. The role of the hydrogen bond and water in biological processes. *J. Mol. Struct.,* **1994**, *322*, 21-25.
[http://dx.doi.org/10.1016/0022-2860(94)87017-9]

[21] Tóth, G.; Bowers, S.G; Truong, A.P; Probst, G. The role and significance of unconventional hydrogen bonds in small molecule recognition by biological receptors of pharmaceutical relevance. *Curr. Pharm. Des.,* **2007**, *13*(34), 3476-3493.
[http://dx.doi.org/10.2174/138161207782794284] [PMID: 18220785]

[22] Winterbourn, C.C. The biological chemistry of hydrogen peroxide. *Meth. Enzy.,* **2013**, *528*, 3-25.
[http://dx.doi.org/10.1016/B978-0-12-405881-1.00001-X] [PMID: 23849856]

[23] Černý, M.; Habánová, H.; Berka, M.; Luklová, M.; Brzobohatý, B. Hydrogen peroxide: Its role in plant biology and crosstalk with signalling networks. *Int. J. Mol. Sci.,* **2018**, *19*(9), 2812.
[http://dx.doi.org/10.3390/ijms19092812] [PMID: 30231521]

[24] Ochoa, E.L.M. Lithium as a neuroprotective agent for bipolar disorder: An overview. *Cell. Mol. Neurobiol.,* **2022**, *42*(1), 85-97.
[http://dx.doi.org/10.1007/s10571-021-01129-9] [PMID: 34357564]

[25] Fountoulakis, K.N.; Tohen, M.; Zarate, Jr, C.A. Lithium treatment of Bipolar disorder in adults: A systematic review of randomized trials and meta-analyses. *Eur. Neuropsychopharmacol.,* **2022**, *54*, 100-115.
[http://dx.doi.org/10.1016/j.euroneuro.2021.10.003] [PMID: 34980362]

[26] Gomes-da-Costa, S.; Marx, W.; Corponi, F.; Anmella, G.; Murru, A.; Pons-Cabrera, M.T.; Giménez-Palomo, A.; Gutiérrez-Arango, F.; Llach, C.D.; Fico, G.; Kotzalidis, G.D.; Verdolini, N.; Valentí, M.; Berk, M.; Vieta, E.; Pacchiarotti, I. Lithium therapy and weight change in people with bipolar

disorder: A systematic review and meta-analysis. *Neurosci. Biobehav. Rev.,* **2022**, *134*, 104266.
[http://dx.doi.org/10.1016/j.neubiorev.2021.07.011] [PMID: 34265322]

[27]   Sigel, A.; Sigel, H.; Sigel, R.K.O., Eds. *The Alkali Metal Ions: Their Role for Life, MILS-16*; Springer International Publishing: Cham, Switzerland, **2016**.
[http://dx.doi.org/10.1007/978-3-319-21756-7]

[28]   Pohl, H.R.; Wheeler, J.S.; Murray, H.E. Sodium and potassium in health and disease. In: *Interrelations between essential metal ions and human diseases*; Sigel, A.; Sigel, H.; Sigel, R.K.O., Eds.; Dordrecht, The Netherlands: Springer Science and Business Media B.V., **2013**.
[http://dx.doi.org/10.1007/978-94-007-7500-8_2]

[29]   Bertini, I.; Sigel, A.; Sigel, H., Eds. *Handbook on Metalloproteins*; Marcel Dekker, Inc.: New York and Basel, **2001**.
[http://dx.doi.org/10.1201/9781482270822]

[30]   Seay, N.W.; Lehrich, R.W.; Greenberg, A. Diagnosis and management of disorders of body tonicity—hyponatremia and hypernatremia: Core curriculum 2020. *Am. J. Kidney Dis.,* **2020**, *75*(2), 272-286.
[http://dx.doi.org/10.1053/j.ajkd.2019.07.014] [PMID: 31606238]

[31]   Adrogué, H.J.; Tucker, B.M.; Madias, N.E. Diagnosis and management of hyponatremia: A review. *JAMA,* **2022**, *328*(3), 280-291.
[http://dx.doi.org/10.1001/jama.2022.11176] [PMID: 35852524]

[32]   Hunter, R.W.; Bailey, M.A. Hyperkalemia: Pathophysiology, risk factors and consequences. *Nephrol. Dial. Transplant.,* **2019**, *34* Suppl. 3, iii2-iii11.
[http://dx.doi.org/10.1093/ndt/gfz206] [PMID: 31800080]

[33]   Palmer, B.F.; Clegg, D.J. Physiology and pathophysiology of potassium homeostasis: Core curriculum 2019. *Am. J. Kidney Dis.,* **2019**, *74*(5), 682-695.
[http://dx.doi.org/10.1053/j.ajkd.2019.03.427] [PMID: 31227226]

[34]   Relman, A.S. The physiological behavior of rubidium and cesium in relation to that of potassium. *Yale J. Biol. Med.,* **1956**, *29*(3), 248-262.
[PMID: 13409924]

[35]   Pais, I.; Jones, J.B. *The handbook of trace elements*; CRC Press: Boca Raton, FL, **1997**.

[36]   Wang, Y.; Dai, S. Structural basis of metal hypersensitivity. *Immunol. Res.,* **2013**, *55*(1-3), 83-90.
[http://dx.doi.org/10.1007/s12026-012-8351-1] [PMID: 22983897]

[37]   Müller, M.; Buchner, M.R. Beryllium complexes with bio-relevant functional groups: Coordination geometries and binding affinities. *Angew. Chem. Int. Ed.,* **2018**, *57*(29), 9180-9184.
[http://dx.doi.org/10.1002/anie.201803667] [PMID: 29682869]

[38]   Thierse, H.J.; Gamerdinger, K.; Junkes, C.; Guerreiro, N.; Weltzien, H.U. T cell receptor (TCR) interaction with haptens: Metal ions as non-classical haptens. *Toxicology,* **2005**, *209*(2), 101-107.
[http://dx.doi.org/10.1016/j.tox.2004.12.015] [PMID: 15767020]

[39]   Fontenot, A.P.; Maier, L.A. Genetic susceptibility and immune-mediated destruction in beryllium-induced disease. *Trends Immunol.,* **2005**, *26*(10), 543-549.
[http://dx.doi.org/10.1016/j.it.2005.08.004] [PMID: 16099719]

[40]   Dai, S.; Falta, M.T.; Bowerman, N.A.; McKee, A.S.; Fontenot, A.P. T cell recognition of beryllium. *Curr. Opin. Immunol.,* **2013**, *25*(6), 775-780.
[http://dx.doi.org/10.1016/j.coi.2013.07.012] [PMID: 23978481]

[41]   Dai, S.; Murphy, G.A.; Crawford, F.; Mack, D.G.; Falta, M.T.; Marrack, P.; Kappler, J.W.; Fontenot, A.P. Crystal structure of HLA-DP2 and implications for chronic beryllium disease. *Proc. Natl. Acad. Sci.,* **2010**, *107*(16), 7425-7430.
[http://dx.doi.org/10.1073/pnas.1001772107] [PMID: 20356827]

[42]   Falta, M.T.; Pinilla, C.; Mack, D.G.; Tinega, A.N.; Crawford, F.; Giulianotti, M.; Santos, R.; Clayton, G.M.; Wang, Y.; Zhang, X.; Maier, L.A.; Marrack, P.; Kappler, J.W.; Fontenot, A.P. Identification of beryllium-dependent peptides recognized by CD4+ T cells in chronic beryllium disease. *J. Exp. Med.,* **2013**, *210*(7), 1403-1418.
[http://dx.doi.org/10.1084/jem.20122426] [PMID: 23797096]

[43]   Bathellier, C.; Tcherkez, G.; Lorimer, G.H.; Farquhar, G.D. Rubisco is not really so bad. *Plant Cell Environ.,* **2018**, *41*(4), 705-716.
[http://dx.doi.org/10.1111/pce.13149] [PMID: 29359811]

[44]   Erb, T.J.; Zarzycki, J. A short history of RubisCO: The rise and fall (?) of Nature's predominant CO_2 fixing enzyme. *Curr. Opin. Biotechnol.,* **2018**, *49*, 100-107.
[http://dx.doi.org/10.1016/j.copbio.2017.07.017] [PMID: 28843191]

[45]   Romani, A.M.P. Magnesium in health and disease. *Met. Ions Life Sci.,* **2013**, *13*, 49-79.
[http://dx.doi.org/10.1007/978-94-007-7500-8_3] [PMID: 24470089]

[46]   Hartwig, A. Role of magnesium in genomic stability. *Mutat. Res.,* **2001**, *475*(1-2), 113-121.
[http://dx.doi.org/10.1016/S0027-5107(01)00074-4] [PMID: 11295157]

[47]   Klein, D.J.; Moore, P.B.; Steitz, T.A. The contribution of metal ions to the structural stability of the large ribosomal subunit. *RNA,* **2004**, *10*(9), 1366-1379.
[http://dx.doi.org/10.1261/rna.7390804] [PMID: 15317974]

[48]   Selmer, M.; Dunham, C.M.; Murphy, F.V., IV; Weixlbaumer, A.; Petry, S.; Kelley, A.C.; Weir, J.R.; Ramakrishnan, V. Structure of the 70S ribosome complexed with mRNA and tRNA. *Science,* **2006**, *313*(5795), 1935-1942.
[http://dx.doi.org/10.1126/science.1131127] [PMID: 16959973]

[49]   Beaven, G.H.; Parmar, J.; Nash, G.B.; Bennett, P.M.; Gratzer, W.B. Effect of magnesium ions on red cell membrane properties. *J. Membr. Biol.,* **1990**, *118*(3), 251-257.
[http://dx.doi.org/10.1007/BF01868609] [PMID: 2077132]

[50]   Payandeh, J.; Pfoh, R.; Pai, E.F. The structure and regulation of magnesium selective ion channels. *Biochim. Biophys. Acta Biomembr.,* **2013**, *1828*(11), 2778-2792.
[http://dx.doi.org/10.1016/j.bbamem.2013.08.002] [PMID: 23954807]

[51]   Chrysant, S.G.; Chrysant, G.S. Association of hypomagnesemia with cardiovascular diseases and hypertension. *Inter. Jnl. Cardio. Hyper.,* **2019**, *1*, 100005.
[http://dx.doi.org/10.1016/j.ijchy.2019.100005] [PMID: 33447739]

[52]   Van Laecke, S. Hypomagnesemia and hypermagnesemia. *Acta Clin. Belg.,* **2019**, *74*(1), 41-47.
[http://dx.doi.org/10.1080/17843286.2018.1516173] [PMID: 30220246]

[53]   Brini, M.; Ottolini, D.; Calì, T.; Carafoli, E. Calcium in health and disease. *Met. Ions Life Sci.,* **2013**, *13*, 81-137.
[http://dx.doi.org/10.1007/978-94-007-7500-8_4] [PMID: 24470090]

[54]   Brini, M.; Calì, T.; Ottolini, D.; Carafoli, E. The plasma membrane calcium pump in health and disease. *FEBS J.,* **2013**, *280*(21), 5385-5397.
[http://dx.doi.org/10.1111/febs.12193] [PMID: 23413890]

[55]   Brini, M.; Calì, T.; Ottolini, D.; Carafoli, E. Intracellular calcium homeostasis and signaling. *Met. Ions Life Sci.,* **2013**, *12*, 119-168.
[http://dx.doi.org/10.1007/978-94-007-5561-1_5] [PMID: 23595672]

[56]   Pepe, J.; Colangelo, L.; Biamonte, F.; Sonato, C.; Danese, V.C.; Cecchetti, V.; Occhiuto, M.; Piazzolla, V.; De Martino, V.; Ferrone, F.; Minisola, S.; Cipriani, C. Diagnosis and management of hypocalcemia. *Endocrine,* **2020**, *69*(3), 485-495.
[http://dx.doi.org/10.1007/s12020-020-02324-2] [PMID: 32367335]

[57]   Motlaghzadeh, Y.; Bilezikian, J.P.; Sellmeyer, D.E. Rare causes of hypercalcemia: 2021 update. *J.*

Clin. Endocrinol. Metab., **2021**, *106*(11), 3113-3128.
[http://dx.doi.org/10.1210/clinem/dgab504] [PMID: 34240162]

[58] Meunier, P.J.; Roux, C.; Seeman, E.; Ortolani, S.; Badurski, J.E.; Spector, T.D.; Cannata, J.; Balogh, A.; Lemmel, E.M.; Pors-Nielsen, S.; Rizzoli, R.; Genant, H.K.; Reginster, J.Y. The effects of strontium ranelate on the risk of vertebral fracture in women with postmenopausal osteoporosis. *N. Engl. J. Med.,* **2004**, *350*(5), 459-468.
[http://dx.doi.org/10.1056/NEJMoa022436] [PMID: 14749454]

[59] McKee, M.W.; Jurgens, R.W.Jr. Barium sulfate products for roentgenographic examination of the gastrointestinal tract. *Am. J. Hosp. Pharm,* **1986**, *43*(1), 145-148.
[http://dx.doi.org/10.1093/ajhp/43.1.145] [PMID: 3953584]

[60] Greb, L.; Ebner, F.; Ginzburg, Y.; Sigmund, L.M. Element-ligand cooperativity with p-Block Elements. *Eur. J. Inorg. Chem.,* **2020**, (32), 3030-3047.
[http://dx.doi.org/10.1002/ejic.202000449]

[61] Dinca, L.; Scorei, R. Boron in human nutrition and its regulations use. *J. Nutr. Ther.,* **2013**, *2*, 22-29.

[62] Newnham, R.E. Essentiality of boron for healthy bones and joints. *Environ. Health Perspect.,* **1994**, *102*(Suppl 7) Suppl. 7, 83-85.
[http://dx.doi.org/10.1289/ehp.94102s783] [PMID: 7889887]

[63] Price, C.T.; Langford, J.R.; Liporace, F.A. Essential nutrients for bone health and a review of their availability in the average North American diet. *Open Orthop. J.,* **2012**, *6*(1), 143-149.
[http://dx.doi.org/10.2174/1874325001206010143] [PMID: 22523525]

[64] Dembitsky, V.M.; Smoum, R.; Al-Quntar, A.A.; Ali, H.A.; Pergament, I.; Srebnik, M. Natural occurrence of boron-containing compounds in plants, algae and microorganisms. *Plant Sci.,* **2002**, *163*(5), 931-942.
[http://dx.doi.org/10.1016/S0168-9452(02)00174-7]

[65] Cheng, X.; Li, F.; Liang, L. Boron neutron capture therapy: Clinical application and research progress. *Curr. Oncol.,* **2022**, *29*(10), 7868-7886.
[http://dx.doi.org/10.3390/curroncol29100622] [PMID: 36290899]

[66] Wills, M.R.; Savory, J. Aluminium poisoning: Dialysis encephalopathy, osteomalacia, and anaemia. *Lancet,* **1983**, *322*(8340), 29-34.
[http://dx.doi.org/10.1016/S0140-6736(83)90014-4] [PMID: 6134894]

[67] Kumar, V.; Gill, K.D. Oxidative stress and mitochondrial dysfunction in aluminium neurotoxicity and its amelioration: A review. *Neurotoxicology,* **2014**, *41*, 154-166.
[http://dx.doi.org/10.1016/j.neuro.2014.02.004] [PMID: 24560992]

[68] Exley, C. Aluminum should now be considered a primary etiological factor in alzheimer's Disease. *J. Alzheimers Dis. Rep.,* **2017**, *1*(1), 23-25.
[http://dx.doi.org/10.3233/ADR-170010] [PMID: 30480226]

[69] Virk, S.A.; Eslick, G.D. Occupational Exposure to Aluminum and Alzheimer Disease: A Meta-Analysis. *J. Occup. Environ. Med.,* **2015**, *57*(8), 893-896.
[http://dx.doi.org/10.1097/JOM.0000000000000487] [PMID: 26247643]

[70] Mujika, J.I.; Dalla Torre, G.; Formoso, E.; Grande-Aztatzi, R.; Grabowski, S.J.; Exley, C.; Lopez, X. Aluminum's preferential binding site in proteins: Sidechain of amino acids *versus* backbone interactions. *J. Inorg. Biochem.,* **2018**, *181*, 111-116.
[http://dx.doi.org/10.1016/j.jinorgbio.2017.10.014] [PMID: 29183625]

[71] Pineau, A.; Fauconneau, B.; Sappino, A.P.; Deloncle, R.; Guillard, O. If exposure to aluminium in antiperspirants presents health risks, its content should be reduced. *J. Trace Elem. Med. Biol.,* **2014**, *28*(2), 147-150.
[http://dx.doi.org/10.1016/j.jtemb.2013.12.002] [PMID: 24418462]

[72] Peng, X.X.; Gao, S.; Zhang, J.L. Gallium (III) complexes in cancer chemotherapy. *Eur. J. Inorg.*

Chem., **2022**, *2022*(6), e202100953.

[73]   Beraldo, H. Pharmacological applications of non-radioactive indium(III) complexes: A field yet to be explored. *Coord. Chem. Rev.,* **2020**, *419*, 213375.
[http://dx.doi.org/10.1016/j.ccr.2020.213375]

[74]   Xu, X.; Liu, J.H.; Yuan, C.X.; Xing, Y.M.; Wang, M.; Zhang, Y.H.; Zhou, X.H.; Litvinov, Y.A.; Blaum, K.; Chen, R.J.; Chen, X.C.; Fu, C.Y.; Gao, B.S.; He, J.J.; Kubono, S.; Lam, Y.H.; Li, H.F.; Liu, M.L.; Ma, X.W.; Shuai, P.; Si, M.; Sun, M.Z.; Tu, X.L.; Wang, Q.; Xu, H.S.; Yan, X.L.; Yang, J.C.; Yuan, Y.J.; Zeng, Q.; Zhang, P.; Zhou, X.; Zhan, W.L.; Litvinov, S.; Audi, G.; Naimi, S.; Uesaka, T.; Yamaguchi, Y.; Yamaguchi, T.; Ozawa, A.; Sun, B.H.; Kaneko, K.; Sun, Y.; Xu, F.R. Masses of ground and isomeric states of In 101 and configuration-dependent shell evolution in odd: A indium isotopes. *Phys. Rev. C,* **2019**, *100*(5), 051303.
[http://dx.doi.org/10.1103/PhysRevC.100.051303]

[75]   Eghtesadi, R.; Safavi, S.; Shahmirzayi, F.; Banafshe, H.R.; Omidi, S.; Ghaderi, A. A narrative review of thallium toxicity; preventive measures. *Int. J. Pharm. Res.,* **2019**, *11*(3), 322-330.

[76]   Di Candia, D.; Biehler-Gomez, L.; Giordano, G.; Cattaneo, C. A case of thallium intoxication by walking in a field. *For. Sci. Int. Rep.,* **2020**, *2*, 100102.
[http://dx.doi.org/10.1016/j.fsir.2020.100102]

[77]   Ali, S.R. An overview on greenhouse effect. *Acad. Int. Multidisc. Res. J.,* **2021**, *11*(11), 994-1000.

[78]   Romão, C.C.; Blättler, W.A.; Seixas, J.D.; Bernardes, G.J.L. Developing drug molecules for therapy with carbon monoxide. *Chem. Soc. Rev.,* **2012**, *41*(9), 3571-3583.
[http://dx.doi.org/10.1039/c2cs15317c] [PMID: 22349541]

[79]   Johnson, T.R.; Mann, B.E.; Clark, J.E.; Foresti, R.; Green, C.J.; Motterlini, R. Metal carbonyls: A new class of pharmaceuticals? *Angew. Chem. Int. Ed.,* **2003**, *42*(32), 3722-3729.
[http://dx.doi.org/10.1002/anie.200301634] [PMID: 12923835]

[80]   Mann, B.E.; Motterlini, R. CO and NO in medicine. *Chem. Commun.,* **2007**, *41*(41), 4197-4208.
[http://dx.doi.org/10.1039/b704873d] [PMID: 18217581]

[81]   Malhi, G.S.; Kaur, M.; Kaushik, P. Impact of climate change on agriculture and its mitigation strategies: A review. *Sustainability,* **2021**, *13*(3), 1318.
[http://dx.doi.org/10.3390/su13031318]

[82]   Jugdaohsingh, R. Silicon and bone health. *J. Nutr. Health Aging,* **2007**, *11*(2), 99-110.
[PMID: 17435952]

[83]   Price, C.T.; Koval, K.J.; Langford, J.R. Silicon: A review of its potential role in the prevention and treatment of postmenopausal osteoporosis. *Int. J. Endocrinol.,* **2013**, *2013*, 1-6.
[http://dx.doi.org/10.1155/2013/316783] [PMID: 23762049]

[84]   Sobolev, O.I.; Gutyj, B.V.; Sobolieva, S.V.; Borshch, O.O.; Kushnir, I.M.; Petryshak, R.A.; Vysotskij, A.O. A review of germanium environmental distribution, migration and accumulation. *Ukr. J. Ecol.,* **2020**, *10*(2), 200-208.

[85]   Li, L.; Ruan, T.; Lyu, Y.; Wu, B. Advances in effect of germanium or germanium compounds on animals—a review. *J. Biosci. Med.,* **2017**, *5*(7), 56-73.

[86]   Azam, F.; Volcani, B.E. Germanium-silicon interactions in biological systems. In: *Silicon and siliceous structures in biological systems*; Springer: New York, NY, **1981**; pp. 43-67.
[http://dx.doi.org/10.1007/978-1-4612-5944-2_3]

[87]   Narokha, V.; Nizhenkovska, I.; Kuznetsova, O. Potential of germanium-based compounds in coronavirus infection. *Acta Pharm.,* **2022**, *72*(2), 245-258.
[http://dx.doi.org/10.2478/acph-2022-0016] [PMID: 36651511]

[88]   Nagy, L.; Szorcsik, A.; Kovács, K. Tin compounds in pharmacy and nutrition. *Acta Pharm. Hung.,* **2000**, *70*(2), 53-71.

[PMID: 11192741]

[89]   Aldridge, W.N. The toxicology and biological properties of organotin compounds. In: *Tin as a Vital Nutrient*; CRC Press, **2019**; pp. 245-262.
[http://dx.doi.org/10.1201/9780429280511-26]

[90]   Kucklick, J.R.; Ellisor, M.D. A review of organotin contamination in arctic and subarctic regions. *Emerg. Contamin.*, **2019**, *5*, 150-156.
[http://dx.doi.org/10.1016/j.emcon.2019.04.003]

[91]   Flora, G.; Gupta, D.; Tiwari, A. Toxicity of lead: A review with recent updates. *Interdiscip. Toxicol.*, **2012**, *5*(2), 47-58.
[http://dx.doi.org/10.2478/v10102-012-0009-2] [PMID: 23118587]

[92]   Kumar, A.; Kumar, A.; M M S, C.P.; Chaturvedi, A.K.; Shabnam, A.A.; Subrahmanyam, G.; Mondal, R.; Gupta, D.K.; Malyan, S.K.; S Kumar, S.; A Khan, S.; Yadav, K.K. Lead toxicity: Health hazards, influence on food chain, and sustainable remediation approaches. *Int. J. Environ. Res. Public Health*, **2020**, *17*(7), 2179.
[http://dx.doi.org/10.3390/ijerph17072179] [PMID: 32218253]

[93]   Matović, V.; Buha, A.; Đukić-Ćosić, D.; Bulat, Z. Insight into the oxidative stress induced by lead and/or cadmium in blood, liver and kidneys. *Food Chem. Toxicol.*, **2015**, *78*, 130-140.
[http://dx.doi.org/10.1016/j.fct.2015.02.011] [PMID: 25681546]

[94]   Kumar, V.; Dwivedi, S.K.; Oh, S. A critical review on lead removal from industrial wastewater: Recent advances and future outlook. *J. Water Process Eng.*, **2022**, *45*, 102518.
[http://dx.doi.org/10.1016/j.jwpe.2021.102518]

[95]   Bjørklund, G.; Crisponi, G.; Nurchi, V.M.; Cappai, R.; Buha Djordjevic, A.; Aaseth, J. A review on coordination properties of thiol-containing chelating agents towards mercury, cadmium, and lead. *Molecules*, **2019**, *24*(18), 3247.
[http://dx.doi.org/10.3390/molecules24183247] [PMID: 31489907]

[96]   Patrick, L. Lead toxicity, a review of the literature. Part 1: Exposure, evaluation, and treatment. *Altern. Med. Rev.*, **2006**, *11*(1), 2-22.
[PMID: 16597190]

[97]   DeMartino, A.W.; Kim-Shapiro, D.B.; Patel, R.P.; Gladwin, M.T. Nitrite and nitrate chemical biology and signalling. *Brit. J. Pharmacol.*, **2019**, *176*(2), 228-245.
[http://dx.doi.org/10.1111/bph.14484] [PMID: 30152056]

[98]   Wills, B.K.; Cumpston, K.L.; Downs, J.W.; Rose, S.R. Causative agents in clinically significant methemoglobinemia: A national poison data system study. *Am. J. Therap.*, **2021**, *28*(5), e548-e551.
[http://dx.doi.org/10.1097/MJT.0000000000001277] [PMID: 33416248]

[99]   Farrugia, G.; Szurszewski, J.H. Carbon monoxide, hydrogen sulfide, and nitric oxide as signaling molecules in the gastrointestinal tract. *Gastroenterology*, **2014**, *147*(2), 303-313.
[http://dx.doi.org/10.1053/j.gastro.2014.04.041] [PMID: 24798417]

[100] Röszer, T. *The biology of subcellular nitric oxide*; Dordrecht, The Netherlands: Springer, **2012**.
[http://dx.doi.org/10.1007/978-94-007-2819-6]

[101] Knowles, R.G.; Moncada, S. Nitric oxide synthases in mammals. *Biochem. J.*, **1994**, *298*(2), 249-258.
[http://dx.doi.org/10.1042/bj2980249] [PMID: 7510950]

[102] Kumar, A.; Nautiyal, G. Reactive nitrogen species and its biological effects. *J. Pharmacogn. Phytochem.*, **2019**, *8*(3), 4410-4412.

[103] Ford, P.C.; Miranda, K.M. The solution chemistry of nitric oxide and other reactive nitrogen species. *Nitric Oxide*, **2020**, *103*, 31-46.
[http://dx.doi.org/10.1016/j.niox.2020.07.004] [PMID: 32721555]

[104] Lushchak, V.I.; Lushchak, O. Interplay between reactive oxygen and nitrogen species in living organisms. *Chem. Biol. Interact.,* **2021**, *349*, 109680.
[http://dx.doi.org/10.1016/j.cbi.2021.109680] [PMID: 34606757]

[105] Ahmad, R.; Hussain, A.; Ahsan, H. Peroxynitrite: Cellular pathology and implications in autoimmunity. *J. Immunoassay Immunochem.,* **2019**, *40*(2), 123-138.
[http://dx.doi.org/10.1080/15321819.2019.1583109] [PMID: 30843753]

[106] Dimkpa, C.O.; Fugice, J.; Singh, U.; Lewis, T.D. Development of fertilizers for enhanced nitrogen use efficiency–Trends and perspectives. *Sci. Total Environ.,* **2020**, *731*, 139113.
[http://dx.doi.org/10.1016/j.scitotenv.2020.139113] [PMID: 32438083]

[107] Baker, S.B.; Worthley, L.I. The essentials of calcium, magnesium and phosphate metabolism: Part I. Physiology. *Crit. Care Resusc.,* **2002**, *4*(4), 301-306.
[PMID: 16573443]

[108] Chien, S.H.; Prochnow, L.I.; Tu, S.; Snyder, C.S. Agronomic and environmental aspects of phosphate fertilizers varying in source and solubility: An update review. *Nutr. Cycl. Agroecosyst.,* **2011**, *89*(2), 229-255.
[http://dx.doi.org/10.1007/s10705-010-9390-4]

[109] Amanzadeh, J.; Reilly, R.F.Jr. Hypophosphatemia: An evidence-based approach to its clinical consequences and management. *Nat. Clin. Pract. Nephrol.,* **2006**, *2*(3), 136-148.
[http://dx.doi.org/10.1038/ncpneph0124] [PMID: 16932412]

[110] Hruska, K.A.; Mathew, S.; Lund, R.; Qiu, P.; Pratt, R. Hyperphosphatemia of chronic kidney disease. *Kidney Int.,* **2008**, *74*(2), 148-157.
[http://dx.doi.org/10.1038/ki.2008.130] [PMID: 18449174]

[111] Wilcox, D.E. Arsenic. Can this toxic metalloid sustain life? In: *Interrelations between essential metal ions and human diseases*; Sigel, A.; Sigel, H.; Sigel, R.K.O., Eds.; Springer: Dordrecht, The Netherlands, **2013**.
[http://dx.doi.org/10.1007/978-94-007-7500-8_15]

[112] Prakash, S.; Verma, A.K. Arsenic: it's toxicity and impact on human health. *Inter. Jonl. Bio. Innova.,* **2021**, *3*(1), 38-47.
[http://dx.doi.org/10.46505/IJBI.2021.3102]

[113] Flora, S.J.S. Preventive and therapeutic strategies for acute and chronic human arsenic exposure. In: *Arsenic in drinking water and food*; Springer: The Netherlands, **2020**.
[http://dx.doi.org/10.1007/978-981-13-8587-2_13]

[114] Rajavardhan, R.; Mamadapur, A.; Shyamala, N. Acute arsenic suicidal Poisoning – A rare case. *Inter. J. Dent. Med. Sci.,* **2021**, *10*(1), 1961-1965.
[http://dx.doi.org/10.18311/ijmds/2021/26466]

[115] Naujokas, M.F.; Anderson, B.; Ahsan, H.; Aposhian, H.V.; Graziano, J.H.; Thompson, C.; Suk, W.A. The broad scope of health effects from chronic arsenic exposure: Update on a worldwide public health problem. *Environ. Health Perspect.,* **2013**, *121*(3), 295-302.
[http://dx.doi.org/10.1289/ehp.1205875] [PMID: 23458756]

[116] Thomas, D.J.; Li, J.; Waters, S.B.; Xing, W.; Adair, B.M.; Drobna, Z.; Devesa, V.; Styblo, M. Arsenic (+3 oxidation state) methyltransferase and the methylation of arsenicals. *Exp. Biol. Med.,* **2007**, *232*(1), 3-13.
[http://dx.doi.org/10.3181/00379727-17-2] [PMID: 17202581]

[117] Samikkannu, T.; Chen, C.H.; Yih, L.H.; Wang, A.S.S.; Lin, S.Y.; Chen, T.C.; Jan, K.Y. Reactive oxygen species are involved in arsenic trioxide inhibition of pyruvate dehydrogenase activity. *Chem. Res. Toxicol.,* **2003**, *16*(3), 409-414.
[http://dx.doi.org/10.1021/tx025615j] [PMID: 12641442]

[118] Pi, J.; Horiguchi, S.; Sun, Y.; Nikaido, M.; Shimojo, N.; Hayashi, T.; Yamauchi, H.; Itoh, K.;

Yamamoto, M.; Sun, G.; Waalkes, M.P.; Kumagai, Y. A potential mechanism for the impairment of nitric oxide formation caused by prolonged oral exposure to arsenate in rabbits. *Free Rad. Biol. Med.,* **2003**, *35*(1), 102-113.
[http://dx.doi.org/10.1016/S0891-5849(03)00269-7] [PMID: 12826260]

[119] Nurchi, V.M.; Buha Djordjevic, A.; Crisponi, G.; Alexander, J.; Bjørklund, G.; Aaseth, J. Arsenic toxicity: Molecular targets and therapeutic agents. *Biomolecules,* **2020**, *10*(2), 235.
[http://dx.doi.org/10.3390/biom10020235] [PMID: 32033229]

[120] Saerens, A.; Ghosh, M.; Verdonck, J.; Godderis, L. Risk of cancer for workers exposed to antimony compounds: A systematic review. *Int. J. Environ. Res. Publ. Health,* **2019**, *16*(22), 4474.
[http://dx.doi.org/10.3390/ijerph16224474] [PMID: 31739404]

[121] Sundar, S.; Chakravarty, J. Antimony Toxicity. *Int. J. Environ. Res. Publ. Health,* **2010**, *7*(12), 4267-4277.
[http://dx.doi.org/10.3390/ijerph7124267] [PMID: 21318007]

[122] Liu, Y.; Shen, C.; Zhang, X.; Yu, H.; Wang, F.; Wang, Y.; Zhang, L.W. Exposure and nephrotoxicity concern of bismuth with the occurrence of autophagy. *Toxicol. Ind. Health,* **2018**, *34*(3), 188-199.
[http://dx.doi.org/10.1177/0748233717746810] [PMID: 29506455]

[123] Li, H.; Sun, H. Recent advances in bioinorganic chemistry of bismuth. *Curr. Opin. Chem. Biol.,* **2012**, *16*(1-2), 74-83.
[http://dx.doi.org/10.1016/j.cbpa.2012.01.006] [PMID: 22322154]

[124] Alkim, H.; Koksal, A.R.; Boga, S.; Sen, I.; Alkim, C. Role of bismuth in the eradication of Helicobacter pylori. *Am. J. Therap.,* **2017**, *24*(6), e751-e757.
[http://dx.doi.org/10.1097/MJT.0000000000000389] [PMID: 26808355]

[125] Thomas, F.; Bialek, B.; Hensel, R. Medical use of bismuth: The two sides of the coin. *J. Clin. Toxicol.,* **2011**, S3, 2161-0495.

[126] Ward, J.P.T. Oxygen sensors in context. *Biochim. Biophys. Acta Bioenerg.,* **2008**, *1777*(1), 1-14.
[http://dx.doi.org/10.1016/j.bbabio.2007.10.010] [PMID: 18036551]

[127] Forman, H.J.; Maiorino, M.; Ursini, F. Signaling functions of reactive oxygen species. *Biochemistry,* **2010**, *49*(5), 835-842.
[http://dx.doi.org/10.1021/bi9020378] [PMID: 20050630]

[128] Mach, W.J.; Thimmesch, A.R.; Pierce, J.T.; Pierce, J.D. Consequences of hyperoxia and the toxicity of oxygen in the lung. *Nurs. Res. Pract.,* **2011**, *2011*, 260482.
[http://dx.doi.org/10.1155/2011/260482] [PMID: 21994818]

[129] Michiels, C. Physiological and pathological responses to hypoxia. *Am. J. Pathol.,* **2004**, *164*(6), 1875-1882.
[http://dx.doi.org/10.1016/S0002-9440(10)63747-9] [PMID: 15161623]

[130] Fu, T.M.; Tian, H. Climate change penalty to ozone air quality: Review of current understandings and knowledge gaps. *Curr. Pollut. Rep.,* **2019**, *5*(3), 159-171.
[http://dx.doi.org/10.1007/s40726-019-00115-6]

[131] Rekhate, C.V.; Srivastava, J.K. Recent advances in ozone-based advanced oxidation processes for treatment of wastewater-A review. *Chem. Eng. J. Adv.,* **2020**, *3*, 100031.
[http://dx.doi.org/10.1016/j.ceja.2020.100031]

[132] Afsah-Hejri, L.; Hajeb, P.; Ehsani, R.J. Application of ozone for degradation of mycotoxins in food: A review. *Compr. Rev. Food Sci. Food Saf.,* **2020**, *19*(4), 1777-1808.
[http://dx.doi.org/10.1111/1541-4337.12594] [PMID: 33337096]

[133] Vladilo, G.; Hassanali, A. Hydrogen bonds and life in the universe. *Life,* **2018**, *8*(1), 1.
[http://dx.doi.org/10.3390/life8010001] [PMID: 29301382]

[134] Herschlag, D.; Pinney, M.M. Hydrogen bonds: Simple after all? *Biochemistry,* **2018**, *57*(24), 3338-

3352.
[http://dx.doi.org/10.1021/acs.biochem.8b00217] [PMID: 29678112]

[135] Adhikari, A.; Park, W.W.; Kwon, O.H. Hydrogen-bond dynamics and energetics of biological water. *ChemPlusChem,* **2020**, *85*(12), 2657-2665.
[http://dx.doi.org/10.1002/cplu.202000744] [PMID: 33305536]

[136] Abe, C.; Miyazawa, T.; Miyazawa, T. Current use of fenton reaction in drugs and food. *Molecules,* **2022**, *27*(17), 5451.
[http://dx.doi.org/10.3390/molecules27175451] [PMID: 36080218]

[137] Di Marzo, N.; Chisci, E.; Giovannoni, R. The role of hydrogen peroxide in redox-dependent signaling: Homeostatic and pathological responses in mammalian cells. *Cells,* **2018**, *7*(10), 156.
[http://dx.doi.org/10.3390/cells7100156] [PMID: 30287799]

[138] Checa, J.; Aran, J.M. Reactive oxygen species: Drivers of physiological and pathological processes. *J. Inflamm. Res.,* **2020**, *13*, 1057-1073.
[http://dx.doi.org/10.2147/JIR.S275595] [PMID: 33293849]

[139] Jie, Z.; Liu, J.; Shu, M.; Ying, Y.; Yang, H. Detection strategies for superoxide anion: A review. *Talanta,* **2022**, *236*, 122892.
[http://dx.doi.org/10.1016/j.talanta.2021.122892] [PMID: 34635271]

[140] Fleming, A.M.; Burrows, C.J. On the irrelevancy of hydroxyl radical to DNA damage from oxidative stress and implications for epigenetics. *Chem. Soc. Rev.,* **2020**, *49*(18), 6524-6528.
[http://dx.doi.org/10.1039/D0CS00579G] [PMID: 32785348]

[141] Di Mascio, P.; Martinez, G.R.; Miyamoto, S.; Ronsein, G.E.; Medeiros, M.H.G.; Cadet, J. Singlet molecular oxygen reactions with nucleic acids, lipids, and proteins. *Chem. Rev.,* **2019**, *119*(3), 2043-2086.
[http://dx.doi.org/10.1021/acs.chemrev.8b00554] [PMID: 30721030]

[142] Mourenza, Á.; Gil, J.A.; Mateos, L.M.; Letek, M. Oxidative stress-generating antimicrobials, a novel strategy to overcome antibacterial resistance. *Antioxidants,* **2020**, *9*(5), 361.
[http://dx.doi.org/10.3390/antiox9050361] [PMID: 32357394]

[143] Adwas, A.A.; Elsayed, A.; Azab, A.E.; Quwaydir, F.A. Oxidative stress and antioxidant mechanisms in human body. *J. Appl. Biotechnol. Bioeng.,* **2019**, *6*(1), 43-47.

[144] Surai, P.F. Antioxidant systems in poultry biology: Superoxide dismutase. *Anim. Nutr.,* **2016**, *1*, 8.

[145] Hayes, J.D.; Flanagan, J.U.; Jowsey, I.R. Glutathione transferases. *Annu. Rev. Pharmacol. Toxicol.,* **2005**, *45*(1), 51-88.
[http://dx.doi.org/10.1146/annurev.pharmtox.45.120403.095857] [PMID: 15822171]

[146] Sen, C.K.; Khanna, S.; Roy, S. Tocotrienols: Vitamin E beyond tocopherols. *Life Sci.,* **2006**, *78*(18), 2088-2098.
[http://dx.doi.org/10.1016/j.lfs.2005.12.001] [PMID: 16458936]

[147] Linster, C.L.; Van Schaftingen, E. Vitamin C. Biosynthesis, recycling and degradation in mammals. *FEBS J.,* **2007**, *274*(1), 1-22.
[http://dx.doi.org/10.1111/j.1742-4658.2006.05607.x] [PMID: 17222174]

[148] Karak, P. Biological activities of flavonoids: An overview. *Int. J. Pharm. Sci. Res.,* **2019**, *10*(4), 1567-1574.

[149] Glantzounis, G.K.; Tsimoyiannis, E.C.; Kappas, A.M.; Galaris, D.A. Uric acid and oxidative stress. *Curr. Pharm. Des.,* **2005**, *11*(32), 4145-4151.
[http://dx.doi.org/10.2174/138161205774913255] [PMID: 16375736]

[150] Marí, M.; de Gregorio, E.; de Dios, C.; Roca-Agujetas, V.; Cucarull, B.; Tutusaus, A.; Morales, A.; Colell, A. Mitochondrial glutathione: Recent insights and role in disease. *Antioxidants,* **2020**, *9*(10), 909.

[http://dx.doi.org/10.3390/antiox9100909] [PMID: 32987701]

[151] Ulrich, K.; Jakob, U. The role of thiols in antioxidant systems. *Free Rad. Biol. Med.,* **2019**, *140*, 14-27.
[http://dx.doi.org/10.1016/j.freeradbiomed.2019.05.035] [PMID: 31201851]

[152] Soto Conti, C.P. Bilirubin: The toxic mechanisms of an antioxidant molecule. *Arch. Argent. Pediatr.,* **2021**, *119*(1), e18-e25.
[PMID: 33458986]

[153] Giordano, M.; Prioretti, L. Sulphur and algae: Metabolism, ecology and evolution. In: *The Physiology of Microalgae*; Springer: Cham, **2016**.
[http://dx.doi.org/10.1007/978-3-319-24945-2_9]

[154] Francioso, A.; Baseggio Conrado, A.; Mosca, L.; Fontana, M. Chemistry and biochemistry of sulfur natural compounds: Key intermediates of metabolism and redox biology. *Oxid. Med. Cell. Longev.,* **2020**, *2020*, 8294158.
[http://dx.doi.org/10.1155/2020/8294158] [PMID: 33062147]

[155] Ingenbleek, Y.; Kimura, H. Nutritional essentiality of sulfur in health and disease. *Nutr. Rev.,* **2013**, *71*(7), 413-432.
[http://dx.doi.org/10.1111/nure.12050] [PMID: 23815141]

[156] Pompella, A.; Visvikis, A.; Paolicchi, A.; Tata, V.D.; Casini, A.F. The changing faces of glutathione, a cellular protagonist. *Biochem. Pharmacol.,* **2003**, *66*(8), 1499-1503.
[http://dx.doi.org/10.1016/S0006-2952(03)00504-5] [PMID: 14555227]

[157] Paul, B.D.; Snyder, S.H. H_2S signalling through protein sulfhydration and beyond. *Nat. Rev. Mol. Cell Biol.,* **2012**, *13*(8), 499-507.
[http://dx.doi.org/10.1038/nrm3391] [PMID: 22781905]

[158] Mani, S.; Li, H.; Untereiner, A.; Wu, L.; Yang, G.; Austin, R.C.; Dickhout, J.G.; Lhoták, Š.; Meng, Q.H.; Wang, R. Decreased endogenous production of hydrogen sulfide accelerates atherosclerosis. *Circulation,* **2013**, *127*(25), 2523-2534.
[http://dx.doi.org/10.1161/CIRCULATIONAHA.113.002208] [PMID: 23704252]

[159] Xu, S.; Liu, Z.; Liu, P. Targeting hydrogen sulfide as a promising therapeutic strategy for atherosclerosis. *Int. J. Cardiol.,* **2014**, *172*(2), 313-317.
[http://dx.doi.org/10.1016/j.ijcard.2014.01.068] [PMID: 24491853]

[160] Hariharan, S.; Dharmaraj, S. Selenium and selenoproteins: It's role in regulation of inflammation. *Inflammopharmacol.,* **2020**, *28*(3), 667-695.
[http://dx.doi.org/10.1007/s10787-020-00690-x] [PMID: 32144521]

[161] Kurokawa, S.; Berry, M.J. Selenium. Role of the essential metalloid in health. In: *Interrelations between essential metal ions and human diseases*; Sigel, A.; Sigel, H.; Sigel, R.K.O., Eds.; Dordrecht, The Netherlands: Springer Science and Business Media B.V., **2013**.
[http://dx.doi.org/10.1007/978-94-007-7500-8_16]

[162] Zwolak, I. The role of selenium in arsenic and cadmium toxicity: An updated review of scientific literature. *Biol. Trace Elem. Res.,* **2020**, *193*(1), 44-63.
[http://dx.doi.org/10.1007/s12011-019-01691-w] [PMID: 30877523]

[163] Wang, H.; Chen, B.; He, M.; Yu, X.; Hu, B. Selenocystine against methyl mercury cytotoxicity in HepG2 cells. *Sci. Rep.,* **2017**, *7*(1), 147.
[http://dx.doi.org/10.1038/s41598-017-00231-7] [PMID: 28273949]

[164] Hu, W.; Zhao, C.; Hu, H.; Yin, S. Food sources of selenium and its relationship with chronic diseases. *Nutrients,* **2021**, *13*(5), 1739.
[http://dx.doi.org/10.3390/nu13051739] [PMID: 34065478]

[165] Stolwijk, J.M.; Garje, R.; Sieren, J.C.; Buettner, G.R.; Zakharia, Y. Understanding the redox biology of selenium in the search of targeted cancer therapies. *Antioxidants,* **2020**, *9*(5), 420.
[http://dx.doi.org/10.3390/antiox9050420] [PMID: 32414091]

[166] Hosnedlova, B.; Kepinska, M.; Skalickova, S.; Fernandez, C.; Ruttkay-Nedecky, B.; Peng, Q.; Baron, M.; Melcova, M.; Opatrilova, R.; Zidkova, J.; Bjørklund, G.; Sochor, J.; Kizek, R. Nano-selenium and its nanomedicine applications: A critical review. *Int. J. Nanomed.*, **2018**, *13*, 2107-2128.
[http://dx.doi.org/10.2147/IJN.S157541] [PMID: 29692609]

[167] Vávrová, S.; Struhárňanská, E.; Turňa, J.; Stuchlík, S. Tellurium: A rare element with influence on prokaryotic and eukaryotic biological systems. *Int. J. Mol. Sci.*, **2021**, *22*(11), 5924.
[http://dx.doi.org/10.3390/ijms22115924] [PMID: 34072929]

[168] Wang, H.; Chai, L.; Xie, Z.; Zhang, H. Recent advance of tellurium for biomedical applications. *Chem. Res. Chin. Univ.*, **2020**, *36*(4), 551-559.
[http://dx.doi.org/10.1007/s40242-020-0193-0]

[169] Everett, E.T. Fluoride's effects on the formation of teeth and bones, and the influence of genetics. *J. Dent. Res.*, **2011**, *90*(5), 552-560.
[http://dx.doi.org/10.1177/0022034510384626] [PMID: 20929720]

[170] Buzalaf, M.A.R.; Whitford, G.M. Fluoride metabolism. In: *Fluoride and the oral environment*; Buzalaf, M.A.R., Ed.; Karger: Basel, Switzerland, **2011**; pp. 20-36.
[http://dx.doi.org/10.1159/000325107]

[171] Li, L. The biochemistry and physiology of metallic fluoride: action, mechanism, and implications. *Crit. Rev. Oral Biol. Med.*, **2003**, *14*(2), 100-114.
[http://dx.doi.org/10.1177/154411130301400204] [PMID: 12764073]

[172] Han, J.; Kiss, L.; Mei, H.; Remete, A.M.; Ponikvar-Svet, M.; Sedgwick, D.M.; Roman, R.; Fustero, S.; Moriwaki, H.; Soloshonok, V.A. Chemical aspects of human and environmental overload with fluorine. *Chem. Rev.*, **2021**, *121*(8), 4678-4742.
[http://dx.doi.org/10.1021/acs.chemrev.0c01263] [PMID: 33723999]

[173] Kettle, A.J.; Albrett, A.M.; Chapman, A.L.; Dickerhof, N.; Forbes, L.V.; Khalilova, I.; Turner, R. Measuring chlorine bleach in biology and medicine. *Biochim. Biophys. Acta, Gen. Subj.*, **2014**, *1840*(2), 781-793.
[http://dx.doi.org/10.1016/j.bbagen.2013.07.004] [PMID: 23872351]

[174] Serdar, B.; LeBlanc, W.G.; Norris, J.M.; Dickinson, L.M. Potential effects of polychlorinated biphenyls (PCBs) and selected organochlorine pesticides (OCPs) on immune cells and blood biochemistry measures: A cross-sectional assessment of the NHANES 2003-2004 data. *Environ. Health*, **2014**, *13*(1), 1-12.
[http://dx.doi.org/10.1186/1476-069X-13-114] [PMID: 25515064]

[175] Aldridge, R.E.; Chan, T.; van Dalen, C.J.; Senthilmohan, R.; Winn, M.; Venge, P.; Town, G.I.; Kettle, A.J. Eosinophil peroxidase produces hypobromous acid in the airways of stable asthmatics. *Free Radic. Biol. Med.*, **2002**, *33*(6), 847-856.
[http://dx.doi.org/10.1016/S0891-5849(02)00976-0] [PMID: 12208372]

[176] Zbigniew, S. Role of iodine in metabolism. *Rec. Pat. Endocr. Metab. Immune Drug Discov.*, **2017**, *10*(2), 123-126.
[http://dx.doi.org/10.2174/1872214811666170119110618] [PMID: 28103777]

[177] Dohán, O.; De la Vieja, A.; Paroder, V.; Riedel, C.; Artani, M.; Reed, M.; Ginter, C.S.; Carrasco, N. The sodium/iodide Symporter (NIS): Characterization, regulation, and medical significance. *Endocr. Rev.*, **2003**, *24*(1), 48-77.
[http://dx.doi.org/10.1210/er.2001-0029] [PMID: 12588808]

[178] Hatch-McChesney, A.; Lieberman, H.R. Iodine and iodine deficiency: A comprehensive review of a re-emerging issue. *Nutrients*, **2022**, *14*(17), 3474.
[http://dx.doi.org/10.3390/nu14173474] [PMID: 36079737]

[179] Barreto, R.; Barrois, B.; Lambert, J.; Malhotra-Kumar, S.; Santos-Fernandes, V.; Monstrey, S. Addressing the challenges in antisepsis: Focus on povidone iodine. *Int. J. Antimicrob. Agents*, **2020**,

56(3), 106064.
[http://dx.doi.org/10.1016/j.ijantimicag.2020.106064] [PMID: 32599228]

[180] Nasir, S.A.; Othman, S.A.; Nordin, N.I.M. Health risk from radioactive iodine (RAI) therapy and medical imaging: A short review. *Malays. J. Appl. Sci.,* **2022,** *7*(2), 44-52.

[181] Kim, B.W. Does radioactive iodine therapy for hyperthyroidism cause cancer? *J. Clin. Endocrin. Metab.,* **2022,** *107*(2), e448-e457.
[http://dx.doi.org/10.1210/clinem/dgab700] [PMID: 34555150]

[182] Makvandi, M.; Dupis, E.; Engle, J.W.; Nortier, F.M.; Fassbender, M.E.; Simon, S.; Birnbaum, E.R.; Atcher, R.W.; John, K.D.; Rixe, O.; Norenberg, J.P. Alpha-emitters and targeted alpha therapy in oncology: From basic science to clinical investigations. *Targ. Oncol.,* **2018,** *13*(2), 189-203.
[http://dx.doi.org/10.1007/s11523-018-0550-9] [PMID: 29423595]

[183] Guerra Liberal, F.D.C.; O'Sullivan, J.M.; McMahon, S.J.; Prise, K.M. Targeted alpha therapy: Current clinical applications. *Cancer Biother. Radiopharm.,* **2020,** *35*(6), 404-417.
[http://dx.doi.org/10.1089/cbr.2020.3576] [PMID: 32552031]

[184] Zalutsky, M.R. Radioactive noble gases for medical applications. In: *Radiotracers for Medical Applications*; CRC Press, **2019**; pp. 95-118.
[http://dx.doi.org/10.1201/9780429278785-2]

[185] Koziakova, M.; Harris, K.; Edge, C.J.; Franks, N.P.; White, I.L.; Dickinson, R. Noble gas neuroprotection: Xenon and argon protect against hypoxic–ischaemic injury in rat hippocampus *in vitro via* distinct mechanisms. *Brit. J. Anaesth.,* **2019,** *123*(5), 601-609.
[http://dx.doi.org/10.1016/j.bja.2019.07.010] [PMID: 31470983]

[186] Zhang, J.; Liu, W.; Bi, M.; Xu, J.; Yang, H.; Zhang, Y. Noble Gases Therapy in Cardiocerebrovascular Diseases: The Novel Stars? *Front. Cardiovasc. Med.,* **2022,** *9,* 802783.
[http://dx.doi.org/10.3389/fcvm.2022.802783] [PMID: 35369316]

[187] Munteanu, C.; Dogaru, G.; Rotariu, M.; Onose, G. Therapeutic gases used in balneotherapy and rehabilitation medicine - scientific relevance in the last ten years (2011 – 2020) - Synthetic literature review. *Balneo and PRM Research Journal,* **2021,** *12*(Vol.12, no.2), 111-122.
[http://dx.doi.org/10.12680/balneo.2021.430]

[188] Blum, J.D.; Erel, Y. Radiogenic isotopes in weathering and hydrology. *Treat. Geochem.,* **2003,** *5,* 605.

[189] Dong, X.Z.; Ritterbusch, F.; Yuan, D.F.; Yan, J.W.; Chen, W.T.; Jiang, W.; Lu, Z-T.; Wang, J.S.; Wang, X-A.; Yang, G-M. Generation of metastable krypton using a 124-nm laser. *Phys. Rev. A,* **2022,** *105*(3), L031101.
[http://dx.doi.org/10.1103/PhysRevA.105.L031101]

[190] Harris, K.; Armstrong, S.P.; Campos-Pires, R.; Kiru, L.; Franks, N.P.; Dickinson, R. Neuroprotection against traumatic brain injury by xenon, but not argon, is mediated by inhibition at the N-methyl-D-aspartate receptor glycine site. *Anesthesiology,* **2013,** *119*(5), 1137-1148.
[http://dx.doi.org/10.1097/ALN.0b013e3182a2a265] [PMID: 23867231]

[191] Ojo, T.J.; Ajayi, I.R. A review on environmental radon and its potential health risk on humans. *J. Environ. Sci. Toxicol. Food Technol.,* **2014,** *8,* 1-8.

[192] Kaim, W.; Schwederski, B. Cooperation of metals with electroactive ligands of biochemical relevance: Beyond metalloporphyrins. *Pure Appl. Chem.,* **2004,** *76*(2), 351-364.
[http://dx.doi.org/10.1351/pac200476020351]

[193] Aaseth, J.; Crisponi, G.; Anderson, O. *Chelation therapy in the treatment of metal intoxication*; Academic Press: Cambridge, MA, USA, **2016.**

[194] Nurchi, V.; Crespo-Alonso, M.; Toso, L.; Lachowicz, J.; Crisponi, G. Chelation therapy for metal intoxication: Comments from a thermodynamic viewpoint. *Mini Rev. Med. Chem.,* **2013,** *13*(11), 1541-1549.
[http://dx.doi.org/10.2174/13895575113139990077] [PMID: 23895193]

[195] Nierengarten, J.F. In My Element: Copper. *Chem. Eur. J.,* **2019**, *25*(1), 16-18.
[http://dx.doi.org/10.1002/chem.201805277]

[196] Scheiber, I.; Dringen, R.; Mercer, J.F.B. Copper: effects of deficiency and overload. *Met. Ions Life Sci.,* **2013**, *13*, 359-387.
[http://dx.doi.org/10.1007/978-94-007-7500-8_11] [PMID: 24470097]

[197] Gaggelli, E.; Kozlowski, H.; Valensin, D.; Valensin, G. Copper homeostasis and neurodegenerative disorders (Alzheimer's, prion, and Parkinson's diseases and amyotrophic lateral sclerosis). *Chem. Rev.,* **2006**, *106*(6), 1995-2044.
[http://dx.doi.org/10.1021/cr040410w] [PMID: 16771441]

[198] Altarelli, M.; Ben-Hamouda, N.; Schneider, A.; Berger, M.M. Copper deficiency: Causes, manifestations, and treatment. *Nutr. Clin. Pract.,* **2019**, *34*(4), 504-513.
[http://dx.doi.org/10.1002/ncp.10328] [PMID: 31209935]

[199] Mulligan, C.; Bronstein, J.M. Wilson disease: an overview and approach to management. *Neurol. Clin.,* **2020**, *38*(2), 417-432.
[http://dx.doi.org/10.1016/j.ncl.2020.01.005] [PMID: 32279718]

[200] Galdiero, S.; Falanga, A.; Vitiello, M.; Cantisani, M.; Marra, V.; Galdiero, M. Silver nanoparticles as potential antiviral agents. *Molecules,* **2011**, *16*(10), 8894-8918.
[http://dx.doi.org/10.3390/molecules16108894] [PMID: 22024958]

[201] Yuan, Q.; Zhao, Y.; Cai, P.; He, Z.; Gao, F.; Zhang, J.; Gao, X. Dose-dependent efficacy of gold clusters on rheumatoid arthritis therapy. *ACS Omega,* **2019**, *4*(9), 14092-14099.
[http://dx.doi.org/10.1021/acsomega.9b02003] [PMID: 31497728]

[202] Lopez, J.; Ramchandani, D.; Vahdat, L. Copper depletion as a therapeutic strategy in cancer. *Met. Ions Life Sci.,* **2019**, *19*, 303-330.
[http://dx.doi.org/10.1515/9783110527872-012] [PMID: 30855113]

[203] Kochańczyk, T.; Drozd, A.; Krężel, A. Relationship between the architecture of zinc coordination and zinc binding affinity in proteins-insights into zinc regulation. *Metallomics,* **2015**, *7*(2), 244-257.
[http://dx.doi.org/10.1039/C4MT00094C] [PMID: 25255078]

[204] Yang, Y.; Joshi, M.; Takahashi, Y.H.; Ning, Z.; Qu, Q.; Brunzelle, J.S.; Skiniotis, G.; Figeys, D.; Shilatifard, A.; Couture, J.F. A non-canonical monovalent zinc finger stabilizes the integration of Cfp1 into the H3K4 methyltransferase complex COMPASS. *Nucl. Acids Res.,* **2020**, *48*(1), 421-431.
[PMID: 31724694]

[205] Grüngreiff, K.; Gottstein, T.; Reinhold, D. Zinc deficiency—an independent risk factor in the pathogenesis of haemorrhagic stroke? *Nutrients,* **2020**, *12*(11), 3548.
[http://dx.doi.org/10.3390/nu12113548] [PMID: 33228216]

[206] Salzman, M.B.; Smith, E.M.; Koo, C. Excessive oral zinc supplementation. *J. Pediatr. Hematol. Oncol.,* **2002**, *24*(7), 582-584.
[http://dx.doi.org/10.1097/00043426-200210000-00020] [PMID: 12368702]

[207] Genchi, G.; Sinicropi, M.S.; Lauria, G.; Carocci, A.; Catalano, A. The effects of cadmium toxicity. *Envir. Res. Publ.,* **2020**, *17*(11), 3782.
[http://dx.doi.org/10.3390/ijerph17113782] [PMID: 32466586]

[208] Mahmood, Q.; Asif, M.; Shaheen, S.; Hayat, M.T.; Ali, S. Cadmium contamination in water and soil. In: *Cadmium toxicity and tolerance in plants*; Academic Press, **2019**; pp. 141-161.
[http://dx.doi.org/10.1016/B978-0-12-814864-8.00006-1]

[209] Fatima, G.; Raza, A.M.; Hadi, N.; Nigam, N.; Mahdi, A.A. Cadmium in human diseases: It's more than just a mere metal. *Ind. J. Clin. Biochem.,* **2019**, *34*(4), 371-378.
[http://dx.doi.org/10.1007/s12291-019-00839-8] [PMID: 31686724]

[210] Kumar, S.; Sharma, A. Cadmium toxicity: Effects on human reproduction and fertility. *Rev. Environ.*

Health, **2019**, *34*(4), 327-338.
[http://dx.doi.org/10.1515/reveh-2019-0016] [PMID: 31129655]

[211] Unsal, V.; Dalkiran, T.; Çiçek, M.; Kölükçü, E. The role of natural antioxidants against reactive oxygen species produced by cadmium toxicity: A review. *Adv. Pharm. Bull.,* **2020**, *10*(2), 184-202.
[http://dx.doi.org/10.34172/apb.2020.023] [PMID: 32373487]

[212] Cui, Z.G.; Ahmed, K.; Zaidi, S.F.; Muhammad, J.S. Ins and outs of cadmium-induced carcinogenesis: Mechanism and prevention. *Cancer Treat. Res. Commun.,* **2021**, *27*, 100372.
[http://dx.doi.org/10.1016/j.ctarc.2021.100372] [PMID: 33865114]

[213] Domingo-Relloso, A.; Riffo-Campos, A.L.; Haack, K.; Rentero-Garrido, P.; Ladd-Acosta, C.; Fallin, D.M.; Tang, W.Y.; Herreros-Martinez, M.; Gonzalez, J.R.; Bozack, A.K.; Cole, S.A.; Navas-Acien, A.; Tellez-Plaza, M. Cadmium, smoking, and human blood DNA methylation profiles in adults from the strong heart study. *Environ. Health Perspect.,* **2020**, *128*(6), 067005.
[http://dx.doi.org/10.1289/EHP6345] [PMID: 32484362]

[214] Ajsuvakova, O.P.; Tinkov, A.A.; Aschner, M.; Rocha, J.B.T.; Michalke, B.; Skalnaya, M.G.; Skalny, A.V.; Butnariu, M.; Dadar, M.; Sarac, I.; Aaseth, J.; Bjørklund, G. Sulfhydryl groups as targets of mercury toxicity. *Coord. Chem. Rev.,* **2020**, *417*, 213343.
[http://dx.doi.org/10.1016/j.ccr.2020.213343] [PMID: 32905350]

[215] Magowska, A. The natural history of the concept of antidote. *Toxicol. Rep.,* **2021**, *8*, 1305-1309.
[http://dx.doi.org/10.1016/j.toxrep.2021.06.019] [PMID: 34195019]

[216] Ahmad, S.; Mahmood, R. Mercury chloride toxicity in human erythrocytes: enhanced generation of ROS and RNS, hemoglobin oxidation, impaired antioxidant power, and inhibition of plasma membrane redox system. *Environ. Sci. Pollut. Res.,* **2019**, *26*(6), 5645-5657.
[http://dx.doi.org/10.1007/s11356-018-04062-5] [PMID: 30612358]

[217] Ukale, D.; Lönnberg, T. Organomercury nucleic acids: Past, present and future. *ChemBioChem,* **2021**, *22*(10), 1733-1739.
[http://dx.doi.org/10.1002/cbic.202000821] [PMID: 33410571]

[218] Mikolajczak, R.; Huclier-Markai, S.; Alliot, C.; Haddad, F.; Szikra, D.; Forgacs, V.; Garnuszek, P. Production of scandium radionuclides for theranostic applications: Towards standardization of quality requirements. *EJNMMI Radiopharm. Chem.,* **2021**, *6*(1), 19.
[http://dx.doi.org/10.1186/s41181-021-00131-2] [PMID: 34036449]

[219] Ghosh, A.; Dhiman, S.; Gupta, A.; Jain, R. Process evaluation of scandium production and its environmental impact. *Environments,* **2022**, *10*(1), 8.
[http://dx.doi.org/10.3390/environments10010008]

[220] Shin, S.H.; Kim, H.O.; Rim, K.T. Worker safety in the rare earth elements recycling process from the review of toxicity and issues. *Saf. Health Work,* **2019**, *10*(4), 409-419.
[http://dx.doi.org/10.1016/j.shaw.2019.08.005] [PMID: 31890323]

[221] Kim, K.T.; Eo, M.Y.; Nguyen, T.T.H.; Kim, S.M. General review of titanium toxicity. *Int. J. Implant Dent.,* **2019**, *5*(1), 1-12.
[http://dx.doi.org/10.1186/s40729-019-0162-x] [PMID: 30854575]

[222] Lee, D.B.N.; Roberts, M.; Bluchel, C.G.; Odell, R.A. Zirconium: biomedical and nephrological applications. *ASAIO J.,* **2010**, *56*(6), 550-556.
[http://dx.doi.org/10.1097/MAT.0b013e73f20] [PMID: 21245802]

[223] Hu, Z.; Wang, Y.; Zhao, D. The chemistry and applications of hafnium and cerium(IV) metal–organic frameworks. *Chem. Soc. Rev.,* **2021**, *50*(7), 4629-4683.
[http://dx.doi.org/10.1039/D0CS00920B] [PMID: 33616126]

[224] Tulcan, R.X.S.; Ouyang, W.; Lin, C.; He, M.; Wang, B. Vanadium pollution and health risks in marine ecosystems: Anthropogenic sources over natural contributions. *Water Res.,* **2021**, *207*, 117838.
[http://dx.doi.org/10.1016/j.watres.2021.117838] [PMID: 34775169]

[225] Rehder, D. Vanadium. Its role for humans. In: *Interrelations between essential metal ions and human diseases*; Sigel, A.; Sigel, H.; Sigel, R.K.O., Eds.; , **2013**; pp. 139-169.
[http://dx.doi.org/10.1007/978-94-007-7500-8_5]

[226] Ścibior, A.; Pietrzyk, Ł.; Plewa, Z.; Skiba, A. Vanadium: risks and possible benefits in the light of a comprehensive overview of its pharmacotoxicological mechanisms and multi-applications with a summary of further research trends. *J. Tr. Elem. Med. Biol.*, **2020**, *61*, 126508.
[http://dx.doi.org/10.1016/j.jtemb.2020.126508] [PMID: 32305626]

[227] Anke, M. Vanadium-an element both essential and toxic to plants, animals and humans. *Anal. Real. Acad. Nac. Farm.*, **2004**, *70*, 961-999.

[228] Prasad, K.S.; Ramachandrappa, S.U. Potential medicinal applications of vanadium and its coordination compounds in current research prospects: A review. *Curr. Bioact. Comp.*, **2020**, *16*(3), 201-209.
[http://dx.doi.org/10.2174/1573407214666181115111357]

[229] Olivares-Navarrete, R.; Olaya, J.J.; Ramírez, C.; Rodil, S.E. Biocompatibility of niobium coatings. *Coatings*, **2011**, *1*(1), 72-87.
[http://dx.doi.org/10.3390/coatings1010072]

[230] Zhou, Y.L.; Niinomi, M.; Akahori, T.; Nakai, M.; Fukui, H. Comparison of various properties between titanium-tantalum alloy and pure titanium for biomedical applications. *Mater. Transact.*, **2007**, *48*(3), 380-384.
[http://dx.doi.org/10.2320/matertrans.48.380]

[231] Rydzynski, K.; Pakulska, D. Vanadium, niobium, and tantalum. *Patty's Toxicol*; , **2001**, pp. 511-564.

[232] Pavesi, T.; Moreira, J.C. Mechanisms and individuality in chromium toxicity in humans. *J. Appl. Toxicol.*, **2020**, *40*(9), 1183-1197.
[http://dx.doi.org/10.1002/jat.3965] [PMID: 32166774]

[233] DesMarias, T.L.; Costa, M. Mechanisms of chromium-induced toxicity. *Curr. Opin. Toxicol.*, **2019**, *14*, 1-7.
[http://dx.doi.org/10.1016/j.cotox.2019.05.003] [PMID: 31511838]

[234] Maret, W. Chromium supplementation in human health, metabolic syndrome, and diabetes. *Met. Ions Life Sci.*, **2019**, *19*, 231.
[http://dx.doi.org/10.1515/9783110527872-009] [PMID: 30855110]

[235] Prasad, S.; Yadav, K.K.; Kumar, S.; Gupta, N.; Cabral-Pinto, M.M.S.; Rezania, S.; Radwan, N.; Alam, J. Chromium contamination and effect on environmental health and its remediation: A sustainable approaches. *J. Envir. Manag.*, **2021**, *285*, 112174.
[http://dx.doi.org/10.1016/j.jenvman.2021.112174] [PMID: 33607566]

[236] Halmi, M.I.E.; Ahmad, S.A. Chemistry, biochemistry, toxicity and pollution of molybdenum: A mini review. *J. Microbiol. Biotechnol*, **2014**, *2*(1), 1-6.
[http://dx.doi.org/10.54987/jobimb.v2i1.122]

[237] Schwarz, G. Molybdenum cofactor and human disease. *Curr. Opin. Chem. Biol.*, **2016**, *31*, 179-187.
[http://dx.doi.org/10.1016/j.cbpa.2016.03.016] [PMID: 27055119]

[238] Mendel, R.R.; Bittner, F. Cell biology of molybdenum. *Biochim. Biophys. Acta (BBA)- Mol. Cell Res.*, **2006**, *1763*(7), 621-635.

[239] Hille, R.; Nishino, T.; Bittner, F. Molybdenum enzymes in higher organisms. *Coord. Chem. Rev.*, **2011**, *255*(9-10), 1179-1205.
[http://dx.doi.org/10.1016/j.ccr.2010.11.034] [PMID: 21516203]

[240] Rana, M.; Bhantana, P.; Sun, X.C.; Imran, M.; Shaaban, M.; Moussa, M.; Hu, C.X. Molybdenum as an essential element for crops: An overview. *Int. J. Sci. Res. Growth*, **2020**, *24*, 18535.

[241] Ferreira, C.R.; Gahl, W.A. Disorders of metal metabolism. *Transl. Sci. Rare Dis.*, **2017**, *2*(3-4), 101-139.

[http://dx.doi.org/10.3233/TRD-170015] [PMID: 29354481]

[242] Ghasemzadeh, N.; Karimi-Nazari, E.; Yaghoubi, F.; Zarei, S.; Azadmanesh, F.; Zavar Reza, J.; Sargazi, S. Molybdenum cofactor biology and disorders related to its deficiency; a review study. *J. Nutr. Food Secur.*, **2019**, *4*(3), 206-217.
[http://dx.doi.org/10.18502/jnfs.v4i3.1313]

[243] Novotny, J.A.; Peterson, C.A. Molybdenum. *Adv. Nutr.*, **2018**, *9*(3), 272-273.
[http://dx.doi.org/10.1093/advances/nmx001] [PMID: 29767695]

[244] Crawford, A.M.; Cotelesage, J.J.; Prince, R.C.; George, G.N. The catalytic mechanisms of the molybdenum and tungsten enzymes. In: *Metallocofactors that Activate Small Molecules. Structure and Bonding*; Ribbe, M., Ed.; Springer: Cham, **2018**. Vol. 179.
[http://dx.doi.org/10.1007/430_2018_30]

[245] Iksat, N.N.; Zhangazin, S.B.; Madirov, A.A.; Omarov, R.T. Effect of molybdenum on the activity of molybdoenzymes. *Eurasian J. Appl. Biotechnol.*, **2020**, *2*(2), 1-13.
[http://dx.doi.org/10.11134/btp.2.2020.2]

[246] Bolt, A.M.; Mann, K.K. Tungsten: an emerging toxicant, alone or in combination. *Curr. Environ. Health Rep.*, **2016**, *3*(4), 405-415.
[http://dx.doi.org/10.1007/s40572-016-0106-z] [PMID: 27678292]

[247] Erikson, K.M.; Aschner, M. Manganese: its role in disease and health. *Met. Ions Life Sci.*, **2019**, *19*, 253-266.
[http://dx.doi.org/10.1515/9783110527872-010] [PMID: 30855111]

[248] Millaleo, R.; Reyes-Díaz, M.; Ivanov, A.G.; Mora, M.L.; Alberdi, M. Manganese as essential and toxic element for plants: Transport, accumulation and resistance mechanisms. *J. Soil Sci. Plant Nutr.*, **2010**, *10*(4), 470-481.
[http://dx.doi.org/10.4067/S0718-95162010000200008]

[249] Lingappa, U.F.; Monteverde, D.R.; Magyar, J.S.; Valentine, J.S.; Fischer, W.W. How manganese empowered life with dioxygen *(and vice versa)*. *Free Rad. Biol. Med.*, **2019**, *140*, 113-125.
[http://dx.doi.org/10.1016/j.freeradbiomed.2019.01.036] [PMID: 30738765]

[250] Anagianni, S.; Tuschl, K. Genetic disorders of manganese metabolism. *Curr. Neurol. Neurosci. Rep.*, **2019**, *19*(6), 1-10.
[http://dx.doi.org/10.1007/s11910-019-0942-y] [PMID: 31089831]

[251] Martins, A.C.; Krum, B.N.; Queirós, L.; Tinkov, A.A.; Skalny, A.V.; Bowman, A.B.; Aschner, M. Manganese in the diet: Bioaccessibility, adequate intake, and neurotoxicological effects. *J. Agricult. Food Chem.*, **2020**, *68*(46), 12893-12903.
[http://dx.doi.org/10.1021/acs.jafc.0c00641] [PMID: 32298096]

[252] Cloyd, R.A.; Koren, S.A.; Abisambra, J.F. Manganese-enhanced magnetic resonance imaging: Overview and central nervous system applications with a focus on neurodegeneration. *Front. Aging Neurosci.*, **2018**, *10*, 403.
[http://dx.doi.org/10.3389/fnagi.2018.00403] [PMID: 30618710]

[253] Ruth, T.J. The shortage of technetium-99m and possible solutions. *Annu. Rev. Nucl. Part. Sci.*, **2020**, *70*(1), 77-94.
[http://dx.doi.org/10.1146/annurev-nucl-032020-021829]

[254] Haase, A.A.; Bauer, E.B.; Kühn, F.E.; Crans, D.C. Speciation and toxicity of rhenium salts, organometallics and coordination complexes. *Coord. Chem. Rev.*, **2019**, *394*, 135-161.
[http://dx.doi.org/10.1016/j.ccr.2019.05.012]

[255] Bauer, E.B.; Haase, A.A.; Reich, R.M.; Crans, D.C.; Kühn, F.E. Organometallic and coordination rhenium compounds and their potential in cancer therapy. *Coord. Chem. Rev.*, **2019**, *393*, 79-117.
[http://dx.doi.org/10.1016/j.ccr.2019.04.014]

[256] Rouault, T.A. The role of iron regulatory proteins in mammalian iron homeostasis and disease. *Nat.*

Chem. Biol., **2006**, *2*(8), 406-414.
[http://dx.doi.org/10.1038/nchembio807] [PMID: 16850017]

[257] Hider, R.C.; Kong, X. Iron: Effect of overload and deficiency. *Met. Ions Life Sci.,* **2013**, *13*, 229-294.
[http://dx.doi.org/10.1007/978-94-007-7500-8_8] [PMID: 24470094]

[258] Santucci, R.; Sinibaldi, F.; Cozza, P.; Polticelli, F.; Fiorucci, L. Cytochrome c: An extreme
multifunctional protein with a key role in cell fate. *Int. J. Biol. Macromol.,* **2019**, *136*, 1237-1246.
[http://dx.doi.org/10.1016/j.ijbiomac.2019.06.180] [PMID: 31252007]

[259] Ruckpaul, K.; Rein, H., Eds. Cytochrome P-450: Structural and functional relationships biochemical
and physicochemical aspects of mixed function oxidases. Walter de Gruyter GmbH & Co KG, **2022**.

[260] Eggenreich, B.; Willim, M.; Wurm, D.J.; Herwig, C.; Spadiut, O. Production strategies for active
heme-containing peroxidases from E. coli inclusion bodies–a review. *Biotechnol. Rep.,* **2016**, *10*, 75-
83.
[http://dx.doi.org/10.1016/j.btre.2016.03.005] [PMID: 28352527]

[261] Howard, J.B.; Rees, D.C. Perspectives on non-heme iron protein chemistry. *Adv. Prot. Chem.,* **1991**,
42, 199-280.
[http://dx.doi.org/10.1016/S0065-3233(08)60537-9] [PMID: 1793006]

[262] Kawabata, H. Transferrin and transferrin receptors update. *Free Rad. Biol. Med.,* **2019**, *133*, 46-54.
[http://dx.doi.org/10.1016/j.freeradbiomed.2018.06.037] [PMID: 29969719]

[263] Gervason, S.; Larkem, D.; Mansour, A.B.; Botzanowski, T.; Müller, C.S.; Pecqueur, L.; Le Pavec, G.;
Delaunay-Moisan, A.; Brun, O.; Agramunt, J.; Grandas, A.; Fontecave, M.; Schünemann, V.;
Cianférani, S.; Sizun, C.; Tolédano, M.B.; D'Autréaux, B. Physiologically relevant reconstitution of
iron-sulfur cluster biosynthesis uncovers persulfide-processing functions of ferredoxin-2 and frataxin.
Nat. Commun., **2019**, *10*(1), 3566.
[http://dx.doi.org/10.1038/s41467-019-11470-9] [PMID: 31395877]

[264] Albelda-Berenguer, M.; Monachon, M.; Joseph, E. Siderophores: From natural roles to potential
applications. *Adv. Appl. Microbiol.,* **2019**, *106*, 193-225.
[http://dx.doi.org/10.1016/bs.aambs.2018.12.001] [PMID: 30798803]

[265] Zhang, H.; Zhabyeyev, P.; Wang, S.; Oudit, G.Y. Role of iron metabolism in heart failure: From iron
deficiency to iron overload. *Biochim. Biophys. Acta (BBA)-Mol. Basis Dis.,* **2019**, *1865*(7), 1925-1937.
[http://dx.doi.org/10.1016/j.bbadis.2018.08.030] [PMID: 31109456]

[266] Pasricha, S.R.; Tye-Din, J.; Muckenthaler, M.U.; Swinkels, D.W. Iron deficiency. *Lancet,* **2021**,
397(10270), 233-248.
[http://dx.doi.org/10.1016/S0140-6736(20)32594-0] [PMID: 33285139]

[267] Camaschella, C. Iron deficiency. *Blood J. Am. Soc. Hematol.,* **2019**, *133*(1), 30-39.
[http://dx.doi.org/10.1182/blood-2018-05-815944] [PMID: 30401704]

[268] van de Lagemaat, E.E.; de Groot, L.C.; van den Heuvel, E. Vitamin B12 in relation to oxidative stress:
A systematic review. *Nutrients,* **2019**, *11*(2), 482.
[http://dx.doi.org/10.3390/nu11020482] [PMID: 30823595]

[269] Obeid, R.; Heil, S.G.; Verhoeven, M.M.A.; van den Heuvel, E.G.H.M.; de Groot, L.C.P.G.M.; Eussen,
S.J.P.M. Vitamin B12 intake from animal foods, biomarkers, and health aspects. *Front. Nutr.,* **2019**, *6*,
93.
[http://dx.doi.org/10.3389/fnut.2019.00093] [PMID: 31316992]

[270] Azzini, E.; Raguzzini, A.; Polito, A. A brief review on vitamin B12 deficiency looking at some case
study reports in adults. *Int. J. Mol. Sci.,* **2021**, *22*(18), 9694.
[http://dx.doi.org/10.3390/ijms22189694] [PMID: 34575856]

[271] Mahey, S.; Kumar, R.; Sharma, M.; Kumar, V.; Bhardwaj, R. A critical review on toxicity of cobalt
and its bioremediation strategies. *SN Appl. Sci.,* **2020**, *2*(7), 1279.
[http://dx.doi.org/10.1007/s42452-020-3020-9]

[272] Umar, M.; Sultan, A.; Jahangir, N.; Saeed, Z. Cobalt Toxicity. In: *Metal Toxicology Handbook*; CRC Press, **2020**; pp. 287-301.
[http://dx.doi.org/10.1201/9780429438004-22]

[273] Azarakhsh, M.R.; Asrar, Z.; Mansouri, H. Effects of seed and vegetative stage cysteine treatments on oxidative stress response molecules and enzymes in *Ocimum basilicum* L. under cobalt stress. *J. Soil Sci. Plant Nutr.*, **2015**, *15*, 651-662.
[http://dx.doi.org/10.4067/S0718-95162015005000044]

[274] Gharavian, S.; Hosseini-Giv, N.; Rafat-Motavalli, L.; Abdollahi, S.; Bahrami, A.R.; Miri-Hakimabad, H.; Matin, M.M. Assessing the relative biological effectiveness of high-dose rate 60Co brachytherapy alone and in combination with cisplatin treatment on a cervical cancer cell line (HeLa). *Rad. Phys. Chem.*, **2021**, *184*, 109465.
[http://dx.doi.org/10.1016/j.radphyschem.2021.109465]

[275] Enger, S.A.; Lundqvist, H.; D'Amours, M.; Beaulieu, L. Exploring ^{57}Co as a new isotope for brachytherapy applications. *Med. Phys.*, **2012**, *39*(5), 2342-2345.
[http://dx.doi.org/10.1118/1.3700171] [PMID: 22559604]

[276] Begum, W.; Rai, S.; Banerjee, S.; Bhattacharjee, S.; Mondal, M.H.; Bhattarai, A.; Saha, B. A comprehensive review on the sources, essentiality and toxicological profile of nickel. *RSC Adv.*, **2022**, *12*(15), 9139-9153.
[http://dx.doi.org/10.1039/D2RA00378C] [PMID: 35424851]

[277] Genchi, G.; Carocci, A.; Lauria, G.; Sinicropi, M.S.; Catalano, A. Nickel: Human health and environmental toxicology. *Int. J. Envir. Res. Publ. Health.*, **2020**, *17*(3), 679.
[http://dx.doi.org/10.3390/ijerph17030679] [PMID: 31973020]

[278] Zambelli, B.; Uversky, V.N.; Ciurli, S. Nickel impact on human health: An intrinsic disorder perspective. *Biochim. Biophys. Acta (BBA)-Prot. Proteom.*, **2016**, *1864*(12), 1714-1731.
[http://dx.doi.org/10.1016/j.bbapap.2016.09.008] [PMID: 27645710]

[279] Dudek-Adamska, D.; Lech, T.; Konopka, T.; Kościelniak, P. Nickel content in human internal organs. *Biol. Trace Elem. Res.*, **2021**, *199*(6), 2138-2144.
[http://dx.doi.org/10.1007/s12011-020-02347-w] [PMID: 32839915]

[280] Hassan, M.U.; Chattha, M.U.; Khan, I.; Chattha, M.B.; Aamer, M.; Nawaz, M.; Ali, A.; Khan, M.A.U.; Khan, T.A. Nickel toxicity in plants: Reasons, toxic effects, tolerance mechanisms, and remediation possibilities—a review. *Environ. Sci. Pollut. Res.*, **2019**, *26*(13), 12673-12688.
[http://dx.doi.org/10.1007/s11356-019-04892-x] [PMID: 30924044]

[281] Alfano, M.; Cavazza, C. Structure, function, and biosynthesis of nickel-dependent enzymes. *Prot. Sci.*, **2020**, *29*(5), 1071-1089.
[http://dx.doi.org/10.1002/pro.3836] [PMID: 32022353]

[282] Klein, C.B.; Costa, M.A.X. In Handbook on the Toxicology of Metals Academic Press, **2022**; pp. 615-637.

[283] Buxton, S.; Garman, E.; Heim, K.E.; Lyons-Darden, T.; Schlekat, C.E.; Taylor, M.D.; Oller, A.R. Concise review of nickel human health toxicology and ecotoxicology. *Inorganics*, **2019**, *7*(7), 89.
[http://dx.doi.org/10.3390/inorganics7070089]

[284] Guo, H.; Liu, H.; Wu, H.; Cui, H.; Fang, J.; Zuo, Z.; Deng, J.; Li, Y.; Wang, X.; Zhao, L. Nickel carcinogenesis mechanism: DNA damage. *Int. J. Mol. Sci.*, **2019**, *20*(19), 4690.
[http://dx.doi.org/10.3390/ijms20194690] [PMID: 31546657]

[285] Kenny, R.G.; Marmion, C.J. Toward multi-targeted platinum and ruthenium drugs—a new paradigm in cancer drug treatment regimens? *Chem. Rev.*, **2019**, *119*(2), 1058-1137.
[http://dx.doi.org/10.1021/acs.chemrev.8b00271] [PMID: 30640441]

[286] Sundar, H.; Padmini, S.; Devi, P.B. Bioremediation of nuclear waste effluent using different communities of microbes. In: *Metagenomics to Bioremediation*; Academic Press, **2023**.

[http://dx.doi.org/10.1016/B978-0-323-96113-4.00007-X]

[287] Zuba, I.; Zuba, M.; Piotrowski, M.; Pawlukojć, A. Ruthenium as an important element in nuclear energy and cancer treatment. *Appl. Rad. Isot.,* **2020,** *162,* 109176.
[http://dx.doi.org/10.1016/j.apradiso.2020.109176] [PMID: 32310093]

[288] Sahu, A.K.; Dash, D.K.; Mishra, K.; Mishra, S.P.; Yadav, R.; Kashyap, P. Properties and applications of ruthenium. In: *Noble and Precious Metals-Properties*; Nanoscale Effects and Applications. IntechOpen, **2018.**
[http://dx.doi.org/10.5772/intechopen.76393]

[289] Li, F.; Collins, J.G.; Keene, F.R. Ruthenium complexes as antimicrobial agents. *Chem. Soc. Rev.,* **2015,** *44*(8), 2529-2542.
[http://dx.doi.org/10.1039/C4CS00343H] [PMID: 25724019]

[290] Jain, A.; Garrett, N.T.; Malone, Z.P. Ruthenium-based photoactive metalloantibiotics. *Photochem. Photobiol.,* **2022,** *98*(1), 6-16.
[http://dx.doi.org/10.1111/php.13435] [PMID: 33882620]

[291] Clarke, M.J. Ruthenium metallopharmaceuticals. *Coord. Chem. Rev.,* **2002,** *232*(1-2), 69-93.
[http://dx.doi.org/10.1016/S0010-8545(02)00025-5]

[292] Coverdale, J.; Laroiya-McCarron, T.; Romero-Canelón, I. Designing ruthenium anticancer drugs: What have we learnt from the key drug candidates? *Inorganics,* **2019,** *7*(3), 31.
[http://dx.doi.org/10.3390/inorganics7030031]

[293] Liu, J.; Zhang, C.; Rees, T.W.; Ke, L.; Ji, L.; Chao, H. Harnessing ruthenium(II) as photodynamic agents: Encouraging advances in cancer therapy. *Coord. Chem. Rev.,* **2018,** *363,* 17-28.
[http://dx.doi.org/10.1016/j.ccr.2018.03.002]

[294] Sohrabi, M.; Saeedi, M.; Larijani, B.; Mahdavi, M. Recent advances in biological activities of rhodium complexes: Their applications in drug discovery research. *Eur. J. Med. Chem.,* **2021,** *216,* 113308.
[http://dx.doi.org/10.1016/j.ejmech.2021.113308] [PMID: 33713976]

[295] Ohata, J.; Ball, Z.T. Rhodium at the chemistry–biology interface. *Dalton Trans.,* **2018,** *47*(42), 14855-14860.
[http://dx.doi.org/10.1039/C8DT03032D] [PMID: 30234200]

[296] Loreto, D.; Merlino, A. The interaction of rhodium compounds with proteins: A structural overview. *Coord. Chem. Rev.,* **2021,** *442,* 213999.
[http://dx.doi.org/10.1016/j.ccr.2021.213999]

[297] Rushforth, R. Palladium in restorative dentistry. *Platin. Met. Rev.,* **2004,** *48*(1), 30-31.

[298] Kielhorn, J.; Melber, C.; Keller, D.; Mangelsdorf, I. Palladium – A review of exposure and effects to human health. *Int. J. Hyg. Environ. Health,* **2002,** *205*(6), 417-432.
[http://dx.doi.org/10.1078/1438-4639-00180] [PMID: 12455264]

[299] Scattolin, T.; Voloshkin, V.A.; Visentin, F.; Nolan, S.P. A critical review of palladium organometallic anticancer agents. *Cell Rep. Phys. Sci.,* **2021,** *2*(6), 100446.
[http://dx.doi.org/10.1016/j.xcrp.2021.100446]

[300] Olesya, S.; Alexander, P. Antimicrobial activity of mono-and polynuclear platinum and palladium complexes. *Foods and Raw Materials,* **2020,** *8*(2), 298-311.
[http://dx.doi.org/10.21603/2308-4057-2020-2-298-311]

[301] Jahromi, E.Z.; Divsalar, A.; Saboury, A.A.; Khaleghizadeh, S.; Mansouri-Torshizi, H.; Kostova, I. Palladium complexes: New candidates for anti-cancer drugs. *J. Iran. Chem. Soc.,* **2016,** *13*(5), 967-989.
[http://dx.doi.org/10.1007/s13738-015-0804-8]

[302] Carneiro, T.J.; Martins, A.S.; Marques, M.P.M.; Gil, A.M. Metabolic aspects of palladium (II) potential anti-cancer drugs. *Front. Oncol.,* **2020,** *10,* 590970.

[http://dx.doi.org/10.3389/fonc.2020.590970] [PMID: 33154950]

[303]   Pelclova, D. In: *Handbook on the Toxicology of Metals*. Academic Press, **2022**, pp. 639-647.

[304]   Nkomo, D.; Mwamba, A. Beneficiation opportunities for osmium: A review. In IOP Conference Series. In: *Materials Science and Engineering*; IOP Publishing, **2020**; 839, pp. (1)012-014.
[http://dx.doi.org/10.1088/1757-899X/839/1/012014]

[305]   Hanif, M.; Babak, M.V.; Hartinger, C.G. Development of anticancer agents: Wizardry with osmium. *Drug Discov. Today,* **2014**, *19*(10), 1640-1648.
[http://dx.doi.org/10.1016/j.drudis.2014.06.016] [PMID: 24955838]

[306]   Quinson, J. Osmium and OsOx nanoparticles: An overview of syntheses and applications. *Open Res. Eur.,* **2022**, *2*, 39.
[http://dx.doi.org/10.12688/openreseurope.14595.2]

[307]   Ohriner, E.K. Processing of iridium and iridium alloys. *Platin. Met. Rev.,* **2008**, *52*(3), 186-197.
[http://dx.doi.org/10.1595/147106708X333827]

[308]   Sharma, A.; Sudhindra, P.; Roy, N.; Paira, P. Advances in novel iridium (III) based complexes for anticancer applications: A review. *Inorg. Chim. Acta.,* **2020**, *513*, 119925.
[http://dx.doi.org/10.1016/j.ica.2020.119925]

[309]   Liang, J.; Sun, D.; Yang, Y.; Li, M.; Li, H.; Chen, L. Discovery of metal-based complexes as promising antimicrobial agents. *Eur. J. Med. Chem.,* **2021**, *224*, 113696.
[http://dx.doi.org/10.1016/j.ejmech.2021.113696] [PMID: 34274828]

[310]   Quinson, J. Iridium and IrOx nanoparticles: An overview and review of syntheses and applications. Adv. Colloid Interf. Sci., **2022**; p. 102643.

[311]   Singh, S.B. Iridium chemistry and its catalytic applications: A Brief. *Green Chem. Technol. Lett.,* **2016**, *2*(206), 456-518.
[http://dx.doi.org/10.18510/gctl.2016.247]

[312]   Walker, M.; Smith, J.R. Iridium-192: A literature review for further referencing the isotope, its activity units, and dosimetry techniques. *Vet. Radiol.,* **1990**, *31*(6), 281-292.
[http://dx.doi.org/10.1111/j.1740-8261.1990.tb00802.x]

[313]   Hartmann, J.T.; Lipp, H.P. Toxicity of platinum compounds. *Exp. Opin. Pharmacother.,* **2003**, *4*(6), 889-901.
[http://dx.doi.org/10.1517/14656566.4.6.889] [PMID: 12783586]

[314]   Odularu, A.T.; Ajibade, P.A.; Mbese, J.Z.; Oyedeji, O.O. Developments in platinum-group metals as dual antibacterial and anticancer agents. *J. Chem.,* **2019**, *2019*, 1-18.
[http://dx.doi.org/10.1155/2019/5459461]

[315]   Rajendran, S.; Prabha, S.S.; Rathish, R.J.; Singh, G.; Al-Hashem, A. Antibacterial activity of platinum nanoparticles. In: *Nanotoxicity*; Elsevier, **2020**; pp. 275-281.
[http://dx.doi.org/10.1016/B978-0-12-819943-5.00012-9]

[316]   Tavares, O.A.P.; Medeiros, E.L. Natural and artificial alpha radioactivity of platinum isotopes. *Phys. Scr.,* **2011**, *84*(4), 045202.
[http://dx.doi.org/10.1088/0031-8949/84/04/045202]

[317]   Chistoserdova, L. New pieces to the lanthanide puzzle. *Mol. Microbiol.,* **2019**, *111*(5), 1127-1131.
[http://dx.doi.org/10.1111/mmi.14210] [PMID: 30673122]

[318]   Rim, K.T.; Koo, K.H.; Park, J.S. Toxicological evaluations of rare earths and their health impacts to workers: A literature review. *Saf. Health Work,* **2013**, *4*(1), 12-26.
[http://dx.doi.org/10.5491/SHAW.2013.4.1.12] [PMID: 23516020]

[319]   Farnaby, J.H.; Chowdhury, T.; Horsewill, S.J.; Wilson, B.; Jaroschik, F. Lanthanides and actinides: Annual survey of their organometallic chemistry covering the year 2019. *Coord. Chem. Rev.,* **2021**, *437*, 213830.

[http://dx.doi.org/10.1016/j.ccr.2021.213830]

[320] Li, Y.; Li, B.; Chen, L.; Dong, J.; Xia, Z.; Tian, Y. Chelating decorporation agents for internal contamination by actinides: Designs, mechanisms, and advances. *J. Inorg. Biochem.,* **2022**, *238,* 112034.
[http://dx.doi.org/10.1016/j.jinorgbio.2022.112034] [PMID: 36306597]

[321] Bunzli, J.C.G.; Pecharsky, V.K. In: *Handbook on the Physics and Chemistry of Rare Earths.* Elsevier, **2016**.

[322] Featherston, E.R.; Cotruvo, J.A.Jr. The biochemistry of lanthanide acquisition, trafficking, and utilization. *Biochim. Biophys. Acta (BBA)-Mol. Cell Res.,* **2021**, *1868*(1), 118864.
[http://dx.doi.org/10.1016/j.bbamcr.2020.118864] [PMID: 32979423]

[323] Götzke, L.; Schaper, G.; März, J.; Kaden, P.; Huittinen, N.; Stumpf, T.; Kammerlander, K.K.K.; Brunner, E.; Hahn, P.; Mehnert, A.; Kersting, B.; Henle, T.; Lindoy, L.F.; Zanoni, G.; Weigand, J.J. Coordination chemistry of f-block metal ions with ligands bearing bio-relevant functional groups. *Coord. Chem. Rev.,* **2019**, *386*, 267-309.
[http://dx.doi.org/10.1016/j.ccr.2019.01.006]

[324] Cotton, S.A.; Harrowfield, J.M. Lanthanides: Biological activity and medical applications. In: *Encyclopedia of Inorganic and Bioinorganic Chemistry*; John Wiley & Sons, **2011**.

[325] Valcheva-Traykova, M.; Saso, L.; Kostova, I. Involvement of lanthanides in the free radicals homeostasis. *Curr. Top. Med. Chem.,* **2014**, *14*(22), 2508-2519.
[http://dx.doi.org/10.2174/1568026614666141203123620] [PMID: 25478885]

[326] Eliseeva, S.V.; Bünzli, J.C.G. Rare earths: Jewels for functional materials of the future. *New J. Chem.,* **2011**, *35*(6), 1165-1176.
[http://dx.doi.org/10.1039/c0nj00969e]

[327] Matthews, A.; Zhu, X-K.; O'Nions, K. Kinetic iron stable isotope fractionation between iron (-II) and (-III) complexes in solution. *Earth Planet. Sci. Lett.,* **2001**, *192*(1), 81-92.
[http://dx.doi.org/10.1016/S0012-821X(01)00432-0]

[328] Zhu, X.K.; Guo, Y.; Williams, R.J.P.; O'Nions, R.K.; Matthews, A.; Belshaw, N.S.; Canters, G.W.; de Waal, E.C.; Weser, U.; Burgess, B.K.; Salvato, B. Mass fractionation processes of transition metal isotopes. *Earth Planet. Sci. Lett.,* **2002**, *200*(1-2), 47-62.
[http://dx.doi.org/10.1016/S0012-821X(02)00615-5]

[329] Gant, T.G. Using deuterium in drug discovery: Leaving the label in the drug. *J. Med. Chem.,* **2014**, *57*(9), 3595-3611.
[http://dx.doi.org/10.1021/jm4007998] [PMID: 24294889]

[330] Dawson, E.B. The relationship of tap water and physiological levels of lithium to mental hospital admission and homicide in Texas. In: *Lithium in biology and medicine*; Schrauzer, G.N.; Klippel, K.F., Eds.; VCH: Weinheim, Germany, **1991**; pp. 171-187.

[331] Birch, N.J. Lithium in medicine. In: *Handbook of metal-ligand interactions in biological fluids*; Berthon, G., Ed.; Marcel Dekker: New York, NY, **1995**; pp. 1274-1281.

[332] Gould, T.D.; Manji, H.K. Glycogen synthase kinase-3: A putative molecular target for lithium mimetic drugs. *Neuropsychopharmacol.,* **2005**, *30*(7), 1223-1237.
[http://dx.doi.org/10.1038/sj.npp.1300731] [PMID: 15827567]

[333] Chen, C.H.; Lee, C.S.; Lee, M.T.M.; Ouyang, W.C.; Chen, C.C.; Chong, M.Y.; Wu, J.Y.; Tan, H.K.L.; Lee, Y.C.; Chuo, L.J.; Chiu, N.Y.; Tsang, H.Y.; Chang, T.J.; Lung, F.W.; Chiu, C.H.; Chang, C.H.; Chen, Y.S.; Hou, Y.M.; Chen, C.C.; Lai, T.J.; Tung, C.L.; Chen, C.Y.; Lane, H.Y.; Su, T.P.; Feng, J.; Lin, J.J.; Chang, C.J.; Teng, P.R.; Liu, C.Y.; Chen, C.K.; Liu, I.C.; Chen, J.J.; Lu, T.; Fan, C.C.; Wu, C.K.; Li, C.F.; Wang, K.H.T.; Wu, L.S.H.; Peng, H.L.; Chang, C.P.; Lu, L.S.; Chen, Y.T.; Cheng, A.T.A. Variant GADL1 and response to lithium therapy in bipolar I disorder. *N. Engl. J. Med.,* **2014**, *370*(2), 119-128.

[http://dx.doi.org/10.1056/NEJMoa1212444] [PMID: 24369049]

[334] Hottinger, D.G.; Beebe, D.S.; Belani, K.G.; Prielipp, R.C.; Kozhimannil, T. Sodium nitroprusside in 2014: A clinical concepts review. *J. Anaesth. Clin. Pharmacol.,* **2014**, *30*(4), 462-471.
[http://dx.doi.org/10.4103/0970-9185.142799] [PMID: 25425768]

[335] Ripeckyj, A.; Kosmopoulos, M.; Shekar, K.; Carlson, C.; Kalra, R.; Rees, J.; Aufderheide, T.P.; Bartos, J.A.; Yannopoulos, D. Sodium nitroprusside–enhanced cardiopulmonary resuscitation improves blood flow by pulmonary vasodilation leading to higher oxygen requirements. *JACC: Basic Transl. Sci.,* **2020**, *5*(2), 183-192.
[http://dx.doi.org/10.1016/j.jacbts.2019.11.010] [PMID: 32140624]

[336] Tout, D.; Tonge, C.M.; Muthu, S.; Arumugam, P. Assessment of a protocol for routine simultaneous myocardial blood flow measurement and standard myocardial perfusion imaging with rubidium-82 on a high count rate positron emission tomography system. *Nucl. Med. Commun.,* **2012**, *33*(11), 1202-1211.
[http://dx.doi.org/10.1097/MNM.0b013e3283567554] [PMID: 22760302]

[337] Beller, G.; Bergmann, S.R. Myocardial perfusion imaging agents: SPECT and PET. *J. Nucl. Cardiol.,* **2004**, *11*(1), 71-86.
[http://dx.doi.org/10.1016/j.nuclcard.2003.12.002] [PMID: 14752475]

[338] Palmisciano, P.; Haider, A.S.; Balasubramanian, K.; D'Amico, R.S.; Wernicke, A.G. The role of cesium-131 brachytherapy in brain tumors: A scoping review of the literature and ongoing clinical trials. *J. Neuro-Oncol.,* **2022**, *159*(1), 117-133.
[http://dx.doi.org/10.1007/s11060-022-04050-3] [PMID: 35696019]

[339] Schwalfenberg, G.K.; Genuis, S.J. The importance of magnesium in clinical healthcare. *Scientifica,* **2017**, *2017*, 1-14.
[http://dx.doi.org/10.1155/2017/4179326] [PMID: 29093983]

[340] Glasdam, S.M.; Glasdam, S.; Peters, G.H. The Importance of Magnesium in the Human Body: A Systematic Literature Review. *Adv. Clin. Chem.,* **2016**, *73*, 169-193.
[http://dx.doi.org/10.1016/bs.acc.2015.10.002] [PMID: 26975973]

[341] Case, D.R.; Zubieta, J.; P Doyle, R. The coordination chemistry of bio-relevant ligands and their magnesium complexes. *Molecules,* **2020**, *25*(14), 3172-3195.
[http://dx.doi.org/10.3390/molecules25143172] [PMID: 32664540]

[342] Aiello, D.; Carnamucio, F.; Cordaro, M.; Foti, C.; Napoli, A.; Giuffrè, O. Ca^{2+} complexation with relevant bioligands in aqueous solution: A speciation study with implications for biological fluids. *Front Chem.,* **2021**, *9*, 640219.
[http://dx.doi.org/10.3389/fchem.2021.640219] [PMID: 33718329]

[343] Surdacka, A.; Stopa, J.; Torlinski, L. In Situ effect of strontium toothpaste on artificially decalcified human enamel. *Biol. Trace Elem. Res.,* **2007**, *116*, 147-153.
[http://dx.doi.org/10.1007/BF02685927] [PMID: 17646684]

[344] Pors Nielsen, S. The biological role of strontium. *Bone,* **2004**, *35*(3), 583-588.
[http://dx.doi.org/10.1016/j.bone.2004.04.026] [PMID: 15336592]

[345] Querido, W.; Campos, A.P.C.; Martins Ferreira, E.H.; San Gil, R.A.S.; Rossi, A.M.; Farina, M. Strontium ranelate changes the composition and crystal structure of the biological bone-like apatite produced in osteoblast cell cultures. *Cell Tissue Res.,* **2014**, *357*, 793-801.
[http://dx.doi.org/10.1007/s00441-014-1901-1] [PMID: 24859219]

[346] Hahn, G.S. Strontium is a potent and selective inhibitor of sensory irritation. *Dermatol. Surg.,* **1999**, *25*(9), 689-694.
[http://dx.doi.org/10.1046/j.1524-4725.1999.99099.x] [PMID: 10491058]

[347] Tomblyn, M. The role of bone-seeking radionuclides in the palliative treatment of patients with painful osteoblastic skeletal metastases. *Cancer Contr.,* **2012**, *19*(2), 137-144.

[http://dx.doi.org/10.1177/107327481201900208] [PMID: 22487976]

[348] Blake, G.M.; Zivanovic, M.A.; Blaquiere, R.M.; Fine, D.R.; McEwan, A.J.; Ackery, D.M. Strontium-89 therapy: Measurement of absorbed dose to skeletal metastases. *J. Nucl. Med.,* **1988**, *29*(4), 549-557.
[PMID: 3351609]

[349] Fuster, D.; Herranz, R.; Vidal-Sicart, S.; Muñoz, M.; Conill, C.; Mateos, J.J.; Martín, F.; Pons, F. Usefulness of strontium-89 for bone pain palliation in metastatic breast cancer patients. *Nucl. Med. Commun.,* **2000**, *21*(7), 623-626.
[http://dx.doi.org/10.1097/00006231-200007000-00004] [PMID: 10994664]

[350] Gunawardana, D.H.; Lichtenstein, M.; Better, N.; Rosenthal, M. Results of strontium-89 therapy in patients with prostate cancer resistant to chemotherapy. *Clin. Nucl. Med.,* **2004**, *29*(2), 81-85.
[http://dx.doi.org/10.1097/01.rlu.0000109721.58471.44] [PMID: 14734902]

[351] Oskarsson, A. In: *Handbook on the Toxicology of Metals.* Academic Press, **2022**, pp. 91-100.

[352] Bruland, Ø.S.; Nilsson, S.; Fisher, D.R.; Larsen, R.H. High-linear energy transfer irradiation targeted to skeletal metastases by the α-emitter ^{223}Ra: Adjuvant or alternative to conventional modalities? *Clin. Cancer Res.,* **2006**, *12*(20), 6250s-6257s.
[http://dx.doi.org/10.1158/1078-0432.CCR-06-0841] [PMID: 17062709]

[353] Lewington, V.J. Bone-seeking radionuclides for therapy. *J. Nucl. Med.,* **2005**, *46* Suppl. 1, 38S-47S.
[PMID: 15653650]

[354] Henriksen, G.; Breistøl, K.; Bruland, O.S.; Fodstad, Ø.; Larsen, R.H. Significant antitumor effect from bone-seeking, α-particle-emitting-^{223}Ra demonstrated in an experimental skeletal metastases model. *Cancer Res.,* **2002**, *62*(11), 3120-3125.
[PMID: 12036923]

[355] Henriksen, G.; Fisher, D.R.; Roeske, J.C.; Bruland, O.S.; Larsen, R.H. Targeting of osseous sites with α-emitting ^{223}Ra: Comparison with the beta-emitter ^{89}Sr in mice. *J. Nucl. Med.,* **2003**, *44*(2), 252-259.
[PMID: 12571218]

[356] Larsen, R.H.; Saxtorph, H.; Skydsgaard, M.; Borrebaek, J.; Jonasdottir, T.J.; Bruland, O.S.; Klastrup, S.; Harling, R.; Ramdahl, T. Radiotoxicity of the alpha-emitting bone-seeker ^{223}Ra injected intravenously into mice: histology, clinical chemistry and hematology. *In Vivo,* **2006**, *20*(3), 325-331.
[PMID: 16724665]

[357] Nilsson, S.; Strang, P.; Aksnes, A.K.; Franzèn, L.; Olivier, P.; Pecking, A.; Staffurth, J.; Vasanthan, S.; Andersson, C.; Bruland, Ø.S. A randomized, dose–response, multicenter phase II study of radium-223 chloride for the palliation of painful bone metastases in patients with castration-resistant prostate cancer. *Eur. J. Cancer,* **2012**, *48*(5), 678-686.
[http://dx.doi.org/10.1016/j.ejca.2011.12.023] [PMID: 22341993]

[358] Baker, S.J.; Tomsho, J.W.; Benkovic, S.J. Boron-containing inhibitors of synthetases. *Chem. Soc. Rev.,* **2011**, *40*(8), 4279-4285.
[http://dx.doi.org/10.1039/c0cs00131g] [PMID: 21298158]

[359] Kohno, J.; Kawahata, T.; Otake, T.; Morimoto, M.; Mori, H.; Ueba, N.; Nishio, M.; Kinumaki, A.; Komatsubara, S.; Kawashima, K. Boromycin, an anti-HIV antibiotic. *Biosci. Biotechnol. Biochem.,* **1996**, *60*(6), 1036-1037.
[http://dx.doi.org/10.1271/bbb.60.1036] [PMID: 8695905]

[360] Soriano-Ursúa, M.A.; Das, B.C.; Trujillo-Ferrara, J.G. Boron-containing compounds: Chemico-biological properties and expanding medicinal potential in prevention, diagnosis and therapy. *Expert Opin. Ther. Pat.,* **2014**, *24*(5), 485-500.
[http://dx.doi.org/10.1517/13543776.2014.881472] [PMID: 24456081]

[361] Ciaravino, V.; Plattner, J.; Chanda, S. An assessment of the genetic toxicology of novel boron-containing therapeutic agents. *Environ. Mol. Mutagen.,* **2013**, *54*(5), 338-346.
[http://dx.doi.org/10.1002/em.21779] [PMID: 23625818]

[362] Nedunchezhian, K.; Aswath, N.; Thiruppathy, M.; Thirugnanamurthy, S. Boron neutron capture therapy - A literature review. *J. Clin. Diagn. Res.,* **2016**, *10*(12), ZE01.
[http://dx.doi.org/10.7860/JCDR/2016/19890.9024] [PMID: 28209015]

[363] Kohli, S.K.; Kaur, H.; Khanna, K.; Handa, N.; Bhardwaj, R.; Rinklebe, J.; Ahmad, P. Boron in plants: Uptake, deficiency and biological potential. *Plant Growth Regul.,* **2022**, 1-16.

[364] García, A.; De Sanctis, J.B. An overview of adjuvant formulations and delivery systems. *APMIS,* **2014**, *122*(4), 257-267.
[http://dx.doi.org/10.1111/apm.12143] [PMID: 23919674]

[365] Tomljenovic, L.; Shaw, C.A. Aluminum vaccine adjuvants: Are they safe? *Curr. Med. Chem.,* **2011**, *18*(17), 2630-2637.
[http://dx.doi.org/10.2174/092986711795933740] [PMID: 21568886]

[366] Verron, E.; Bouler, J.M.; Scimeca, J.C. Gallium as a potential candidate for treatment of osteoporosis. *Drug Discov. Today,* **2012**, *17*(19-20), 1127-1132.
[http://dx.doi.org/10.1016/j.drudis.2012.06.007] [PMID: 22710367]

[367] Chitambar, C.R. Medical applications and toxicities of gallium compounds. *Int. J. Environ. Res. Public Health,* **2010**, *7*(5), 2337-2361.
[http://dx.doi.org/10.3390/ijerph7052337] [PMID: 20623028]

[368] Leyland-Jones, B. Treating cancer-related hypercalcemia with gallium nitrate. *J. Support. Oncol.,* **2004**, *2*(6), 509-516.
[PMID: 15605917]

[369] Hoffman, L.R.; Ramsey, B.W. Cystic fibrosis therapeutics: The road ahead. *Chest,* **2013**, *143*(1), 207-213.
[http://dx.doi.org/10.1378/chest.12-1639] [PMID: 23276843]

[370] Todorov, L.; Kostova, I.; Traykova, M. Lanthanum, gallium and their impact on oxidative stress. *Curr. Med. Chem.,* **2019**, *26*(22), 4280-4295.
[http://dx.doi.org/10.2174/0929867326666190104165311] [PMID: 31438825]

[371] Wilke, N.L.; Abodo, L.O.; Frias, C.; Frias, J.; Baas, J.; Jakupec, M.A.; Keppler, B.K.; Prokop, A. The gallium complex KP46 sensitizes resistant leukemia cells and overcomes Bcl-2-induced multidrug resistance in lymphoma cells *via* upregulation of Harakiri and downregulation of XIAP *in vitro*. *Biomed. Pharmacother.,* **2022**, *156*, 113974.
[http://dx.doi.org/10.1016/j.biopha.2022.113974] [PMID: 36411649]

[372] Hreusova, M.; Novohradsky, V.; Markova, L.; Kostrhunova, H.; Potočňák, I.; Brabec, V.; Kasparkova, J. Gallium (III) complex with cloxyquin ligands induces ferroptosis in cancer cells and is a potent agent against both differentiated and tumorigenic cancer stem rhabdomyosarcoma cells. *Bioinorg. Chem. Appl.,* **2022**.

[373] Chitambar, C.R.; Antholine, W.E. Iron-targeting antitumor activity of gallium compounds and novel insights into triapine ® -metal complexes. *Antiox. Red. Signal.,* **2013**, *18*(8), 956-972.
[http://dx.doi.org/10.1089/ars.2012.4880] [PMID: 22900955]

[374] Lessa, J.A.; Parrilha, G.L.; Beraldo, H. Gallium complexes as new promising metallodrug candidates. *Inorg. Chim. Acta,* **2012**, *393*, 53-63.
[http://dx.doi.org/10.1016/j.ica.2012.06.003]

[375] Chitambar, C.R. Gallium-containing anticancer compounds. *Fut. Med. Chem.,* **2012**, *4*(10), 1257-1272.
[http://dx.doi.org/10.4155/fmc.12.69] [PMID: 22800370]

[376] Qi, J.; Liu, T.; Zhao, W.; Zheng, X.; Wang, Y. Synthesis, crystal structure and antiproliferative mechanisms of gallium(III) complexes with benzoylpyridine thiosemicarbazones. *RSC Adv.,* **2020**, *10*(32), 18553-18559.
[http://dx.doi.org/10.1039/D0RA02913K] [PMID: 35518317]

[377] dos SS Firmino, G.; André, S.C.; Hastenreiter, Z.; Campos, V.K.; Abdel-Salam, M.A.L.; de Souza-Fagundes, E.M.; Lessa, J.A. *In vitro* assessment of the cytotoxicity of gallium(III) complexes with isoniazid-derived hydrazones: effects on clonogenic survival of hct-116 cells. *Inorg. Chim. Acta,* **2019**, *497*, 119079.
[http://dx.doi.org/10.1016/j.ica.2019.119079]

[378] Robin, P.; Singh, K.; Suntharalingam, K. Gallium(III)-polypyridyl complexes as anti-osteosarcoma stem cell agents. *Chem. Commun.,* **2020**, *56*(10), 1509-1512.
[http://dx.doi.org/10.1039/C9CC08962D] [PMID: 31917383]

[379] Litecká, M.; Hreusová, M.; Kašpárková, J.; Gyepes, R.; Smolková, R.; Obuch, J.; David, T.; Potočňák, I. Low-dimensional compounds containing bioactive ligands. Part XIV: High selective antiproliferative activity of tris (5-chloro-8-quinolinolato) gallium (III) complex against human cancer cell lines. *Bioorg. Med. Chem. Lett.,* **2020**, *30*(13), 127206.
[http://dx.doi.org/10.1016/j.bmcl.2020.127206] [PMID: 32354569]

[380] Banerjee, S.R.; Pomper, M.G. Clinical applications of Gallium-68. *Appl. Radiat. Isot.,* **2013**, *76*, 2-13.
[http://dx.doi.org/10.1016/j.apradiso.2013.01.039] [PMID: 23522791]

[381] Khan, M.U.; Khan, S.; El-Refaie, S.; Win, Z.; Rubello, D.; Al-Nahhas, A. Clinical indications for Gallium-68 positron emission tomography imaging. *Eur. J. Surg. Oncol.,* **2009**, *35*(6), 561-567.
[http://dx.doi.org/10.1016/j.ejso.2009.01.007] [PMID: 19201567]

[382] Nishiyama, Y.; Yamamoto, Y.; Toyama, Y.; Satoh, K.; Nagai, M.; Ohkawa, M. Usefulness of ^{67}Ga scintigraphy in extranodal malignant lymphoma patients. *Ann. Nucl. Med.,* **2003**, *17*(8), 657-662.
[http://dx.doi.org/10.1007/BF02984971] [PMID: 14971607]

[383] Goldsmith, S.J. Targeted radionuclide therapy: A historical and personal review. In: *Seminars in Nuclear Medicine*; WB Saunders, **2020**, *50*(1), 87-97.
[http://dx.doi.org/10.1053/j.semnuclmed.2019.07.006]

[384] Kurdziel, K.A.; Mena, E.; McKinney, Y.; Wong, K.; Adler, S.; Sissung, T.; Lee, J.; Lipkowitz, S.; Lindenberg, L.; Turkbey, B.; Kummar, S.; Milenic, D.E.; Doroshow, J.H.; Figg, W.D.; Merino, M.J.; Paik, C.H.; Brechbiel, M.W.; Choyke, P.L. First-in-human phase 0 study of ^{111}In-CHX-A"-DTPA trastuzumab for HER2 tumor imaging. *J. Transl. Sci.,* **2019**, *5*(2), 10.
[PMID: 30906574]

[385] Banerjee, S.R.; Kumar, V.; Lisok, A.; Plyku, D.; Nováková, Z.; Brummet, M.; Wharram, B.; Barinka, C.; Hobbs, R.; Pomper, M.G. Evaluation of 111In-DOTA-5D3, a surrogate SPECT imaging agent for radioimmunotherapy of prostate-specific membrane antigen. *J. Nucl. Med.,* **2019**, *60*(3), 400-406.
[http://dx.doi.org/10.2967/jnumed.118.214403] [PMID: 30237212]

[386] Campanella, B.; Colombaioni, L.; Benedetti, E.; Di Ciaula, A.; Ghezzi, L.; Onor, M.; D'Orazio, M.; Giannecchini, R.; Petrini, R.; Bramanti, E. Toxicity of thallium at low doses: A review. *Int. J. Environ. Res. Publ. Health,* **2019**, *16*(23), 4732.
[http://dx.doi.org/10.3390/ijerph16234732] [PMID: 31783498]

[387] Genchi, G.; Carocci, A.; Lauria, G.; Sinicropi, M.S.; Catalano, A. Thallium use, toxicity, and detoxification therapy: An overview. *Appl. Sci.,* **2021**, *11*(18), 8322.
[http://dx.doi.org/10.3390/app11188322]

[388] Al Badarin, F.J.; Malhotra, S. Diagnosis and prognosis of coronary artery disease with SPECT and PET. *Curr. Card. Rep.,* **2019**, *21*(7), 57.
[http://dx.doi.org/10.1007/s11886-019-1146-4] [PMID: 31104158]

[389] Ahmad, N.; Gupta, S.; Feyes, D.K.; Mukhtar, H. Involvement of Fas (APO-1/CD-95) during photodynamic-therapy-mediated apoptosis in human epidermoid carcinoma A431 cells. *J. Invest. Dermatol.,* **2000**, *115*(6), 1041-1046.
[http://dx.doi.org/10.1046/j.1523-1747.2000.00147.x] [PMID: 11121139]

[390] Ke, M.S.; Xue, L.Y.; Feyes, D.K.; Azizuddin, K.; Baron, E.D.; McCormick, T.S.; Mukhtar, H.;

Panneerselvam, A.; Schluchter, M.D.; Cooper, K.D.; Oleinick, N.L.; Stevens, S.R. Apoptosis mechanisms related to the increased sensitivity of Jurkat T-cells vs A431 epidermoid cells to photodynamic therapy with the phthalocyanine Pc 4. *Photochem. Photobiol.,* **2008**, *84*(2), 407-414. [http://dx.doi.org/10.1111/j.1751-1097.2007.00278.x] [PMID: 18221452]

[391] Baron, E.D.; Malbasa, C.L.; Santo-Domingo, D.; Fu, P.; Miller, J.D.; Hanneman, K.K.; Hsia, A.H.; Oleinick, N.L.; Colussi, V.C.; Cooper, K.D. Silicon phthalocyanine (pc 4) photodynamic therapy is a safe modality for cutaneous neoplasms: results of a phase 1 clinical trial. *Lasers Surg. Med.,* **2010**, *42*(10), 888-895. [http://dx.doi.org/10.1002/lsm.20984] [PMID: 21246576]

[392] Lo, P.C.; Rodríguez-Morgade, M.S.; Pandey, R.K.; Ng, D.K.P.; Torres, T.; Dumoulin, F. The unique features and promises of phthalocyanines as advanced photosensitisers for photodynamic therapy of cancer. *Chem. Soc. Rev.,* **2020**, *49*(4), 1041-1056. [http://dx.doi.org/10.1039/C9CS00129H] [PMID: 31845688]

[393] Mitra, K.; Hartman, M.C.T. Silicon phthalocyanines: Synthesis and resurgent applications. *Org. Biomol. Chem.,* **2021**, *19*(6), 1168-1190. [http://dx.doi.org/10.1039/D0OB02299C] [PMID: 33475120]

[394] Tao, S.H.; Bolger, P.M. Hazard assessment of germanium supplements. *Regul. Toxicol. Pharmacol.,* **1997**, *25*(3), 211-219. [http://dx.doi.org/10.1006/rtph.1997.1098] [PMID: 9237323]

[395] Sabbioni, E.; Fortaner, S.; Bosisio, S.; Farina, M.; Del Torchio, R.; Edel, J.; Fischbach, M. Metabolic fate of ultratrace levels of $GeCl_4$ in the rat and *in vitro* studies on its basal cytotoxicity and carcinogenic potential in Balb/3T3 and HaCaT cell lines. *J. Appl. Toxicol.,* **2010**, *30*(1), 34-41. [http://dx.doi.org/10.1002/jat.1469] [PMID: 19757410]

[396] Schauss, A.G. Nephrotoxicity in humans by the ultratrace element germanium. *Ren. Fail.,* **1991**, *13*(1), 1-4. [http://dx.doi.org/10.3109/08860229109022139] [PMID: 1924911]

[397] Gerber, G.B.; Léonard, A. Mutagenicity, carcinogenicity and teratogenicity of germanium compounds. *Mutat. Res. Rev. Mutat. Res.,* **1997**, *387*(3), 141-146. [http://dx.doi.org/10.1016/S1383-5742(97)00034-3] [PMID: 9439710]

[398] Gerik, S.; Maypole, J. Overview of biologically based therapies in rehabilitation. In: *Complementary therapies for physical therapy*; Deutsch, J.E.; Anderson, E.Z., Eds.; W.B. Saunders: Saint Louis, MO, **2007**; pp. 156-175. [http://dx.doi.org/10.1016/B978-072160111-3.50016-6]

[399] Menchikov, L.G.; Ignatenko, M.A. Biological activity of organogermanium compounds (a review). *Pharm. Chem. J.,* **2013**, *46*(11), 635-638. [http://dx.doi.org/10.1007/s11094-013-0860-2]

[400] Alama, A.; Tasso, B.; Novelli, F.; Sparatore, F. Organometallic compounds in oncology: Implications of novel organotins as antitumor agents. *Drug Discov. Today,* **2009**, *14*(9-10), 500-508. [http://dx.doi.org/10.1016/j.drudis.2009.02.002] [PMID: 19429510]

[401] Nath, M. Toxicity and the cardiovascular activity of organotin compounds: A review. *Appl. Organomet. Chem.,* **2008**, *22*(10), 598-612. [http://dx.doi.org/10.1002/aoc.1436]

[402] Graisa, A.; Zainulabdeen, K.; Salman, I.; Al-Ani, A.; Mohammed, R.; Hairunisa, N.; Mohammed, S.; Yousif, E. Toxicity and anti-tumour activity of organotin (IV) compounds. *Baghdad J. Biochem. Appl. Biol. Sci.,* **2022**, *3*(2), 99-108. [http://dx.doi.org/10.47419/bjbabs.v3i02.131]

[403] Iornumbe, E.N.; Yiase, S.G.; Sha'Ato, R.; Tor-Anyiin, T.A. Synthesis, characterization and antifungal activity of some organotin (IV) derivatives of octanedioic acid. *Int. J. Sci. Res.,* **2015**, *4*(5), 2095-2101.

[404] Allison, R.R.; Sibata, C.H. Oncologic photodynamic therapy photosensitizers: A clinical review. *Photodiagn. Photodyn. Ther.,* **2010**, *7*(2), 61-75.
[http://dx.doi.org/10.1016/j.pdpdt.2010.02.001] [PMID: 20510301]

[405] Lobinski, R.; Adams, F.C. Lead and organolead compounds. In: *Anal. Contam. Edible Aquat. Resour;* VCH, **1994**; pp. 115-157.

[406] Tan, Z.; Chen, P.; Schneider, N.; Glover, S.; Cui, L.; Torgue, J.; Rixe, O.; Spitz, H.B.; Dong, Z. Significant systemic therapeutic effects of high-LET immunoradiation by 212Pb-trastuzumab against prostatic tumors of androgen-independent human prostate cancer in mice. *Int. J. Oncol.,* **2012**, *40*(6), 1881-1888.
[PMID: 22322558]

[407] Meredith, R.F.; Torgue, J.; Azure, M.T.; Shen, S.; Saddekni, S.; Banaga, E.; Carlise, R.; Bunch, P.; Yoder, D.; Alvarez, R. Pharmacokinetics and imaging of ^{212}Pb-TCMC-trastuzumab after intraperitoneal administration in ovarian cancer patients. *Cancer Biother. Radiopharm.,* **2014**, *29*(1), 12-17.
[http://dx.doi.org/10.1089/cbr.2013.1531] [PMID: 24229395]

[408] Milenic, D.E.; Garmestani, K.; Brady, E.D.; Baidoo, K.E.; Albert, P.S.; Wong, K.J.; Flynn, J.; Brechbiel, M.W. Multimodality therapy: Potentiation of high linear energy transfer radiation with paclitaxel for the treatment of disseminated peritoneal disease. *Clin. Cancer Res.,* **2008**, *14*(16), 5108-5115.
[http://dx.doi.org/10.1158/1078-0432.CCR-08-0256] [PMID: 18698028]

[409] Twiner, M.J.; Hennessy, J.; Wein, R.; Levy, P.D. Nitroglycerin use in the emergency department: Current perspectives. *Open Access Emerg. Med.,* **2022**, *14*, 327-333.
[http://dx.doi.org/10.2147/OAEM.S340513] [PMID: 35847764]

[410] Guo, K.; Gao, H. Physiological roles of nitrite and nitric oxide in bacteria: Similar consequences from distinct cell targets, protection, and Sensing Systems. *Adv. Biol.,* **2021**, *5*(9), 2100773.
[http://dx.doi.org/10.1002/adbi.202100773] [PMID: 34310085]

[411] Harper, P.V.; Schwartz, J.; Beck, R.N.; Lathrop, K.A.; Lembares, N.; Krizek, H.; Gloria, I.; Dinwoodie, R.; McLaughlin, A.; Stark, V.J.; Bekerman, C.; Hoffer, P.B.; Gottschalk, A.; Resnekov, L.; Al-Sadir, J.; Mayorga, A.; Brooks, H.L. Clinical myocardial imaging with nitrogen-13 ammonia. *Radiology,* **1973**, *108*(3), 613-617.
[http://dx.doi.org/10.1148/108.3.613] [PMID: 4723662]

[412] Machac, J. Radiopharmaceuticals for clinical cardiac PET imaging. In: *Cardiac PET and PET/CT imaging;* Di Carli, M.F.; Lipton, M.J., Eds.; Springer: New York, NY, **2007**; pp. 73-82.
[http://dx.doi.org/10.1007/978-0-387-38295-1_5]

[413] Woolfenden, J.M.; Barber, H.B. Radiation detector probes for tumor localization using tumor-seeking radioactive tracers. *Am. J. Roentgenol.,* **1989**, *153*(1), 35-39.
[http://dx.doi.org/10.2214/ajr.153.1.35] [PMID: 2660536]

[414] Antman, K.H. Introduction: The history of arsenic trioxide in cancer therapy. *Oncologist,* **2001**, *6*(S2), 1-2.
[http://dx.doi.org/10.1634/theoncologist.6-suppl_2-1] [PMID: 11331433]

[415] Fang, J.; Chen, S-J.; Tong, J-H.; Wang, Z-G.; Chen, G-Q.; Chen, Z. Treatment of acute promyelocytic leukemia with ATRA and As$_2$O$_3$: A model of molecular. *Cancer Biol. Ther.,* **2002**, *1*(6), 614-620.
[http://dx.doi.org/10.4161/cbt.308] [PMID: 12642682]

[416] Blower, P.J. 30 Inorganic pharmaceuticals. *Annu. Rep. Sect. A Inorg. Chem.,* **2004**, *100*, 633-658.
[http://dx.doi.org/10.1039/B312109G]

[417] Bisser, S.; N'Siesi, F.X.; Lejon, V.; Preux, P.M.; Van Nieuwenhove, S.; Miaka Mia Bilenge, C.; Büscher, P. Equivalence trial of melarsoprol and nifurtimox monotherapy and combination therapy for the treatment of second-stage trypanosoma brucei gambiense sleeping sickness. *J. Infect. Dis.,* **2007**,

195(3), 322-329.
[http://dx.doi.org/10.1086/510534] [PMID: 17205469]

[418] Garnier, N.; Redstone, G.G.J.; Dahabieh, M.S.; Nichol, J.N.; del Rincon, S.V.; Gu, Y.; Bohle, D.S.; Sun, Y.; Conklin, D.S.; Mann, K.K.; Miller, W.H.Jr. The novel arsenical darinaparsin is transported by cystine importing systems. *Mol. Pharmacol.,* **2014**, *85*(4), 576-585.
[http://dx.doi.org/10.1124/mol.113.089433] [PMID: 24431147]

[419] Lloyd, N.C.; Morgan, H.W.; Nicholson, B.K.; Ronimus, R.S. The composition of Ehrlich's salvarsan: Resolution of a century-old debate. *Angew. Chem. Int. Ed.,* **2005**, *44*(6), 941-944.
[http://dx.doi.org/10.1002/anie.200461471] [PMID: 15624113]

[420] Sanders, V.A.; Cutler, C.S. Radioarsenic: A promising theragnostic candidate for nuclear medicine. *Nucl. Med. Biol.,* **2021**, *92*, 184-201.
[http://dx.doi.org/10.1016/j.nucmedbio.2020.03.004] [PMID: 32376084]

[421] Haldar, A.K.; Sen, P.; Roy, S. Use of antimony in the treatment of leishmaniasis: Current status and future directions. *Mol. Biol. Int.,* **2011**, *2011*, 571242.
[http://dx.doi.org/10.4061/2011/571242] [PMID: 22091408]

[422] Frézard, F.; Demicheli, C.; Ribeiro, R.R. Pentavalent antimonials: New perspectives for old drugs. *Molecules,* **2009**, *14*(7), 2317-2336.
[http://dx.doi.org/10.3390/molecules14072317] [PMID: 19633606]

[423] Nühs, A.; Schäfer, C.; Zander, D.; Trübe, L.; Tejera Nevado, P.; Schmidt, S.; Arevalo, J.; Adaui, V.; Maes, L.; Dujardin, J.C.; Clos, J. A novel marker, ARM58, confers antimony resistance to Leishmania spp. *Int. J. Parasitol. Drugs and Drug Resist.,* **2014**, *4*(1), 37-47.
[http://dx.doi.org/10.1016/j.ijpddr.2013.11.004] [PMID: 24596667]

[424] Yan, S.; Li, F.; Ding, K.; Sun, H. Reduction of pentavalent antimony by trypanothione and formation of a binary and ternary complex of antimony(III) and trypanothione. *J. Biol. Inorg. Chem.,* **2003**, *8*(6), 689-697.
[http://dx.doi.org/10.1007/s00775-003-0468-1] [PMID: 12827457]

[425] Yan, S.; Wong, I.L.K.; Chow, L.M.C.; Sun, H. Rapid reduction of pentavalent antimony by trypanothione: Potential relevance to antimonial activation. *Chem. Commun.,* **2003**, *2*, 266-267.
[http://dx.doi.org/10.1039/b210240d] [PMID: 12585423]

[426] Mai, L.M.; Lin, C.Y.; Chen, C.Y.; Tsai, Y.C. Synergistic effect of bismuth subgallate and borneol, the major components of Sulbogin®, on the healing of skin wound. *Biomaterials,* **2003**, *24*(18), 3005-3012.
[http://dx.doi.org/10.1016/S0142-9612(03)00126-1] [PMID: 12895572]

[427] Shiotani, A.; Roy, P.; Lu, H.; Graham, D.Y. *Helicobacter pylori* diagnosis and therapy in the era of antimicrobial stewardship. *Therap. Adv. Gastroenterol.,* **2021**, *14*, 17562848211064080.
[http://dx.doi.org/10.1177/17562848211064080] [PMID: 34987609]

[428] Wang, R.; Li, H.; Ip, T.K.Y.; Sun, H. Bismuth drugs as antimicrobial agents. In: *Advances in Inorganic Chemistry*; Academic Press, **2020**; Vol. 75, pp. 183-205.

[429] Halani, S.; Wu, P.E. Salicylate toxicity from chronic bismuth subsalicylate use. *BMJ Case Rep. CP.,* **2020**, *13*(11), e236929.
[http://dx.doi.org/10.1136/bcr-2020-236929] [PMID: 33257373]

[430] Sun, H.; Li, H.; Sadler, P.J. The biological and medicinal chemistry of bismuth. *Chem. Ber.,* **1997**, *130*(6), 669-681.
[http://dx.doi.org/10.1002/cber.19971300602]

[431] Sadler, P.J.; Li, H.; Sun, H. Coordination chemistry of metals in medicine: Target sites for bismuth. *Coord. Chem. Rev.,* **1999**, *185-186(S2)*, 689-709.
[http://dx.doi.org/10.1016/S0010-8545(99)00018-1]

[432] Xie, Y.; Pan, X.; Li, Y.; Wang, H.; Du, Y.; Xu, J.; Wang, J.; Zeng, Z.; Chen, Y.; Zhang, G.; Wu, K.;

Liu, D.; Lv, N. New single capsule of bismuth, metronidazole and tetracycline given with omeprazole *versus* quadruple therapy consisting of bismuth, omeprazole, amoxicillin and clarithromycin for eradication of *helicobacter pylori* in duodenal ulcer patients: A chinese prospective, randomized, multicentre trial. *J. Antimicrob. Chemother.,* **2018**, *73*(6), 1681-1687.
[http://dx.doi.org/10.1093/jac/dky056] [PMID: 29596646]

[433] Shetu, S.A.; Sanchez-Palestino, L.M.; Rivera, G.; Bandyopadhyay, D. Medicinal bismuth: Bismuth-organic frameworks as pharmaceutically privileged compounds. *Tetrahedron,* **2022**, *129(Suppl 1)*, 133117.
[http://dx.doi.org/10.1016/j.tet.2022.133117]

[434] Kowalik, M.; Masternak, J.; Barszcz, B. Recent research trends on bismuth compounds in cancer chemo-and radiotherapy. *Curr. Med. Chem.,* **2019**, *26*(4), 729-759.
[http://dx.doi.org/10.2174/0929867324666171003113540] [PMID: 28971764]

[435] Yang, N.; Sun, H. Biocoordination chemistry of bismuth: Recent advances. *Coord. Chem. Rev.,* **2007**, *251*(17-20), 2354-2366.
[http://dx.doi.org/10.1016/j.ccr.2007.03.003]

[436] Bartoli, M.; Jagdale, P.; Tagliaferro, A. A short review on biomedical applications of nanostructured bismuth oxide and related Nanomaterials. *Materials,* **2020**, *13*(22), 5234.
[http://dx.doi.org/10.3390/ma13225234] [PMID: 33228140]

[437] Peng, Z.; Tang, J. Intestinal infection of *candida albicans*: preventing the formation of biofilm by *C. albicans* and protecting the intestinal epithelial barrier. *Front. Microbiol.,* **2022**, *12*, 783010.
[http://dx.doi.org/10.3389/fmicb.2021.783010] [PMID: 35185813]

[438] Prakash, M.; Kavitha, H.P.; Abinaya, S.; Vennila, J.P.; Lohita, D. Green synthesis of bismuth based nanoparticles and its applications - A review. *Sust. Chem. Pharm.,* **2022**, *25*, 100547.
[http://dx.doi.org/10.1016/j.scp.2021.100547]

[439] Rosenblat, T.L.; McDevitt, M.R.; Mulford, D.A.; Pandit-Taskar, N.; Divgi, C.R.; Panageas, K.S.; Heaney, M.L.; Chanel, S.; Morgenstern, A.; Sgouros, G.; Larson, S.M.; Scheinberg, D.A.; Jurcic, J.G. Sequential cytarabine and alpha-particle immunotherapy with bismuth-213-lintuzumab (HuM195) for acute myeloid leukemia. *Clin. Cancer Res.,* **2010**, *16*(21), 5303-5311.
[http://dx.doi.org/10.1158/1078-0432.CCR-10-0382] [PMID: 20858843]

[440] Jurcic, J. Alpha-particle therapy for acute myeloid leukemia. *J. Med. Imaging Radiat. Sci.,* **2019**, *50*(4), S86-S87.
[http://dx.doi.org/10.1016/j.jmir.2019.11.063]

[441] Zare, O.; Afzalipour, R.; Golvardi Yazdi, M.S. Review of alloy containing bismuth oxide nanoparticles on x-ray absorption in radiology shields. *Dis. Diagn.,* **2022**, *11*(1), 31-35.
[http://dx.doi.org/10.34172/ddj.2022.07]

[442] Oliaei, S.; SeyedAlinaghi, S.A.; Mehrtak, M.; Karimi, A.; Noori, T.; Mirzapour, P.; Shojaei, A.; MohsseniPour, M.; Mirghaderi, P.; Alilou, S.; Shobeiri, P.; Azadi Cheshmekabodi, H.; Mehraeen, E.; Dadras, O. The effects of hyperbaric oxygen therapy (HBOT) on coronavirus disease-2019 (COVID-19): A systematic review. *Eur. J. Med. Res.,* **2021**, *26*(1), 96.
[http://dx.doi.org/10.1186/s40001-021-00570-2] [PMID: 33388089]

[443] Cattel, F.; Giordano, S.; Bertiond, C.; Lupia, T.; Corcione, S.; Scaldaferri, M.; Angelone, L.; De Rosa, F.G. Ozone therapy in COVID-19: A narrative review. *Virus Res.,* **2021**, *291*, 198207.
[http://dx.doi.org/10.1016/j.virusres.2020.198207] [PMID: 33115670]

[444] Izadi, M.; Cegolon, L.; Javanbakht, M.; Sarafzadeh, A.; Abolghasemi, H.; Alishiri, G.; Zhao, S.; Einollahi, B.; Kashaki, M.; Jonaidi-Jafari, N.; Asadi, M.; Jafari, R.; Fathi, S.; Nikoueinejad, H.; Ebrahimi, M.; Imanizadeh, S.; Ghazale, A.H. Ozone therapy for the treatment of COVID-19 pneumonia: A scoping review. *Int. Immunopharmacol.,* **2021**, *92*, 107307.
[http://dx.doi.org/10.1016/j.intimp.2020.107307] [PMID: 33476982]

[445] Scott, K.A.; Njardarson, J.T. Analysis of US FDA-approved drugs containing sulfur atoms. In: *Sulfur*

Chemistry. Topics in Current Chemistry Collections; Jiang, X., Ed.; Springer: Cham., **2019**; pp. 1-34. [http://dx.doi.org/10.1007/s41061-018-0184-5]

[446] Feng, M.; Tang, B.; Liang, S.H.; Jiang, X. Sulfur containing scaffolds in drugs: Synthesis and application in medicinal chemistry. *Curr. Top. Med. Chem.,* **2016**, *16*(11), 1200-1216. [http://dx.doi.org/10.2174/1568026615666150915111741] [PMID: 26369815]

[447] Tilby, M.J.; Willis, M.C. How do we address neglected sulfur pharmacophores in drug discovery? *Exp. Opin. Drug Discov.,* **2021**, *16*(11), 1227-1231. [http://dx.doi.org/10.1080/17460441.2021.1948008] [PMID: 34212815]

[448] Frings, M.; Bolm, C.; Blum, A.; Gnamm, C. Sulfoximines from a medicinal chemist's perspective: Physicochemical and *in vitro* parameters relevant for drug discovery. *Eur. J. Med. Chem.,* **2017**, *126*, 225-245. [http://dx.doi.org/10.1016/j.ejmech.2016.09.091] [PMID: 27821325]

[449] Wesolowski, L.T.; Semanchik, P.L.; White-Springer, S.H. Beyond antioxidants: Selenium and skeletal muscle mitochondria. *Front. Veter. Sci.,* **2022**, *9*, 1868. [http://dx.doi.org/10.3389/fvets.2022.1011159] [PMID: 36532343]

[450] Parish, L.; Parish, J.; Routh, H. Selenium sulfide in the 21st century. *J. Am. Acad. Dermatol.,* **2008**, *58*, AB72.

[451] Radomska, D.; Czarnomysy, R.; Radomski, D.; Bielawski, K. Selenium compounds as novel potential anticancer agents. *Int. J. Mol. Sci.,* **2021**, *22*(3), 1009. [http://dx.doi.org/10.3390/ijms22031009] [PMID: 33498364]

[452] Medina-Cruz, D.; Tien-Street, W.; Vernet-Crua, A.; Zhang, B.; Huang, X.; Murali, A.; Chen, J.; Liu, Y.; Garcia-Martin, J.M.; Cholula-Díaz, J.L.; Webster, T. Tellurium, the forgotten element: A review of the properties, processes, and biomedical applications of the bulk and nanoscale metalloid. In: *Racing for the Surface*; Li, B.; Moriarty, T.; Webster, T.; Xing, M., Eds.; Springer: Cham, **2020**. [http://dx.doi.org/10.1007/978-3-030-34471-9_26]

[453] Chiaverini, L.; Marzo, T.; La Mendola, D. AS101: An overview on a leading tellurium-based prodrug. *Inorg. Chim. Acta,* **2022**, *540*, 121048. [http://dx.doi.org/10.1016/j.ica.2022.121048]

[454] Halpert, G.; Eitan, T.; Voronov, E.; Apte, R.N.; Rath-Wolfson, L.; Albeck, M.; Kalechman, Y.; Sredni, B. Multifunctional activity of a small tellurium redox immunomodulator compound, AS101, on dextran sodium sulfate-induced murine colitis. *J. Biol. Chem.,* **2014**, *289*(24), 17215-17227. [http://dx.doi.org/10.1074/jbc.M113.536664] [PMID: 24764299]

[455] Filler, R.; Saha, R. Fluorine in medicinal chemistry: A century of progress and a 60-year retrospective of selected highlights. *Fut. Med. Chem.,* **2009**, *1*(5), 777-791. [http://dx.doi.org/10.4155/fmc.09.65] [PMID: 21426080]

[456] Schirmer, M.; Calamia, K.T.; Wenger, M.; Klauser, A.; Salvarani, C.; Moncayo, R. ^{18}F-Fluorodeoxyglucose-positron emission tomography: A new explorative perspective. *Exp. Gerontol.,* **2003**, *38*(4), 463-470. [http://dx.doi.org/10.1016/S0531-5565(02)00267-X] [PMID: 12670633]

[457] Fang, W.Y.; Ravindar, L.; Rakesh, K.P.; Manukumar, H.M.; Shantharam, C.S.; Alharbi, N.S.; Qin, H.L. Synthetic approaches and pharmaceutical applications of chloro-containing molecules for drug discovery: A critical review. *Eur. J. Med. Chem.,* **2019**, *173*, 117-153. [http://dx.doi.org/10.1016/j.ejmech.2019.03.063] [PMID: 30995567]

[458] Jităreanu, A.; Caba, I.C.; Agoroaei, L. Halogenation–a versatile tool for drug synthesis-the importance of developing effective and eco-friendly reaction protocols. *Curr. Ana. Biotechnol.,* **2019**, *2*, 11-25.

[459] Cho, J.Y.; Xing, S.; Liu, X.; Buckwalter, T.L.F.; Hwa, L.; Sferra, T.J.; Chiu, I.M.; Jhiang, S.M. Expression and activity of human Na+/I− symporter in human glioma cells by adenovirus-mediated gene delivery. *Gene Ther.,* **2000**, *7*(9), 740-749.

[http://dx.doi.org/10.1038/sj.gt.3301170] [PMID: 10822300]

[460] Ciarallo, A.; Rivera, J. Radioactive iodine therapy in differentiated thyroid cancer: 2020 update. *AJR Am. J. Roentgenol.*, **2020**, *215*(2), 285-291.
[http://dx.doi.org/10.2214/AJR.19.22626] [PMID: 32551904]

[461] Lindegren, S.; Albertsson, P.; Bäck, T.; Jensen, H.; Palm, S.; Aneheim, E. Realizing clinical trials with astatine-211: The chemistry infrastructure. *Cancer Biother. Radiopharm.*, **2020**, *35*(6), 425-436.
[http://dx.doi.org/10.1089/cbr.2019.3055] [PMID: 32077749]

[462] Zalutsky, M.R.; Pruszynski, M. Astatine-211: Production and availability. *Curr. Radiopharm.*, **2011**, *4*(3), 177-185.
[http://dx.doi.org/10.2174/1874471011104030177] [PMID: 22201707]

[463] Vaidyanathan, G.; Zalutsky, M.R Astatine radiopharmaceuticals: Prospects and problems. *Curr. Radiopharm.*, **2008**, *1*(3), 177-196.
[http://dx.doi.org/10.2174/1874471010801030177] [PMID: 20150978]

[464] Reilly, S.W.; Makvandi, M.; Xu, K.; Mach, R.H. Rapid cu-catalyzed [211At]astatination and [125I]iodination of boronic esters at room temperature. *Org. Lett.*, **2018**, *20*(7), 1752-1755.
[http://dx.doi.org/10.1021/acs.orglett.8b00232] [PMID: 29561158]

[465] Berganza, C.J.; Zhang, J.H. The role of helium gas in medicine. *Med. Gas Res.*, **2013**, *3*(1), 1-7.
[http://dx.doi.org/10.1186/2045-9912-3-18] [PMID: 23916029]

[466] Makarov, D.V.; Kainth, D.; Link, R.E.; Kavoussi, L.R. Physiologic changes during helium insufflation in high-risk patients during laparoscopic renal procedures. *Urology*, **2007**, *70*(1), 35-37.
[http://dx.doi.org/10.1016/j.urology.2007.03.010] [PMID: 17656203]

[467] Schmidt, M.; Byrne, J.M.; Maasilta, I.J. Bio-imaging with the helium-ion microscope: A review. *Beilst. J. Nanotechnol.*, **2021**, *12*(1), 1-23.
[http://dx.doi.org/10.3762/bjnano.12.1] [PMID: 33489663]

[468] Höllig, A.; Schug, A.; Fahlenkamp, A.; Rossaint, R.; Coburn, M.; Brücken, A. Argon: systematic review on neuro-and organoprotective properties of an "inert" gas. *Int. J. Mol. Sci.*, **2014**, *15*(10), 18175-18196.
[http://dx.doi.org/10.3390/ijms151018175] [PMID: 25310646]

[469] Höllig, A.; Coburn, M. Noble gases and neuroprotection: Summary of current evidence. *Curr. Opin. Anaesthesiol.*, **2021**, *34*(5), 603-606.
[http://dx.doi.org/10.1097/ACO.0000000000001033] [PMID: 34224430]

[470] Raiser, J.; Zenker, M. Argon plasma coagulation for open surgical and endoscopic applications: State of the art. *J. Phys. D Appl. Phys.*, **2006**, *39*(16), 3520.
[http://dx.doi.org/10.1088/0022-3727/39/16/S10]

[471] Cleveland, Z.I.; Pavlovskaya, G.E.; Elkins, N.D.; Stupic, K.F.; Repine, J.E.; Meersmann, T. Hyperpolarized 83Kr MRI of lungs. *J. Magn. Reson.*, **2008**, *195*(2), 232-237.
[http://dx.doi.org/10.1016/j.jmr.2008.09.020] [PMID: 18948043]

[472] Henriksen, O.M.; Kruuse, C.; Olesen, J.; Jensen, L.T.; Larsson, H.B.W.; Birk, S.; Hansen, J.M.; Wienecke, T.; Rostrup, E. Sources of variability of resting cerebral blood flow in healthy subjects: A study using 133Xe SPECT measurements. *J. Cereb. Blood Flow Metab.*, **2013**, *33*(5), 787-792.
[http://dx.doi.org/10.1038/jcbfm.2013.17] [PMID: 23403374]

[473] Albert, M.S.; Balamore, D. Development of hyperpolarized noble gas MRI. *Nucl. Instrum. Methods Phys. Res., A*, **1998**, *402*(2-3), 441-453.
[http://dx.doi.org/10.1016/S0168-9002(97)00888-7] [PMID: 11543065]

[474] Maier, A.; Wiedemann, J.; Rapp, F.; Papenfuß, F.; Rödel, F.; Hehlgans, S.; Gaipl, U.S.; Kraft, G.; Fournier, C.; Frey, B. Radon exposure—therapeutic effect and cancer risk. *Int. J. Mol. Sci.*, **2020**, *22*(1), 316.
[http://dx.doi.org/10.3390/ijms22010316] [PMID: 33396815]

[475] Ge, E.J.; Bush, A.I.; Casini, A.; Cobine, P.A.; Cross, J.R.; DeNicola, G.M.; Dou, Q.P.; Franz, K.J.; Gohil, V.M.; Gupta, S.; Kaler, S.G.; Lutsenko, S.; Mittal, V.; Petris, M.J.; Polishchuk, R.; Ralle, M.; Schilsky, M.L.; Tonks, N.K.; Vahdat, L.T.; Van Aelst, L.; Xi, D.; Yuan, P.; Brady, D.C.; Chang, C.J. Connecting copper and cancer: From transition metal signalling to metalloplasia. *Nat. Rev. Cancer.,* **2022**, *22*(2), 102-113.
[http://dx.doi.org/10.1038/s41568-021-00417-2] [PMID: 34764459]

[476] Krasnovskaya, O.; Naumov, A.; Guk, D.; Gorelkin, P.; Erofeev, A.; Beloglazkina, E.; Majouga, A. Copper coordination compounds as biologically active agents. *Int. J. Mol. Sci.,* **2020**, *21*(11), 3965.
[http://dx.doi.org/10.3390/ijms21113965] [PMID: 32486510]

[477] Nímia, H.H.; Carvalho, V.F.; Isaac, C.; Souza, F.Á.; Gemperli, R.; Paggiaro, A.O. Comparative study of Silver Sulfadiazine with other materials for healing and infection prevention in burns: A systematic review and meta-analysis. *Burns,* **2019**, *45*(2), 282-292.
[http://dx.doi.org/10.1016/j.burns.2018.05.014] [PMID: 29903603]

[478] Eckhardt, S.; Brunetto, P.S.; Gagnon, J.; Priebe, M.; Giese, B.; Fromm, K.M. Nanobio silver: Its interactions with peptides and bacteria, and its uses in medicine. *Chem. Rev.,* **2013**, *113*(7), 4708-4754.
[http://dx.doi.org/10.1021/cr300288v] [PMID: 23488929]

[479] Gemmell, C.G.; Edwards, D.I.; Fraise, A.P.; Gould, F.K.; Ridgway, G.L.; Warren, R.E. Guidelines for the prophylaxis and treatment of methicillin-resistant Staphylococcus aureus *(MRSA)* infections in the UK. *J. Antimicrob. Chemother.,* **2006**, *57*(4), 589-608.
[http://dx.doi.org/10.1093/jac/dkl017] [PMID: 16507559]

[480] Soumya, R.S.; Hela, P.G. Nano silver based targeted drug delivery for treatment of cancer. *Der Pharm. Lett.,* **2013**, *5(4)*, 189-197.

[481] Raubenheimer, H.G.; Schmidbaur, H. The late start and amazing upswing in gold chemistry. *J. Chem. Educ.,* **2014**, *91*(12), 2024-2036.
[http://dx.doi.org/10.1021/ed400782p]

[482] Yang, Z.; Jiang, G.; Xu, Z.; Zhao, S.; Liu, W. Advances in alkynyl gold complexes for use as potential anticancer agents. *Coord. Chem. Rev.,* **2020**, *423*, 213492.
[http://dx.doi.org/10.1016/j.ccr.2020.213492]

[483] Che, C.M.; Sun, R.W.Y. Therapeutic applications of gold complexes: Lipophilic gold(III) cations and gold(I) complexes for anti-cancer treatment. *Chem. Commun.,* **2011**, *47*(34), 9554-9560.
[http://dx.doi.org/10.1039/c1cc10860c] [PMID: 21674082]

[484] Nardon, C.; Boscutti, G.; Fregona, D. Beyond platinums: Gold complexes as anticancer agents. *Anticancer Res.,* **2014**, *34*(1), 487-492.
[PMID: 24403506]

[485] Bian, M.; Fan, R.; Jiang, G.; Wang, Y.; Lu, Y.; Liu, W. Halo and pseudohalo gold (I)–NHC complexes derived from 4, 5-diarylimidazoles with excellent *in vitro* and *in vivo* anticancer activities against HCC. *J. Med. Chem.,* **2020**, *63*(17), 9197-9211.
[http://dx.doi.org/10.1021/acs.jmedchem.0c00257] [PMID: 32787098]

[486] Walther, W.; Althagafi, D.; Curran, D.; O'Beirne, C.; Mc Carthy, C.; Ott, I.; Basu, U.; Büttner, B.; Sterner-Kock, A.; Müller-Bunz, H.; Sánchez-Sanz, G.; Zhu, X.; Tacke, M. *In-vitro* and *in-vivo* investigations into the carbene-gold anticancer drug candidates NHC*- Au- SCSNMe2 and NHC*-Au-S- GLUC against advanced prostate cancer PC3. *Anti-Cancer Drugs,* **2020**, *31*(7), 672-683.
[http://dx.doi.org/10.1097/CAD.0000000000000930] [PMID: 32282370]

[487] Gulzar, S.; Ammara, U.; Abid, Z.; Shahid, M.; Ashraf, R.S.; Baig, N.; Kawde, A.N.; Bhatia, G.; Isab, A.A.; Altaf, M. Synthesis, *in vitro* anticancer activity and reactions with biomolecule of gold(I)-NHC carbene complexes. *J. Mol. Struct.,* **2022**, *1255*, 132482.
[http://dx.doi.org/10.1016/j.molstruc.2022.132482]

[488] Alsaeedi, M.S.; Babgi, B.A.; Hussien, M.A.; Abdellattif, M.H.; Humphrey, M.G. DNA-binding and

anticancer activity of binuclear gold (I) alkynyl complexes with a phenanthrenyl bridging ligand. *Molecules,* **2020,** *25*(5), 1033.
[http://dx.doi.org/10.3390/molecules25051033] [PMID: 32106590]

[489] Mármol, I.; Castellnou, P.; Alvarez, R.; Gimeno, M.C.; Rodríguez-Yoldi, M.J.; Cerrada, E. Alkynyl Gold(I) complexes derived from 3-hydroxyflavones as multi-targeted drugs against colon cancer. *Eur. J. Med. Chem.,* **2019,** *183,* 111661.
[http://dx.doi.org/10.1016/j.ejmech.2019.111661] [PMID: 31546196]

[490] Babgi, B.A.; Alsayari, J.; Alenezi, H.M.; Abdellatif, M.H.; Eltayeb, N.E.; Emwas, A.H.M.; Jaremko, M.; Hussien, M.A. Alteration of anticancer and protein-binding properties of gold (I) Alkynyl by phenolic Schiff bases moieties. *Pharmaceutics,* **2021,** *13*(4), 461.
[http://dx.doi.org/10.3390/pharmaceutics13040461] [PMID: 33805337]

[491] Tabrizi, L.; Yang, W.S.; Chintha, C.; Morrison, L.; Samali, A.; Ramos, J.W.; Erxleben, A. Gold(I) complexes with a quinazoline carboxamide alkynyl ligand: Synthesis, cytotoxicity, and mechanistic studies. *Eur. J. Inorg. Chem.,* **2021,** *2021*(20), 1921-1928.
[http://dx.doi.org/10.1002/ejic.202100120] [PMID: 34248416]

[492] Maret, W. Zinc and human disease. In: *Interrelations between essential metal ions and human diseases*; Sigel, A.; Sigel, H.; Sigel, R.K.O., Eds.; Springer Science and Business Media B.V.: Dordrecht, The Netherlands, **2013**; pp. 389-414.
[http://dx.doi.org/10.1007/978-94-007-7500-8_12]

[493] Iqbal, K.; Asmat, M. Uses and effects of mercury in medicine and dentistry. *J. Ayub Med. Coll. Abbottabad,* **2012,** *24*(3-4), 204-207.
[PMID: 24669655]

[494] Erdemli-Köse, S.B.; Yirün, A.; Balci-Özyurt, A.; Erkekoğlu, P. Modification of the toxic effects of methylmercury and thimerosal by testosterone and estradiol in SH-SY5Y neuroblastoma cell line. *J. Appl. Toxicol.,* **2022,** *42*(6), 981-994.
[http://dx.doi.org/10.1002/jat.4269] [PMID: 34874569]

[495] Pniok, M.; Kubíček, V.; Havlíčková, J.; Kotek, J.; Sabatie-Gogová, A.; Plutnar, J.; Huclier-Markai, S.; Hermann, P. Thermodynamic and kinetic study of scandium(III) complexes of DTPA and DOTA: A step toward scandium radiopharmaceuticals. *Chem. Eur. J.,* **2014,** *20*(26), 7944-7955.
[http://dx.doi.org/10.1002/chem.201402041] [PMID: 24838869]

[496] Tickner, B.J.; Stasiuk, G.J.; Duckett, S.B.; Angelovski, G. The use of yttrium in medical imaging and therapy: Historical background and future perspectives. *Chem. Soc. Rev.,* **2020,** *49*(17), 6169-6185.
[http://dx.doi.org/10.1039/C9CS00840C] [PMID: 32701076]

[497] Noumbissi, S.; Scarano, A.; Gupta, S. A literature review study on atomic ions dissolution of titanium and its alloys in implant dentistry. *Materials,* **2019,** *12*(3), 368.
[http://dx.doi.org/10.3390/ma12030368] [PMID: 30682826]

[498] Wang, X.; Zhong, X.; Cheng, L. Titanium-based nanomaterials for cancer theranostics. *Coord. Chem. Rev.,* **2021,** *430,* 213662.
[http://dx.doi.org/10.1016/j.ccr.2020.213662]

[499] Skoupilova, H.; Hrstka, R.; Bartosik, M. Titanocenes as anticancer agents: Recent insights. *Med. Chem.,* **2017,** *13*(4), 334-344.
[http://dx.doi.org/10.2174/1573406412666161228113650] [PMID: 28031018]

[500] Ghosh, S.; Sharma, A.; Talukder, G. Zirconium: an abnormal trace element in biology. *Biol. Trace Elem. Res.,* **1992,** *35*(3), 247-271.
[http://dx.doi.org/10.1007/BF02783770] [PMID: 1283692]

[501] Marill, J.; Anesary, N.M.; Zhang, P.; Vivet, S.; Borghi, E.; Levy, L.; Pottier, A. Hafnium oxide nanoparticles: Toward an *in vitro* predictive biological effect? *Radiat. Oncol.,* **2014,** *9*(1), 1-11.
[http://dx.doi.org/10.1186/1748-717X-9-150] [PMID: 24981953]

[502] Pottier, A.; Borghi, E.; Levy, L. New use of metals as nanosized radioenhancers. *Anticancer Res.,* **2014**, *34*(1), 443-453.
[PMID: 24403500]

[503] Kowalski, S.; Wyrzykowski, D.; Inkielewicz-Stępniak, I. Molecular and cellular mechanisms of cytotoxic activity of vanadium compounds against cancer cells. *Molecules,* **2020**, *25*(7), 1757.
[http://dx.doi.org/10.3390/molecules25071757] [PMID: 32290299]

[504] Treviño, S.; Diaz, A. Vanadium and insulin: Partners in metabolic regulation. *J. Inorg. Biochem.,* **2020**, *208*, 111094.
[http://dx.doi.org/10.1016/j.jinorgbio.2020.111094] [PMID: 32438270]

[505] Crans, D.C.; Henry, L.; Cardiff, G.; Posner, B.I. Developing vanadium as an antidiabetic or anticancer drug: A clinical and historical perspective. *Met. Ions Life Sci.,* **2019**, *19*, 203-230.
[http://dx.doi.org/10.1515/9783110527872-008] [PMID: 30855109]

[506] Nasibi, S.; Alimohammadi, K.; Bazli, L.; Eskandarinezhad, S.; Mohammadi, A.; Sheysi, N. TZNT alloy for surgical implant applications: A systematic review. *J. Compos. Comp.,* **2020**, *2*(3), 61-67.
[http://dx.doi.org/10.29252/jcc.2.2.1]

[507] Huang, G.; Pan, S.T.; Qiu, J.X. The clinical application of porous tantalum and its new development for bone tissue engineering. *Materials,* **2021**, *14*(10), 2647.
[http://dx.doi.org/10.3390/ma14102647] [PMID: 34070153]

[508] Vincent, J.B. Benefits of Trivalent Chromium in Human Nutrition? In: *Metal Toxicology Handbook*; CRC Press, **2020**; pp. 147-160.
[http://dx.doi.org/10.1201/9780429438004-14]

[509] Sugden, K.D.; Stearns, D.M. The role of chromium(V) in the mechanism of chromate-induced oxidative DNA damage and cancer. *J. Environ. Pathol. Toxicol. Oncol.,* **2000**, *19*(3), 215-230.
[PMID: 10983888]

[510] Rieber, M. Cancer pro-oxidant therapy through copper redox cycling: Repurposing disulfiram and tetrathiomolybdate. *Curr. Pharm. Des.,* **2020**, *26*(35), 4461-4466.
[http://dx.doi.org/10.2174/1381612826666200628022113] [PMID: 32600223]

[511] Bertinat, R.; Westermeier, F.; Gatica, R.; Nualart, F. Sodium tungstate: Is it a safe option for a chronic disease setting, such as diabetes? *J. Cell. Physiol.,* **2019**, *234*(1), 51-60.
[http://dx.doi.org/10.1002/jcp.26913] [PMID: 30132852]

[512] Van Rompuy, L.S.; Parac-Vogt, T.N. Interactions between polyoxometalates and biological systems: From drug design to artificial enzymes. *Curr. Opin. Biotechnol.,* **2019**, *58*, 92-99.
[http://dx.doi.org/10.1016/j.copbio.2018.11.013] [PMID: 30529815]

[513] Liu, J.C.; Wang, J.F.; Han, Q.; Shangguan, P.; Liu, L.L.; Chen, L.J.; Zhao, J.W.; Streb, C.; Song, Y.F. Multicomponent self-assembly of a giant heterometallic polyoxotungstate supercluster with antitumor activity. *Angew. Chem. Int. Ed.,* **2021**, *60*(20), 11153-11157.
[http://dx.doi.org/10.1002/anie.202017318] [PMID: 33590971]

[514] Doan, B-T.; Meme, S.; Beloeil, J-C. General Principles of MRI. In: *The Chemistry of Contrast Agents in Medical Magnetic Resonance Imaging,* 2nd ed; Merbach, A.; Helm, L.; Tóth, É., Eds.; John Wiley & Sons Ltd: Chichester, UK, **2013**; Vol. 1, pp. 1-24.
[http://dx.doi.org/10.1002/9781118503652.ch1]

[515] Brandt, M.; Cardinale, J.; Rausch, I.; Mindt, T.L. Manganese in PET imaging: Opportunities and challenges. *J. Label. Comp. Radiopharm.,* **2019**, *62*(8), 541-551.
[http://dx.doi.org/10.1002/jlcr.3754] [PMID: 31115089]

[516] Garda, Z.; Molnár, E.; Kálmán, F.K.; Botár, R.; Nagy, V.; Baranyai, Z.; Brücher, E.; Kovács, Z.; Tóth, I.; Tircsó, G. Effect of the nature of donor atoms on the thermodynamic, kinetic and relaxation properties of Mn(II) complexes formed with some trisubstituted 12-membered macrocyclic ligands. *Front. Chem.,* **2018**, *6*, 232.

[http://dx.doi.org/10.3389/fchem.2018.00232] [PMID: 30151358]

[517] Drahoš, B.; Kotek, J.; Hermann, P.; Lukeš, I.; Tóth, É. Mn2+ complexes with pyridine-containing 15-membered macrocycles: Thermodynamic, kinetic, crystallographic, and 1H/17O relaxation studies. *Inorg. Chem.,* **2010**, *49*(7), 3224-3238.
[http://dx.doi.org/10.1021/ic9020756] [PMID: 20180546]

[518] Drahoš, B.; Lukeš, I.; Tóth, É. Manganese(II) complexes as potential contrast agents for MRI. *Eur. J. Inorg. Chem.,* **2012**, *2012*(12), 1975-1986.
[http://dx.doi.org/10.1002/ejic.201101336]

[519] Zolle, I. Technetium-99m pharmaceuticals: Preparation and quality control in nuclear medicine. Springer: Berlin, Germany, **2007**.
[http://dx.doi.org/10.1007/978-3-540-33990-8]

[520] Mandegaran, R.; Dhillon, S.; Jen, H. Beyond the bones and joints: A review of ligamentous injuries of the foot and ankle on ^{99m}Tc-MDP-SPECT/CT. *Brit. J. Radiol.,* **2019**, *92*(1104), 20190506.
[http://dx.doi.org/10.1259/bjr.20190506] [PMID: 31365277]

[521] Li, Y.; Zhang, J. A Review of ^{99m}Tc-labeled tumor metabolic imaging agents. *Mini Rev. Med. Chem.,* **2022**, *22*(12), 1586-1596.
[http://dx.doi.org/10.2174/1389557521666210521114024] [PMID: 34355682]

[522] Pourhabib, Z.; Ranjbar, H.; Bahrami Samani, A.; Shokri, A.A. Appraisement of 186/188Re-HEDP, a new compositional radiopharmaceutical. *J. Radioanal. Nucl. Chem.,* **2019**, *322*(2), 1133-1138.
[http://dx.doi.org/10.1007/s10967-019-06816-y]

[523] Abubakar, T.A.; Eke, U.B.; Salisu, A. Bioorganometallic ferroquine and related compounds as antimalarial chemotherapeutic agents: A short review. *J. Chem. Soc. Niger.,* **2022**, *47*(3), 573-592.
[http://dx.doi.org/10.46602/jcsn.v47i3.758]

[524] Wang, R.; Chen, H.; Yan, W.; Zheng, M.; Zhang, T.; Zhang, Y. Ferrocene-containing hybrids as potential anticancer agents: Current developments, mechanisms of action and structure-activity relationships. *Eur. J. Med. Chem.,* **2020**, *190*, 112109.
[http://dx.doi.org/10.1016/j.ejmech.2020.112109] [PMID: 32032851]

[525] Chen, C.; Ge, J.; Gao, Y.; Chen, L.; Cui, J.; Zeng, J.; Gao, M. Ultrasmall superparamagnetic iron oxide nanoparticles: A next generation contrast agent for magnetic resonance imaging. *Wiley Interdiscip. Rev. Nanomed. Nanobiotechnol.,* **2022**, *14*(1), e1740.
[http://dx.doi.org/10.1002/wnan.1740] [PMID: 34296533]

[526] Villarreal, E.G.; Flores, S.; Kriz, C.; Iranpour, N.; Bronicki, R.A.; Loomba, R.S. Sodium nitroprusside *versus* nicardipine for hypertension management after surgery: A systematic review and meta-analysis. *J. Card. Surg.,* **2020**, *35*(5), 1021-1028.
[http://dx.doi.org/10.1111/jocs.14513] [PMID: 32176355]

[527] Takpradit, C.; Viprakasit, V.; Narkbunnam, N.; Vathana, N.; Phuakpet, K.; Pongtanakul, B.; Sanpakit, K.; Buaboonnam, J. Using of deferasirox and deferoxamine in refractory iron overload thalassemia. *Pediatr. Int.,* **2021**, *63*(4), 404-409.
[http://dx.doi.org/10.1111/ped.14444] [PMID: 32856363]

[528] Michel, R.; Nolte, M.; Reich, M.; Löer, F. Systemic effects of implanted prostheses made of cobalt-chromium alloys. *Arch. Orthop. Trauma Surg.,* **1991**, *110*(2), 61-74.
[http://dx.doi.org/10.1007/BF00393876] [PMID: 2015136]

[529] Ditrói, F.; Takács, S.; Tárkányi, F.; Smith, R.W.; Baba, M. Investigation of proton and deuteron induced reactions on cobalt. *J. Korean Phys. Soc.,* **2011**, *59*(2), 1697-1700.
[http://dx.doi.org/10.3938/jkps.59.1697]

[530] Kar, K.; Ghosh, D.; Kabi, B.; Chandra, A. A concise review on cobalt Schiff base complexes as anticancer agents. *Polyhedron,* **2022**, *222*, 115890.
[http://dx.doi.org/10.1016/j.poly.2022.115890]

[531] Heffern, M.C.; Yamamoto, N.; Holbrook, R.J.; Eckermann, A.L.; Meade, T.J. Cobalt derivatives as promising therapeutic agents. *Curr. Opin. Chem. Biol.,* **2013**, *17*(2), 189-196.
[http://dx.doi.org/10.1016/j.cbpa.2012.11.019] [PMID: 23270779]

[532] Petrarca, C.; Poma, A.M.; Vecchiotti, G.; Bernardini, G.; Niu, Q.; Cattaneo, A.G.; Di Gioacchino, M.; Sabbioni, E. Cobalt magnetic nanoparticles as theranostics: Conceivable or forgettable? *Nanotechnol. Rev.,* **2020**, *9*(1), 1522-1538.
[http://dx.doi.org/10.1515/ntrev-2020-0111]

[533] Thangavel, P.; Viswanath, B.; Kim, S. Recent developments in the nanostructured materials functionalized with ruthenium complexes for targeted drug delivery to tumors. *Int. J. Nanomed.,* **2017**, *12*, 2749-2758.
[http://dx.doi.org/10.2147/IJN.S131304] [PMID: 28435255]

[534] Yan, Y.K.; Melchart, M.; Habtemariam, A.; Sadler, P.J. Organometallic chemistry, biology and medicine: Ruthenium arene anticancer complexes. *Chem. Commun.,* **2005**, *38*, 4764-4776.
[http://dx.doi.org/10.1039/b508531b] [PMID: 16193110]

[535] Kostova, I. Ruthenium complexes as anticancer agents. *Curr. Med. Chem.,* **2006**, *13*(9), 1085-1107.
[http://dx.doi.org/10.2174/092986706776360941] [PMID: 16611086]

[536] Lee, S.Y.; Kim, C.Y.; Nam, T.G. Ruthenium complexes as anticancer agents: A brief history and perspectives. *Drug Des. Devel. Ther.,* **2020**, *14*, 5375-5392.
[http://dx.doi.org/10.2147/DDDT.S275007] [PMID: 33299303]

[537] Rilak Simović, A.; Masnikosa, R.; Bratsos, I.; Alessio, E. Chemistry and reactivity of ruthenium(II) complexes: DNA/protein binding mode and anticancer activity are related to the complex structure. *Coord. Chem. Rev.,* **2019**, *398*, 113011.
[http://dx.doi.org/10.1016/j.ccr.2019.07.008]

[538] Cole, H.D.; Roque III, J.A.; Lifshits, L.M.; Hodges, R.; Barrett, P.C.; Havrylyuk, D.; Heidary, D.; Ramasamy, E.; Cameron, C.G.; Glazer, E.C.; McFarland, S.A. Fine-feature modifications to strained ruthenium complexes radically alter their hypoxic anticancer activity. *Photochem. Photobiol.,* **2022**, *98*(1), 73-84.
[http://dx.doi.org/10.1111/php.13395] [PMID: 33559191]

[539] Liang, L.; Wu, X.; Shi, C.; Wen, H.; Wu, S.; Chen, J.; Huang, C.; Wang, Y.; Liu, Y. Synthesis and characterization of polypyridine ruthenium(II) complexes and anticancer efficacy studies *in vivo* and *in vitro. J. Inorg. Biochem.,* **2022**, *236*, 111963.
[http://dx.doi.org/10.1016/j.jinorgbio.2022.111963] [PMID: 35988387]

[540] Chen, J.; Tao, Q.; Wu, J.; Wang, M.; Su, Z.; Qian, Y.; Yu, T.; Wang, Y.; Xue, X.; Liu, H.K. A lysosome-targeted ruthenium(II) polypyridyl complex as photodynamic anticancer agent. *J. Inorg. Biochem.,* **2020**, *210*, 111132.
[http://dx.doi.org/10.1016/j.jinorgbio.2020.111132] [PMID: 32569884]

[541] Chen, C.; Xu, C.; Li, T.; Lu, S.; Luo, F.; Wang, H. Novel NHC-coordinated ruthenium(II) arene complexes achieve synergistic efficacy as safe and effective anticancer therapeutics. *Eur. J. Med. Chem.,* **2020**, *203*, 112605.
[http://dx.doi.org/10.1016/j.ejmech.2020.112605] [PMID: 32688202]

[542] Elsayed, S.A.; Harrypersad, S.; Sahyon, H.A.; El-Magd, M.A.; Walsby, C.J. Ruthenium (II)/(III) DMSO-based complexes of 2-aminophenyl benzimidazole with *in vitro* and *in vivo* anticancer activity. *Molecules,* **2020**, *25*(18), 4284.
[http://dx.doi.org/10.3390/molecules25184284] [PMID: 32962014]

[543] Janković, N.; Milović, E.; Jovanović, J.Đ.; Marković, Z.; Vraneš, M.; Stanojković, T.; Matić, I.; Crnogorac, M.Đ.; Klisurić, O.; Cvetinov, M.; Abbas Bukhari, S.N. A new class of half-sandwich ruthenium complexes containing Biginelli hybrids: Anticancer and anti-SARS-CoV-2 activities. *Chem. Biol. Interact.,* **2022**, *363*, 110025.
[http://dx.doi.org/10.1016/j.cbi.2022.110025] [PMID: 35752294]

[544] Kar, B.; Das, U.; De, S.; Pete, S.; Sharma S, A.; Roy, N.; S K, A.K.; Panda, D.; Paira, P. GSH-resistant and highly cytoselective ruthenium(II)-*p*-cymene-(imidazo[4,5-*f*] [1, 10] phenanthrolin-2-yl) complexes as potential anticancer agents. *Dalton Trans.,* **2021**, *50*(30), 10369-10373.
[http://dx.doi.org/10.1039/D1DT01604K] [PMID: 34308466]

[545] Yufanyi, D.M.; Abbo, H.S.; Titinchi, S.J.J.; Neville, T. Platinum(II) and Ruthenium(II) complexes in medicine: Antimycobacterial and Anti-HIV activities. *Coord. Chem. Rev.,* **2020**, *414*, 213285.
[http://dx.doi.org/10.1016/j.ccr.2020.213285]

[546] Rahul, K.; Shekhar, S. Ruthenium based antifungal compounds and their activity. *Res. J. Chem. Environ.,* **2021**, *25*(7), 177-182.
[http://dx.doi.org/10.25303/257rjce17721]

[547] Rospond-Kubiak, I.; Wróblewska-Zierhoffer, M.; Twardosz-Pawlik, H.; Kocięcki, J. Ruthenium brachytherapy for uveal melanoma–single institution experience. *J. Contemp. Brachyther.,* **2017**, *9*(6), 548-552.
[http://dx.doi.org/10.5114/jcb.2017.72606] [PMID: 29441099]

[548] Guidoccio, F.; Mazzarri, S.; Depalo, T.; Orsini, F.; Erba, P.A.; Mariani, G. Novel Radiopharmaceuticals for Therapy. In: *Nuclear Oncology: From Pathophysiology to Clinical Applications*; Springer Intern. Publ.: Cham, **2022**; pp. 217-243.
[http://dx.doi.org/10.1007/978-3-031-05494-5_36]

[549] Koudinova, N.V.; Pinthus, J.H.; Brandis, A.; Brenner, O.; Bendel, P.; Ramon, J.; Eshhar, Z.; Scherz, A.; Salomon, Y. Photodynamic therapy with Pd-bacteriopheophorbide (TOOKAD): Successful *in vivo* treatment of human prostatic small cell carcinoma xenografts. *Int. J. Cancer,* **2003**, *104*(6), 782-789.
[http://dx.doi.org/10.1002/ijc.11002] [PMID: 12640688]

[550] Ravi, A.; Keller, B.M.; Pignol, J.P. A comparison of postimplant dosimetry for ^{103}Pd *versus* ^{131}Cs seeds on a retrospective series of PBSI patients. *Med. Phys.,* **2011**, *38*(11), 6046-6052.
[http://dx.doi.org/10.1118/1.3651633] [PMID: 22047369]

[551] Goldstein, S.; Czapski, G.; Heller, A. Osmium tetroxide, used in the treatment of arthritic joints, is a fast mimic of superoxide dismutase. *Free Rad. Biol. Med.,* **2005**, *38*(7), 839-845.
[http://dx.doi.org/10.1016/j.freeradbiomed.2004.10.027] [PMID: 15749379]

[552] Lu, N.; Deng, Z.; Gao, J.; Liang, C.; Xia, H.; Zhang, P. An osmium-peroxo complex for photoactive therapy of hypoxic tumors. *Nat. Commun.,* **2022**, *13*(1), 2245.
[http://dx.doi.org/10.1038/s41467-022-29969-z] [PMID: 35473926]

[553] Terrani, I.; Scherer Hofmeier, K.; Bircher, A.J. Indium and iridium: Two rare metals with a high rate of contact sensitization. *Contact Dermat.,* **2020**, *83*(2), 94-98.
[http://dx.doi.org/10.1111/cod.13549] [PMID: 32248538]

[554] Ho, P.Y.; Ho, C.L.; Wong, W.Y. Recent advances of iridium(III) metallophosphors for health-related applications. *Coord. Chem. Rev.,* **2020**, *413*, 213267.
[http://dx.doi.org/10.1016/j.ccr.2020.213267]

[555] Ma, D.L.; Wu, C.; Wu, K.J.; Leung, C.H. Iridium (III) complexes targeting apoptotic cell death in cancer cells. *Molecules,* **2019**, *24*(15), 2739.
[http://dx.doi.org/10.3390/molecules24152739] [PMID: 31357712]

[556] Guan, R.; Xie, L.; Ji, L.; Chao, H. Phosphorescent iridium (III) complexes for anticancer applications. *Eur. J. Inorg. Chem.,* **2020**, *2020*(42), 3978-3986.
[http://dx.doi.org/10.1002/ejic.202000754]

[557] Kharitonov, V.B.; Muratov, D.V.; Loginov, D.A. Cyclopentadienyl complexes of group 9 metals in the total synthesis of natural products. *Coord. Chem. Rev.,* **2022**, *471*, 214744.
[http://dx.doi.org/10.1016/j.ccr.2022.214744]

[558] Roussakis, Y.; Anagnostopoulos, G. Physical and dosimetric aspects of the iridium-knife. *Front. Oncol.,* **2021**, *11*, 728452.

[http://dx.doi.org/10.3389/fonc.2021.728452] [PMID: 34858815]

[559] Cowley, A.; Woodward, B. A healthy future: Platinum in medical applications. *Platin. Met. Rev.,* **2011**, *55*(2), 98-107.
[http://dx.doi.org/10.1595/147106711X566816]

[560] Harper, B.W.; Krause-Heuer, A.M.; Grant, M.P.; Manohar, M.; Garbutcheon-Singh, K.B.; Aldrich-Wright, J.R. Advances in platinum chemotherapeutics. *Chem. Eur. J.,* **2010**, *16*(24), 7064-7077.
[http://dx.doi.org/10.1002/chem.201000148] [PMID: 20533453]

[561] Zamble, D.B.; Lippard, S.J. Cisplatin and DNA repair in cancer chemotherapy. *Trends Biochem. Sci.,* **1995**, *20*(10), 435-439.
[http://dx.doi.org/10.1016/S0968-0004(00)89095-7] [PMID: 8533159]

[562] Abed, A.; Derakhshan, M.; Karimi, M.; Shirazinia, M.; Mahjoubin-Tehran, M.; Homayonfal, M.; Hamblin, M.R.; Mirzaei, S.A.; Soleimanpour, H.; Dehghani, S.; Dehkordi, F.F.; Mirzaei, H. Platinum nanoparticles in biomedicine: Preparation, anti-cancer activity, and drug delivery vehicles. *Front. Pharmacol.,* **2022**, *13*, 797804.
[http://dx.doi.org/10.3389/fphar.2022.797804] [PMID: 35281900]

[563] Wheate, N.; Collins, J. Multi-nuclear platinum drugs: A new paradigm in chemotherapy. *Curr. Med. Chem.-Anti-Cancer Agents,* **2005**, *5*(3), 267-279.
[http://dx.doi.org/10.2174/1568011053765994] [PMID: 15992354]

[564] Zhu, Z.; Wang, Z.; Zhang, C.; Wang, Y.; Zhang, H.; Gan, Z.; Guo, Z.; Wang, X. Mitochondrion-targeted platinum complexes suppressing lung cancer through multiple pathways involving energy metabolism. *Chem. Sci.,* **2019**, *10*(10), 3089-3095.
[http://dx.doi.org/10.1039/C8SC04871A] [PMID: 30996891]

[565] He, C.; Majd, M.H.; Shiri, F.; Shahraki, S. Palladium and platinum complexes of folic acid as new drug delivery systems for treatment of breast cancer cells. *J. Mol. Struct.,* **2021**, *1229*, 129806.
[http://dx.doi.org/10.1016/j.molstruc.2020.129806]

[566] Adams, M.; Sullivan, M.P.; Tong, K.K.H.; Goldstone, D.C.; Hanif, M.; Jamieson, S.M.F.; Hartinger, C.G. Mustards-derived Terpyridine–platinum complexes as anticancer agents: DNA alkylation vs coordination. *Inorg. Chem.,* **2021**, *60*(4), 2414-2424.
[http://dx.doi.org/10.1021/acs.inorgchem.0c03317] [PMID: 33497565]

[567] Kutlu, E.; Emen, F.M.; Kismali, G.; Kınaytürk, N.K.; Kılıç, D.; Karacolak, A.I.; Demirdogen, R.E. Pyridine derivative platinum complexes: Synthesis, molecular structure, DFT and initial anticancer activity studies. *J. Mol. Struct.,* **2021**, *1234*, 130191.
[http://dx.doi.org/10.1016/j.molstruc.2021.130191]

[568] Mbugua, S.N.; Sibuyi, N.R.S.; Njenga, L.W.; Odhiambo, R.A.; Wandiga, S.O.; Meyer, M.; Lalancette, R.A.; Onani, M.O. New palladium (II) and platinum (II) complexes based on pyrrole schiff bases: Synthesis, characterization, X-ray structure, and anticancer activity. *ACS Omega,* **2020**, *5*(25), 14942-14954.
[http://dx.doi.org/10.1021/acsomega.0c00360] [PMID: 32637768]

[569] Lozada, I.B.; Huang, B.; Stilgenbauer, M.; Beach, T.; Qiu, Z.; Zheng, Y.; Herbert, D.E. Monofunctional platinum(II) anticancer complexes based on multidentate phenanthridine-containing ligand frameworks. *Dalton Trans.,* **2020**, *49*(20), 6557-6560.
[http://dx.doi.org/10.1039/D0DT01275K] [PMID: 32342084]

[570] Islam, M.K.; Baek, A.R.; Sung, B.; Yang, B.W.; Choi, G.; Park, H.J.; Kim, Y.H.; Kim, M.; Ha, S.; Lee, G.H.; Kim, H.K.; Chang, Y. Synthesis, characterization, and anticancer activity of benzothiazole aniline derivatives and their platinum (II) complexes as new chemotherapy agents. *Pharmaceuticals,* **2021**, *14*(8), 832.
[http://dx.doi.org/10.3390/ph14080832] [PMID: 34451928]

[571] Bai, X.; Ali, A.; Wang, N.; Liu, Z.; Lv, Z.; Zhang, Z.; Zhao, X.; Hao, H.; Zhang, Y.; Rahman, F.U. Inhibition of SREBP-mediated lipid biosynthesis and activation of multiple anticancer mechanisms by

platinum complexes: Ascribe possibilities of new antitumor strategies. *Eur. J. Med. Chem.,* **2022**, *227*, 113920.
[http://dx.doi.org/10.1016/j.ejmech.2021.113920] [PMID: 34742012]

[572]   Zeynali, H.; Keypour, H.; Hosseinzadeh, L.; Gable, R.W. The non-templating synthesis of macro-cyclic Schiff base ligands containing pyrrole and homopiperazine and their binuclear nickel(II), cobalt(II) and mononuclear platinum(II) complexes: X-ray single crystal and anticancer studies. *J. Mol. Struct.,* **2021**, *1244*, 130956.
[http://dx.doi.org/10.1016/j.molstruc.2021.130956]

[573]   Novohradsky, V.; Pracharova, J.; Kasparkova, J.; Imberti, C.; Bridgewater, H.E.; Sadler, P.J.; Brabec, V. Induction of immunogenic cell death in cancer cells by a photoactivated platinum (IV) prodrug. *Inorg. Chem. Front.,* **2020**, *7*(21), 4150-4159.
[http://dx.doi.org/10.1039/D0QI00991A] [PMID: 34540235]

[574]   Bünzli, J.C.G. Lanthanide light for biology and medical diagnosis. *J. Luminesc.,* **2016**, *170*, 866-878.
[http://dx.doi.org/10.1016/j.jlumin.2015.07.033]

[575]   Misra, S.N.; Gagnani, M.A.; M, I.D.; Shukla, R.S. Biological and clinical aspects of Lanthanide coordination compounds. *Bioinorg. Chem. Appl.,* **2004**, *2*(3-4), 155-192.
[http://dx.doi.org/10.1155/S1565363304000111] [PMID: 18365075]

[576]   Zhang, Q.; O'Brien, S.; Grimm, J. Biomedical applications of lanthanide nanomaterials, for imaging, sensing and therapy. *Nanotheranostics,* **2022**, *6*(2), 184-194.
[http://dx.doi.org/10.7150/ntno.65530] [PMID: 34976593]

[577]   Dobrynina, N.; Feofanova, M.; Gorelov, I. Mixed lanthanide complexes in biology and medicine. *J. Inorg. Biochem.,* **1997**, *67*(1-4), 168-168.
[http://dx.doi.org/10.1016/S0162-0134(97)80046-3]

[578]   Armelao, L.; Quici, S.; Barigelletti, F.; Accorsi, G.; Bottaro, G.; Cavazzini, M.; Tondello, E. Design of luminescent lanthanide complexes: From molecules to highly efficient photo-emitting materials *Coordin. Chem. Rev.,* **2010**, *254*(5-6), 487-505.

[579]   Robertson, A.G.; Rendina, L.M. Gadolinium theranostics for the diagnosis and treatment of cancer. *Chem. Soc. Rev.,* **2021**, *50*(7), 4231-4244.
[http://dx.doi.org/10.1039/D0CS01075H] [PMID: 33599224]

[580]   Kostova, I. Lanthanides as anticancer agents. *Chem.-Anti-Cancer Agents,* **2005**, *5*(6), 591-602.
[http://dx.doi.org/10.2174/156801105774574694] [PMID: 16305481]

[581]   Chundawat, N.S.; Jadoun, S.; Zarrintaj, P.; Chauhan, N.P.S. Lanthanide complexes as anticancer agents: A review. *Polyhedron,* **2021**, *207*, 115387.
[http://dx.doi.org/10.1016/j.poly.2021.115387]

[582]   Abdolmaleki, S.; Aliabadi, A.; Ghadermazi, M. Two La(III) complexes containing pyridine-2, 6-dicarboxylate as *in vitro* potent cytotoxic agents toward human lymphocyte cells. *Inorg. Chim. Acta,* **2022**, *542*, 121152.
[http://dx.doi.org/10.1016/j.ica.2022.121152]

[583]   Gainanova, A.A.; Kuz'micheva, G.M.; Terekhova, R.P.; Pashkin, I.I.; Trigub, A.L.; Malysheva, N.E.; Svetogorov, R.D.; Alimguzina, A.R.; Koroleva, A.V. New antimicrobial materials with cerium ions in the composition of salts, solutions, and composite systems based on Ce^{3+} $(NO_3)_3$ × $6H_2O$. *New J. Chem.,* **2022**, *46*(40), 19271-19282.
[http://dx.doi.org/10.1039/D2NJ03691F]

[584]   Demirci, S.; Sahiner, N. Polyethyleneimine based Cerium(III) and $Ce(NO_3)_3$ metal-organic frameworks with blood compatible, antioxidant and antimicrobial properties. *Inorg. Chim. Acta,* **2022**, *534*, 120814.
[http://dx.doi.org/10.1016/j.ica.2022.120814]

[585]   Reese, A.D.; Keyloun, J.W.; Garg, G.; McLawhorn, M.M.; Moffatt, L.T.; Travis, T.E.; Johnson, L.S.;

Shupp, J.W. Compounded cerium nitrate–silver sulfadiazine cream is safe and effective for the treatment of burn wounds: A burn center's 4-year experience. *J. Burn Care Res.,* **2022**, *43*(3), 716-721.
[http://dx.doi.org/10.1093/jbcr/irab180] [PMID: 34543402]

[586] Rajeshkumar, S.; Naik, P. Synthesis and biomedical applications of Cerium oxide nanoparticles – A Review. *Biotechnol. Rep.,* **2018**, *17*, 1-5.
[http://dx.doi.org/10.1016/j.btre.2017.11.008] [PMID: 29234605]

[587] Barker, E.; Shepherd, J.; Asencio, I.O. The use of cerium compounds as antimicrobials for biomedical applications. *Molecules,* **2022**, *27*(9), 2678.
[http://dx.doi.org/10.3390/molecules27092678] [PMID: 35566026]

[588] Vermeulen, K.; Van de Voorde, M.; Segers, C.; Coolkens, A.; Rodriguez Pérez, S.; Daems, N.; Duchemin, C.; Crabbé, M.; Opsomer, T.; Saldarriaga Vargas, C.; Heinke, R.; Lambert, L.; Bernerd, C.; Burgoyne, A.R.; Cocolios, T.E.; Stora, T.; Ooms, M. Exploring the potential of high-molar-activity samarium-153 for targeted radionuclide therapy with [^{153}Sm]Sm-DOTA-TATE. *Pharmaceutics,* **2022**, *14*(12), 2566.
[http://dx.doi.org/10.3390/pharmaceutics14122566] [PMID: 36559060]

[589] Sharma, S.; Singh, B.; Koul, A.; Mittal, B.R. Comparative therapeutic efficacy of ^{153}sm-EDTMP and ^{177}lu-EDTMP for bone pain palliation in patients with skeletal metastases: Patients' pain score analysis and personalized dosimetry. *Front. Med.,* **2017**, *4*, 46.
[http://dx.doi.org/10.3389/fmed.2017.00046] [PMID: 28507988]

[590] Song, B.; Wu, Y.; Yu, M.; Zhao, P.; Zhou, C.; Kiefer, G.E.; Sherry, A.D. A europium(III)-based PARACEST agent for sensing singlet oxygen by MRI. *Dalton Trans.,* **2013**, *42*(22), 8066-8069.
[http://dx.doi.org/10.1039/c3dt50194a] [PMID: 23575743]

[591] Leguerrier, D.M.D.; Barré, R.; Molloy, J.K.; Thomas, F. Lanthanide complexes as redox and ROS/RNS probes: A new paradigm that makes use of redox-reactive and redox non-innocent ligands. *Coord. Chem. Rev.,* **2021**, *446*, 214133.
[http://dx.doi.org/10.1016/j.ccr.2021.214133]

[592] Kuriyan, N.S.; Sabeena, M. Luminescence studies of Eu3+ doped calcium magnesium silicate phosphor prepared at different annealing temperatures for fine color tunability. *J. Lumin.,* **2022**, *249*, 119038.
[http://dx.doi.org/10.1016/j.jlumin.2022.119038]

[593] Blumfield, E.; Swenson, D.W.; Iyer, R.S.; Stanescu, A.L. Gadolinium-based contrast agents — review of recent literature on magnetic resonance imaging signal intensity changes and tissue deposits, with emphasis on pediatric patients. *Pediatr. Radiol.,* **2019**, *49*(4), 448-457.
[http://dx.doi.org/10.1007/s00247-018-4304-8] [PMID: 30923876]

[594] Clough, T.J.; Jiang, L.; Wong, K.L.; Long, N.J. Ligand design strategies to increase stability of gadolinium-based magnetic resonance imaging contrast agents. *Nat. Commun.,* **2019**, *10*(1), 1420.
[http://dx.doi.org/10.1038/s41467-019-09342-3] [PMID: 30926784]

[595] Peters, J.A.; Huskens, J.; Raber, D.J. Lanthanide induced shifts and relaxation rate enhancements. *Prog. Nucl. Magn. Reson. Spectrosc.,* **1996**, *28*(3-4), 283-350.
[http://dx.doi.org/10.1016/0079-6565(95)01026-2]

[596] Lux, F.; Roux, S.; Perriat, P.; Tillement, O. Biomedical applications of nanomaterials containing gadolinium. *Curr. Inorg. Chem.,* **2011**, *1*(1), 117-129.
[http://dx.doi.org/10.2174/1877944111101010117]

[597] Rodríguez-Galván, A.; Rivera, M.; García-López, P.; Medina, L.A.; Basiuk, V.A. Gadolinium-containing carbon nanomaterials for magnetic resonance imaging: Trends and challenges. *J. Cell. Mol. Med.,* **2020**, *24*(7), 3779-3794.
[http://dx.doi.org/10.1111/jcmm.15065] [PMID: 32154648]

[598] Khalil, G.E.; Thompson, E.K.; Gouterman, M.; Callis, J.B.; Dalton, L.R.; Turro, N.J.; Jockusch, S.

NIR luminescence of gadolinium porphyrin complexes. *Chem. Phys. Lett.,* **2007**, *435*(1-3), 45-49.
[http://dx.doi.org/10.1016/j.cplett.2006.12.042]

[599] Burke, M. Filling the promethium gap. *Chem. Ind.,* **2019**, *83*, 15.

[600] Elkina, V.; Kurushkin, M. Promethium: To strive, to seek, to find and not to yield. *Front Chem.,* **2020**, *8*, 588.
[http://dx.doi.org/10.3389/fchem.2020.00588] [PMID: 32754576]

[601] Studer, D.; Heinitz, S.; Heinke, R.; Naubereit, P.; Dressler, R.; Guerrero, C.; Köster, U.; Schumann, D.; Wendt, K. Atomic transitions and the first ionization potential of promethium determined by laser spectroscopy. *Phys. Rev. A,* **2019**, *99*(6), 062513.
[http://dx.doi.org/10.1103/PhysRevA.99.062513]

[602] Kim, S.H.; Choi, S.I. Uses of rare earth elements for hair improvement. *U.S. Patent* No. 8715714B2, 2014.

[603] Shirmardi, S.P.; Saniei, E.; Das, T.; Noorvand, M.; Erfani, M.; Bagheri, R. Internal dosimetry studies of ^{170}Tm-EDTMP complex, as a bone pain palliation agent, in human tissues based on animal data. *Appl. Rad. Isot.,* **2020**, *166*, 109396.
[http://dx.doi.org/10.1016/j.apradiso.2020.109396] [PMID: 32889376]

[604] Klaassen, N.J.M.; Arntz, M.J.; Gil Arranja, A.; Roosen, J.; Nijsen, J.F.W. The various therapeutic applications of the medical isotope holmium-166: A narrative review. *EJNMMI Radiopharm. Chem.,* **2019**, *4*(1), 1-26.
[http://dx.doi.org/10.1186/s41181-019-0066-3] [PMID: 31659560]

[605] Bakker, R.C.; van Es, R.J.J.; Rosenberg, A.J.W.P.; van Nimwegen, S.A.; Bastiaannet, R.; de Jong, H.W.A.M.; Nijsen, J.F.W.; Lam, M.G.E.H. Intratumoral injection of radioactive holmium-166 microspheres in recurrent head and neck squamous cell carcinoma. *Nucl. Med. Commun.,* **2018**, *39*(3), 213-221.
[http://dx.doi.org/10.1097/MNM.0000000000000792] [PMID: 29309367]

[606] Diniz, M.F.; Ferreira, D.M.; de Lima, W.G.; Pedrosa, M.L.; Silva, M.E.; de Almeida Araujo, S.; Sampaio, K.H.; de Campos, T.P.R.; Siqueira, S.L. Biodegradable seeds of holmium don't change neurological function after implant in brain of rats. *Rep. Pract. Oncol. Radiother.,* **2017**, *22*(4), 319-326.
[http://dx.doi.org/10.1016/j.rpor.2017.03.003] [PMID: 28663714]

[607] Munaweera, I.; Shi, Y.; Koneru, B.; Saez, R.; Aliev, A.; Di Pasqua, A.J.; Balkus, K.J.Jr. Chemoradiotherapeutic magnetic nanoparticles for targeted treatment of nonsmall cell lung cancer. *Mol. Pharm.,* **2015**, *12*(10), 3588-3596.
[http://dx.doi.org/10.1021/acs.molpharmaceut.5b00304] [PMID: 26325115]

[608] Safarzadeh, L. ^{175}Yb-TTHMP as a good candidate for bone pain palliation and substitute of other radiopharmaceuticals. *Ind. J. Nucl. Med.,* **2014**, *29*(3), 135-139.
[http://dx.doi.org/10.4103/0972-3919.136555] [PMID: 25210277]

[609] Patel, N.S.; Fan, P.; Chiu-Tsao, S.T.; Ravi, K.; Sherman, W.; Quon, H.; Pisch, J.; Tsao, H.S.; Harrison, L.B. Ytterbium-169: A promising new radionuclide for intravascular brachytherapy. *Cardiovasc. Rad. Med.,* **2001**, *2*(3), 173-180.
[http://dx.doi.org/10.1016/S1522-1865(01)00085-3] [PMID: 11786324]

[610] Collares, F.M.; Ogliari, F.A.; Lima, G.S.; Fontanella, V.R.C.; Piva, E.; Samuel, S.M.W. Ytterbium trifluoride as a radiopaque agent for dental cements. *Int. Endodont. J.,* **2010**, *43*(9), 792-797.
[http://dx.doi.org/10.1111/j.1365-2591.2010.01746.x] [PMID: 20579134]

[611] Banerjee, S.; Pillai, M.R.A.; Knapp, F.F.R. Lutetium-177 therapeutic radiopharmaceuticals: Linking chemistry, radiochemistry, and practical applications. *Chem. Rev.,* **2015**, *115*(8), 2934-2974.
[http://dx.doi.org/10.1021/cr500171e] [PMID: 25865818]

[612] Chakravarty, R.; Chakraborty, S. A review of advances in the last decade on targeted cancer therapy

using ^{177}Lu: Focusing on ^{177}Lu produced by the direct neutron activation route. *Am. J. Nucl. Med. Mol. Imaging,* **2021**, *11*(6), 443-475.
[PMID: 35003885]

[613] Askari, E.; Harsini, S.; Vahidfar, N.; Divband, G.; Sadeghi, R. ^{177}Lu-EDTMP for metastatic bone pain palliation: A systematic review and meta-analysis. *Cancer Biother. Radiopharm.,* **2021**, *36*(5), 383-390.
[http://dx.doi.org/10.1089/cbr.2020.4323] [PMID: 33259726]

[614] Dash, A.; Pillai, M.R.A.; Knapp, F.F.Jr. Production of ^{177}Lu for targeted radionuclide therapy: Available options. *Nucl. Med. Mol. Imaging,* **2015**, *49*(2), 85-107.
[http://dx.doi.org/10.1007/s13139-014-0315-z] [PMID: 26085854]

[615] van der Doelen, M.J.; Mehra, N.; Smits, M.; van Oort, I.M.; Janssen, M.J.R.; Haberkorn, U.; Kratochwil, C.; Gerritsen, W. Clinical experience with PSMA-Actinium-225 (Ac-225) radioligand therapy (RLT) in end-stage metastatic castration-resistant prostate cancer (mCRPC) patients. *J. Clin. Oncol.,* **2018**, *36*(6_suppl), 344.
[http://dx.doi.org/10.1200/JCO.2018.36.6_suppl.344]

[616] Jurcic, J.G.; Levy, M.Y.; Park, J.H.; Ravandi, F.; Perl, A.E.; Pagel, J.M.; Smith, B.D.; Estey, E.H.; Kantarjian, H.; Cicic, D.; Scheinberg, D.A. Phase I trial of targeted alpha-particle therapy with actinium-225 (225Ac)-lintuzumab and low-dose cytarabine (LDAC) in patients age 60 or older with untreated acute myeloid leukemia (AML). *Blood,* **2016**, *128*(22), 4050.
[http://dx.doi.org/10.1182/blood.V128.22.4050.4050]

[617] Dustin, J.S.; Borrelli, R.A. Assessment of alternative radionuclides for use in a radioisotope thermoelectric generator. *Nucl. Eng. Des.,* **2021**, *385*, 111475.
[http://dx.doi.org/10.1016/j.nucengdes.2021.111475]

[618] Jonckheer, M.H.; Deconinck, F., Eds. *X-ray fluorescent scanning of the thyroid.* Springer Science & Business Media, **2012**. Vol 3.

[619] Maruyama, Y.; van Nagell, J.R.; Yoneda, J.; Donaldson, E.S.; Gallion, H.H.; Powell, D.; Kryscio, R.J. A review of californium-252 neutron brachytherapy for cervical cancer. *Cancer,* **1991**, *68*(6), 1189-1197.
[http://dx.doi.org/10.1002/1097-0142(19910915)68:6<1189::AID-CNCR2820680602>3.0.CO;2-F] [PMID: 1873769]

SUBJECT INDEX

A

Absorption 37, 44, 57, 69, 70, 114, 141, 153, 188, 198, 255, 263
  of manganese 153
  skin-contact 141
Acid(s) 18, 19, 21, 26, 35, 38, 50, 51, 60, 66, 68, 83, 88, 89, 105, 121, 147, 149, 150, 151, 167, 198, 202, 203, 204, 214, 216, 226, 254, 255, 280
  acetoacetic 255
  adenosine triphosphoric 203
  alpha-lipoic 89
  aminocarboxylic 254
  ascorbic 19, 60, 88, 147, 226
  asparagine 38
  aspartic 35
  carbonic 26, 50, 51, 198
  carboxylic 21, 121, 150, 167
  dihydrolipoic 89
  diphosphoric 68
  ferulic 88
  fumaric 18
  glutamine 38
  hydrocyanic 202, 214, 216
  hypohalous 105
  lactic 18
  phosphoric 66, 68, 204
  tetramethylene-phosphonic 280
  uric 83, 88, 149, 150, 151
Acidic stomach reaction 213
Acidosis 22, 23, 32, 36, 51, 103, 112, 185, 198
  diabetic 36
Actinic keratosis 199
Activators, transcription 240
Activity 60, 64, 74, 88, 95, 107, 110, 132, 146, 166, 171, 193, 210, 212, 218, 219, 226, 262, 270, 272, 273, 274, 275, 276, 283
  anti-HIV 193
  anti-inflammatory 270

anti-metastasis 272
anti-metastatic 171
antiapoptotic 218
antibacterial 132, 212
antifungal 60
antimicrobial 74, 107, 210, 262, 273
antimicrobic 275
antioxidant 88, 95, 166, 274, 276
  diagnostic 283
  germicide 226
  hypnotic 219
  hypoglycemic 146
  immunomodulatory 275
  luminescence 273
  neuroprotective 110
  vasodilatation 64
Acute 101, 110, 139, 204, 214, 218, 227, 248, 283, 285, 288
  intestinal symptoms 139
  ischemic stroke 110
  myeloid leukemia (AML) 214, 218, 227, 283, 285, 288
  oral toxic effects 248
  promyelocytic leukemia (APL) 204
  toxicity symptoms 101
Addison's disease 31
  acute 31
Agents 45, 68, 85, 171, 188, 192, 194, 198, 202, 212, 226, 235, 272
  anti-inflammatory 45, 192, 212
  anti neoplastic 235
  anti-ulcer 188, 194
  antibiotic 171, 272
  anticonvulsant 188
  cardiovascular 202
  diuretic 226
  energy transfer 68
  enzyme antioxidant 85
  renal medullary imaging 198
Alcohol dehydrogenase 134, 135
Allergic skin 176

www.ingramcontent.com/pod-product-compliance
Lightning Source LLC
Chambersburg PA
CBHW050806220326

41598CB00006B/127